www.harcourt

Bringing you products fro
companies including Baill
Mosby and W.B. Saunders

- **Browse** for latest information on new books, journals and electronic products

- **Search** for information on over 20 000 published titles with full product information including tables of contents and sample chapters

- **Keep up to date** with our extensive publishing programme in your field by registering with **eAlert** or requesting postal updates

- **Secure online ordering** with prompt delivery, as well as full contact details to order by phone, fax or post

- **News** of special features and promotions

If you are based in the following countries, please visit the country-specific site to receive full details of product availability and local ordering information

USA: www.harcourthealth.com

Canada: www.harcourtcanada.com

Australia: www.harcourt.com.au

Baillière Tindall   CHURCHILL LIVINGSTONE   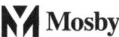 Mosby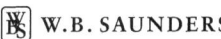

Handbook of Small Animal Radiological Differential Diagnosis

SMALL ANIMAL RADIOLOGICAL DIFFERENTIAL DIAGNOSIS

For W. B. Saunders

Commissioning Editor: Serena Bureau
Project Development Manager: Paul Fam
Project Manager: Scott Millar
Production Manager: Mark Sanderson
Designer: Jayne Jones

Handbook of Small Animal Radiological Differential Diagnosis

by
Ruth Dennis MA, VetMB, DVR, DipECVDI, MRCVS
Centre for Small Animal Studies
The Animal Health Trust
Newmarket
UK

Robert M Kirberger BVSc, MMedVet (Rad), DipECVDI
Onderstepoort Veterinary Academic Hospital
University of Pretoria
Pretoria
Republic of South Africa

Robert H Wrigley BVSc, MS, DVR, MRCVS, DipACVR
Veterinary Teaching Hospital
Colorado State University
Fort Collins
Colorado
USA

Frances J Barr MA, VetMB, PhD, DVR, DipECVDI, MRCVS
School of Veterinary Science
University of Bristol
Bristol
UK

With illustrations by
Jonathan Clayton-Jones BA(HONS)
Northiam
East Sussex
UK

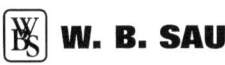
LONDON • EDINBURGH • NEW YORK • PHILADELPHIA • ST LOUIS • SYDNEY • TORONTO 2001

WB SAUNDERS
An imprint of Harcourt Publishers Limited

© Harcourt Publishers Limited 2001

[K] is a registered trademark of Harcourt Publishers Limited

The right of Ruth Dennis, Robert Kirberger, Robert Wrigley and Frances Barr to be identified as authors of this work has been asserted by them in accordance with the Copyright, Designs and Patents Act 1988

All rights reserved. No part of this publication may be reproduced, stored in a retrieval system, or transmitted in any form or by any means, electronic, mechanical, photocopying, recording or otherwise, without either the prior permission of the publishers (Harcourt Publishers Limited, Harcourt Place, 32 Jamestown Road, London NW1 7BY), or a licence permitting restricted copying in the United Kingdom issued by the Copyright Licensing Agency, 90 Tottenham Court Road, London W1P 0LP.

First published 2001

ISBN 0-7020-2485-6

British Library Cataloguing in Publication Data
A catalogue record for this book is available from the British Library

Library of Congress Cataloging in Publication Data
A catalog record for this book is available from the Library of Congress

Note
Medical knowledge is constantly changing. As new information becomes available, changes in treatment, procedures, equipment and the use of drugs become necessary. The editors, contributors and publishers have, as far as it is possible, taken care to ensure that the information given in this text is accurate and up to date. However, readers are strongly advised to confirm that the information, especially with regard to drug usage, complies with the latest legislation and standards of practice.

Transferred to digital printing 2005

Printed and bound by Antony Rowe Ltd, Eastbourne

Contents

Foreword		ix
Preface		xi
1.	Skeletal system: general	1
2.	Joints	31
3.	Appendicular skeleton	39
4.	Head and neck	64
5.	Spine	83
6.	Lower respiratory tract	103
7.	Cardiovascular system	125
8.	Other thoracic structures – pleural cavity, mediastinum, thoracic oesophagus, thoracic wall	143
9.	Gastrointestinal tract	164
10.	Urogenital tract	185
11.	Other abdominal structures – abdominal wall, peritoneal and retroperitoneal cavities, parenchymal organs	209
12.	Soft tissues	236
Appendix:		
	Radiographic faults	242
	Ultrasound terminology and artefacts	244
	Geographic distributions of diseases	246
Index		251

Foreword

I have been intrigued by imaging since 1968 when my veterinary school mentor, Dr Robert E. Lewis, introduced me to the fascination of problem solving by visual examination. Throughout veterinary school, my residency and well into my professional career as an academic radiologist, I vividly remember struggling with discrimination of normal from abnormal, and categorisation of abnormal findings based on Roentgen signs, only to realise that the battle had just begun. Just when I thought the problem was solved, it seemed that someone would always want to know what the Roentgen sign description really meant. Taking imaging abnormalities from the descriptive to the interpretive is the essence of maturing as a radiologist. It is this critical step that separates the truly effective radiologist from a reader of Roentgen signs. Attending clinicians have a hard time deciding how to proceed with the declaration that the patient has 'ventrally located alveolar infiltrate', but when placed in the context of 'probable bacterial pneumonia' the plan of action becomes more easily defined. The process of learning how to reach this final step in competence is often under-emphasised in tutorials or textbooks. This new work, 'Handbook of Small Animal Radiological Differential Diagnosis' is a major step in facilitating completion of the process of becoming a competent interpreter of images

It is a pleasure for me to submit the foreword for this innovative work produced by an International team of esteemed radiologists. Drs Dennis, Kirberger, Wrigley and Barr have assimilated a comprehensive bank of information in a format that is easy to use. Contrary to existing books, the information in this work is designed to order one's thought processes after the radiographic or sonographic abnormalities have been categorised. In other words, once imaging abnormalities have been identified, lists of considerations are provided for each sign. These considerations can then be compared to the history, signalment and physical and clinical findings allowing rational prioritisation of real diseases. This prioritisation can then be used to tailor further diagnostic tests or therapeutic interventions.

This book is not an all-inclusive imaging text, nor will it be useful without some pre-existing experience in imaging interpretation. However, this does not detract from the value of this work – on the contrary, this resourceful publication fills a much-needed gap by enhancing the maturation of the image interpreter. It has been said that the job of a radiologist is to reduce the level of uncertainty surrounding a patient. Information contained herein facilitates taking imaging abnormalities from the descriptive to the interpretive and indeed the inability to complete this process is a major cause of lingering uncertainty. I predict those who use this book religiously will experience a quick and significant reduction in uncertainty, at least as such relates to imaging!

Donald E. Thrall, DVM, PhD
Professor of Radiology
College of Veterinary Medicine
North Carolina State University
Raleigh, NC, USA

Preface

Body systems can only respond to disease or injury in a limited number of ways and therefore it is often impossible to make a specific diagnosis based on a single test, such as radiography. Successful interpretation of radiographs and ultrasonograms depends on the recognition of abnormalities (often called 'Roentgen signs' in radiology), the formulation of lists of possible causes for those abnormalities and a plan for further diagnostic tests, if appropriate. This handbook is intended as an aide memoire of differential diagnoses and other useful information in small animal radiology and ultrasound, in order to assist the radiologist to compile as complete a list of differential diagnoses as possible.

The authors hope that this book will prove useful to all users of small animal diagnostic imaging, from radiologists through general practitioners to veterinary students. However, it is intended to supplement, rather than replace, the many excellent standard textbooks available and a certain degree of experience in the interpretation of images is presupposed. Schematic line drawings of many of the conditions are included, to supplement the text.

The book is divided into sections representing body systems, and for various radiographic and ultrasonographic abnormalities possible diagnoses are listed in approximate order of likelihood. Conditions which principally or exclusively occur in cats are indicated as such, although many of the other diseases listed may occur in cats as well as in dogs. Infectious and parasitic diseases that are not ubiquitous but are confined to certain parts of the world are indicated by an asterisk *, and the reader should consult the table of geographic distribution in the Appendix for further information. Lists of references for further reading are given at the end of each chapter and it is hoped that these will prove helpful to the reader seeking further information about a particular condition.

A book such as this can never hope to be complete, as new conditions are constantly being recognised and described. The authors apologise for any omissions there may be and would welcome comments from our colleagues for possible future editions.

Our thanks go to Professor Don Thrall for kindly agreeing to write the foreword. We are also indebted to our artist, Jonathan Clayton-Jones, for his excellent diagrammatic reproduction of the radiographs and ultrasonograms, and to the many people at Harcourt Health Sciences in London who have supported us throughout this project.

Ruth Dennis
Newmarket, U.K.
December 2000

Skeletal system: general

GENERAL

1.1 Radiographic technique for the skeletal system
1.2 Anatomy of bone – general principles
1.3 Ossification and growth plate closures
1.4 Response of bone to disease or injury
1.5 Patterns of focal bone loss (osteolysis)
1.6 Patterns of osteogenesis – periosteal reactions
1.7 Principles of interpretation
1.8 Features of aggressive and non-aggressive bone lesions
1.9 Fractures – radiography, classification, assessment of healing

BONES

1.10 Altered shape of long bones
1.11 Dwarfism
1.12 Delayed ossification or growth plate closure
1.13 Increased radio-opacity within bone
1.14 Periosteal reactions
1.15 Bony masses
1.16 Osteopenia
1.17 Coarse trabecular pattern
1.18 Osteolytic lesions
1.19 Mixed osteolytic/osteogenic lesions
1.20 Multifocal diseases
1.21 Lesions affecting epiphyses
1.22 Lesions affecting physes
1.23 Lesions affecting metaphyses
1.24 Lesions affecting diaphyses

GENERAL

1.1 Radiographic technique for the skeletal system

The skeletal system lends itself well to radiography but it must be remembered that only the mineralised components of bone are visible. The osteoid matrix of bone is of soft tissue radio-opacity and cannot be assessed radiographically; this comprises 30–35% of adult bone. Articular cartilage is also of soft tissue opacity and is not seen on plain radiographs (see 2.1). Lesions in the skeletal system may be radiographically subtle, and so attention to good radiographic technique is essential:

1. Highest definition film/screen combination consistent with thickness of area and required speed; no grid necessary except for upper limbs and spine in larger dogs.
2. Accurate positioning and centring with a small object/film distance to minimise geometric distortion.
3. Close collimation to enhance radiographic definition and safety.
4. Correct exposure factors to allow examination of soft tissue as well as bone.
5. Beware of hair coat debris creating artefactual shadows.
6. Radiograph the opposite limb for comparison if necessary.
7. Use wedge filtration techniques if a whole limb view required (e.g. for angular limb deformity); use a special wedge filter or intravenous fluid bags.
8. Good processing technique to optimise contrast and definition.
9. Optimum viewing conditions – dry films, darkened room, bright light and dimmer facility, glare around periphery of film masked off.
10. Use a magnifying glass for fine detail; use bone specimens, a film library and radiographic atlases.

1.2 Anatomy of bone – general principles

Apophysis – Non-articular bony protuberance for attachment of tendons and ligaments; a separate centre of ossification.

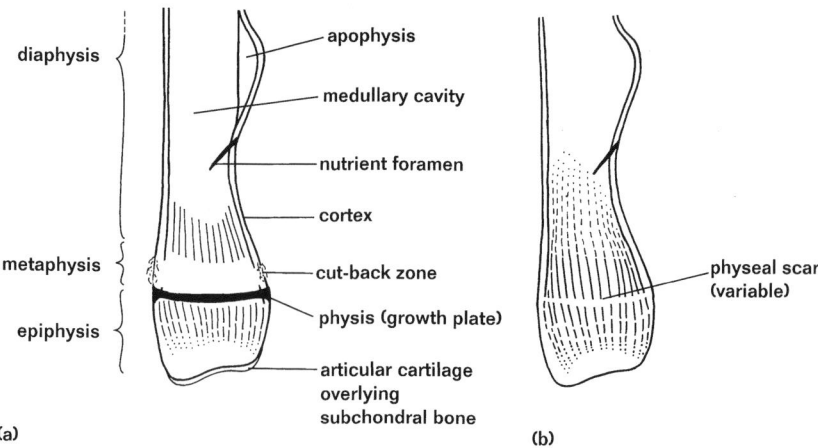

Figure 1.1 (a) Anatomical features of an immature long bone; (b) anatomical features of a mature long bone.

Articular cartilage – Soft tissue opacity, therefore appears radiolucent compared with bones (unless mineralising through disease). Provides longitudinal growth of epiphyses.

Cancellous bone – Spongy bone consisting of a meshwork of bony trabeculae; found in epiphyses, metaphyses and small bones. A coarse trabecular pattern is seen where forces are constant and a fine trabecular pattern where they are variable. The greater surface area compared with cortical bone results in a 40 times greater rate of remodelling in response to disease or injury. The cancellous bone of skull is called *diploë*.

Cortex – Compact, lamellar bone formed by intramembranous ossification from periosteum. Uniformly radio-opaque. Thickest where the circumference of the bone is smallest, where attached soft tissues exert stress or on the concave side of a curved bone.

Diaphysis – The shaft of a long bone; a tube of cortical bone surrounding a medullary cavity and cancellous bone.

Endosteum – Similar to periosteum but thinner. Lines large medullary cavities. May produce bone in some circumstances (e.g. fractures).

Epiphysis – The end of a long bone bearing the articular surface, which forms from a separate centre of ossification; cancellous bone with a denser subchondral layer.

Metaphysis – Between the physis and diaphysis; cancellous bone. In the young animal it remodels bone from the growth plate into the diaphyseal cortex, hence its external surface may be irregular, especially in large dogs; this is known as the *cut-back zone*.

Medullary cavity – Fatty bone marrow space in the mid-diaphysis; radiolucent and homogeneous.

Nutrient foramen – A radiolucent line running obliquely through the cortex and carrying a major blood vessel; its consistent location in long bones reflects relative growth in length from the two ends of the bone (it originates centrally in the foetus). Occasionally it may be in an aberrant location.

Periosteum – Fibroelastic connective tissue surrounding bone except at articular surfaces; its inner layer produces bone by intramembranous ossification.

Physis – Cartilaginous growth plate present in young animals and seen radiographically as a radiolucent band. Its width reduces with progressing ossification; after skeletal maturity it may be seen as a sclerotic line or "physeal scar". It provides longitudinal growth of metaphyses and diaphyses.

Sesamoids – Small bony structures lacking periosteum which form in tendons near joints; thought to reduce friction at sites of direction changes.

Subchondral bone – Thin, dense layer of bone beneath articular cartilage; appears more radio-opaque than adjacent bone.

1.3 Ossification and growth plate closures

Development of bone

- Skeletal mineralisation in dogs and cats begins about two-thirds of the way through pregnancy.

1 SKELETAL SYSTEM – GENERAL

Growth plate closure times (dog)

Scapular tuberosity	4–7 months
Proximal humerus:	
greater tubercle to humeral head	4 months
proximal epiphysis	10–13 months
Distal humerus:	
medial to lateral part of condyle	6 weeks
medial epicondyle	6 months
condyles to diaphysis	5–8 months
Proximal radius	5–11 months
Distal radius	6–12 months
Proximal ulna:	
olecranon	5–10 months
anconeal process	3–5 months
Distal ulna	6–12 months
Accessory carpal bone physis	10 weeks–5 months
Proximal metacarpal I	6 months
Distal metacarpal II–V	5–7 months
Phalanges (distal P1, proximal P2)	4–6 months
Pelvis:	
acetabulum	4–6 months
iliac crest	1–2 years (or may remain open permanently)
tuber ischii	8–10 months
Proximal femur:	
femoral neck	6–11 months
greater trochanter	6–10 months
lesser trochanter	8–13 months
Distal femur	6–11 months
Proximal tibia:	
medial to lateral condyle	6 weeks
tibial tuberosity to condyles	6–8 months
tuberosity and condyles to diaphysis	6–12 months
Distal tibia:	
main physis	5–11 months
medial malleolus of distal tibia	5 months
Proximal fibula	6–12 months
Distal fibula	5–12 months
Tuber calcis	11 weeks–8 months
Vertebral end plates	6–9 months

In the cat, growth plate closure times are more variable and later, especially in neutered animals. (Data from Ticer, J.W. (1975) *Radiograhic Technique in Small Animal Practice*; Philadelphia: W.B. Saunders and Sumner-Smith, G. (1966) Observations on epiphyseal fusion of the canine appendicular skeleton. *J. Small Animal Pract.* 7: 303–312)

- This occurs in a preformed cartilage matrix by endochondral and intramembranous ossification.
- At birth, ossification is seen only in diaphyses and skull bones; joints appear wide because epiphyses are still cartilaginous and therefore radiolucent.
- Subsequent ossification centres appear in epiphyses, apophyses and small bones.
- These secondary ossification centres show ragged margination as ossification progresses.
- As skeletal maturity approaches, secondary ossification centres enlarge and become smoother and physes and "joint spaces" become narrower.

1.4 Response of bone to disease or injury

Regardless of cause, the pathology of bone response is essentially the same. There are only two responses: bone loss (osteolysis) and bone production (osteogenesis). A combination of both processes can occur.

Bone loss (see 1.5)

- Recognised radiographically after approximately 7 days.
- Only the mineralised component of bone is visible radiographically, and 30–60% of mineral content must be lost before it can be detected radiographically.
- Radiography is thus not a sensitive tool for detecting minor bone loss.
- It is easier to see focal bone loss than diffuse bone loss.
- Loss is easier to see in cortical bone than in cancellous bone.
- *Osteopenia* is a radiological term describing a generalised reduction in bone radio-opacity. It is due to two different pathological processes:
  a. *osteomalacia* – insufficient or abnormal mineralisation of organic osteoid
  b. *osteoporosis* – normal proportions of osteoid and mineral component, but reduced amounts.
- Technical factors, such as radiographic exposure, must be taken into account when diagnosing osteopenia (compare with soft tissue opacity).

Bone production (see 1.6)

Sclerosis is a radiological term describing increased bone radio-opacity. It is due to two different pathological processes:
a. increased density of bone (e.g. sequestrum/involucrum, subchondral compaction, enlargement of trabeculae)
b. superimposed periosteal or endosteal reaction

SMALL ANIMAL RADIOLOGICAL DIFFERENTIAL DIAGNOSIS

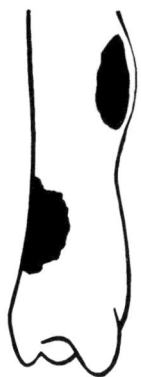

Figure 1.2 Geographic osteolysis

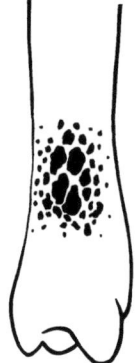

Figure 1.3 Moth-eaten osteolysis

Apparent sclerosis may also be caused by superimposition of bones – e.g. overlapping fracture fragments.

Mixed reactions

- Many lesions combine osteolysis and new bone production to variable degrees.
- New bone may predominate and obscure underlying minor osteolysis.
- Conversely, superimposition of irregular new bone may create areas of relative radiolucency which mimic osteolysis.

1.5 Patterns of focal bone loss (osteolysis)

Bone loss may be recognised 7–10 days after an insult. It is easier to recognise in cortical than trabecular bone and is more obvious if focal. Categorising the type of lysis helps in differential diagnosis by suggesting the "aggressiveness" or activity of the disease process (see 1.8).

Geographic osteolysis (Figure 1.2)

- Single, large area or confluence of several smaller areas, usually over 10 mm in diameter.
- Clearly marginated, i.e. there is a narrow zone of transition to normal bone.
- Sclerotic margins may be present if the body is attempting to wall off the lesion.
- Usually affects the medullary cavity.
- The overlying cortex may be interrupted, or thinned and displaced outwards ("expansile lesion").
- Usually a benign or non-aggressive low-grade lesion such as a bone cyst, pressure atrophy or benign dental tumour.

Moth-eaten osteolysis (Figure 1.3)

- Multiple areas of osteolysis, often varying in size (usually 3–10 mm in diameter).
- May coalesce to form geographic osteolysis in the centre of the lesion.
- Less well defined, with a wider zone of transition to normal bone.
- The cortex is more often irregularly eroded.
- More aggressive disease process – e.g. malignant tumour, osteomyelitis, multiple myeloma.

Permeative osteolysis (Figure 1.4)

- Numerous small pinpoint areas of osteolysis, 1–2 mm in diameter.
- Poorly defined, with a wide zone of transition to normal bone – areas of osteolysis are more spread out at the periphery.

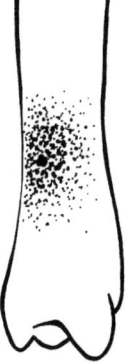

Figure 1.4 Permeative osteolysis

1 SKELETAL SYSTEM – GENERAL

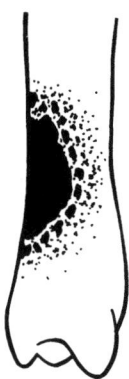

Figure 1.5 Mixed pattern of osteolysis

- Mainly recognised in the cortex (difficult to see in the medulla because of its trabecular pattern); cortex irregularly eroded.
- Highly aggressive disease process such as very active malignant tumour or fulminant osteomyelitis.

Mixed pattern of osteolysis (Figure 1.5)

Often more than one type of osteolysis is recognised – for example, central geographic osteolysis surrounded by moth-eaten and permeative zones. The nature of the lesion is denoted by the most aggressive type of osteolysis present.

Osteopenia (diffuse reduction in bone radio-opacity – see also 1.16)

- Due to osteomalacia or osteoporosis (see 1.4).

- Differential diagnosis (DDx) overexposure, overdevelopment, other causes of fogging.
- Radio-opacity of bone reduced compared with soft tissues ("ghostly bones").
- Thin, shell-like cortices.
- Coarse trabecular pattern as smaller trabeculae are resorbed.
- Apparent sclerosis of subchondral bone, especially in vertebral end plates, as these are relatively spared.
- "Double cortical line" due to intracortical bone resorption (unusual).
- If occurring in a limb due to disuse, mainly affects the epiphyses and small bones.
- Pathological folding fractures may occur, seen as sclerotic lines.

1.6 Patterns of osteogenesis – periosteal reactions

Periosteal new bone is also usually recognised 7–10 days after an insult (earlier in young animals). Identifying its nature helps in differential diagnosis by suggesting the "aggressiveness" of the disease process (see 1.8).

There are two main groups of periosteal reactions, continuous and interrupted.

Continuous periosteal reactions (Figure 1.6)

- A slow disease process, allowing new bone to form in an orderly fashion.
- Uniform in radio-opacity.
- Fairly constant in depth.
- Represent a benign process: non-aggressive, low grade or healed more aggressive disease (or the edge of a more aggressive lesion).

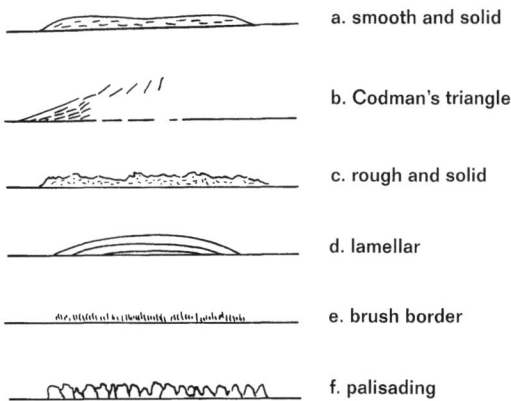

a. smooth and solid

b. Codman's triangle

c. rough and solid

d. lamellar

e. brush border

f. palisading

Figure 1.6 Continuous periosteal reactions

TYPES

- Smooth and solid – e.g. chronic mild trauma, remodelled new bone, healed subperiosteal haematoma.
- Codman's triangle – solid triangle of new bone at the edge of a more active lesion, due to infilling beneath an advancing periosteal elevation. Often at the diaphyseal edge of a primary malignant bone tumour.
- Rough and solid – e.g. trauma, adjacent soft tissue inflammation.
- Lamellar ("onion skin") – due to recurrent episodes of periosteal elevation such as metaphyseal osteopathy (hypertrophic osteodystrophy).
- Brush border ("hair on end") – adjacent soft tissue inflammation, some cases of hypertrophic osteopathy.
- Palisading – solid chunks of new bone develop perpendicular to the cortex – for example, hypertrophic osteopathy, craniomandibular osteopathy. Less aggressive than brush border reaction.

Interrupted periosteal reactions (Figure 1.7)

- Rapidly changing lesions breaching the cortex and periosteum with no time for orderly repair.
- Variable in radio-opacity and depth.
- May be in short, disconnected segments.
- Often associated with underlying cortical lysis.
- Represents an aggressive disease process such as malignant neoplasia or osteomyelitis.

TYPES

- Spicular – wisps of new bone extending out into soft tissue, roughly perpendicular to the cortex.
- "Sunburst" – radiating spicular pattern, deepest centrally; indicates a focal lesion erupting through the cortex and extending into soft tissues.
- Amorphous – fragments of new bone variable in size, shape and orientation; DDx remnants of original bone; tumour bone produced by osteosarcomas (tend to be further out in soft tissues than periosteal new bone).

1.7 Principles of interpretation

Bone has a limited response to disease or insult so lesions with different aetiologies may look similar and radiographs may not give a definitive diagnosis. The radiologist must examine radiographs methodically, learn to recognise patterns and then formulate lists of differential diagnoses. Patient type, history, clinical signs, blood parameters, geographic location (current or previous), change of the lesion over time and response to treatment must all be considered. Films should be oriented consistently on the viewer and bone specimens and radiographic atlases used for reference.

Features to consider when interpreting skeletal radiographs include the following:

1. *DISTRIBUTION OF LESIONS*
   a. Generalised or diffuse changes:
      - metabolic or nutritional disease
      - neoplasia (e.g. widespread osteolysis – multiple myeloma; widespread sclerosis – lymphosarcoma)
   b. Whole limb:
      - disuse.
   c. Focal lesions:
      - congenital or developmental
      - trauma
      - infection/inflammation
      - neoplasia.

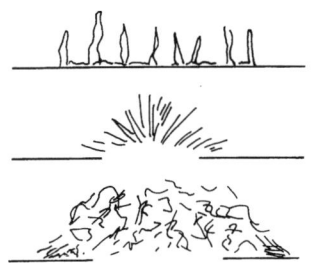

a. spicular

b. sunburst

c. amorphous
(+/– tumour bone and remnants of original bone)

Figure 1.7 Interrupted periosteal reactions.

1 SKELETAL SYSTEM – GENERAL

d. Symmetrical lesions:
   - metabolic disease
   - haematogenous osteomyelitis
   - metaphyseal osteopathy (hypertrophic osteodystrophy)
   - bilateral trauma
   - metastatic tumours.

2. **NUMBER OF LESIONS**
   a. Mono-ostotic:
      - congenital or developmental
      - trauma
      - localised infection (trauma, iatrogenic)
      - neoplasia (primary bone tumour, soft tissue tumour distant from joint, solitary metastasis).
   b. polyostotic (see 1.20).

3. **LOCATION OF LESIONS** (see 1.21–1.24)
   a. Epiphysis – e.g. various arthritides, chondrodysplasias, osteochondrosis (OC), soft tissue tumours.
   b. Physis – mainly young animals – e.g. haematogenous osteomyelitis, trauma, premature closures, rickets.
   c. Metaphysis – e.g. haematogenous osteomyelitis, metaphyseal osteopathy (hypertrophic osteodystrophy), primary malignant bone tumours.
   d. Diaphysis – e.g. trauma, panosteitis, hypertrophic osteopathy, metastatic tumours.

4. **PRESENCE AND TYPE OF OSTEOLYSIS** (see 1.5).

5. **PRESENCE AND TYPE OF OSTEOGENESIS** (see 1.6)
   a. Periosteal.
   b. Endosteal.
   c. Trabecular.
   d. Neoplastic.
   e. Heterotopic.
   f. Dystrophic.

6. **ZONE OF TRANSITION BETWEEN LESION AND NORMAL BONE**
   a. Short – well demarcated lesion, abrupt transition to normal bone; usually benign or non-aggressive disease.
   b. Long – poorly demarcated lesions, gradual transition to normal bone; usually aggressive disease.

7. **SOFT TISSUE CHANGES**
   a. Muscle wastage.
   b. Soft tissue swelling.
   c. Joint effusions.
   d. Displacement or obliteration of fascial planes.
   e. Soft tissue emphysema.
   f. Soft tissue mineralisation.
   g. Radio-opaque foreign bodies.
   h. Abnormalities in other body systems (e.g. lung metastases).

8. **RATE OF CHANGE ON SEQUENTIAL RADIOGRAPHS +/– RESPONSE TO TREATMENT.**

1.8 Features of aggressive and non-aggressive bone lesions

An aggressive lesion is one which extends rapidly into adjacent normal bone with no, or minimal, host response attempting to confine the lesion.

Non-aggressive	Aggressive
Example: uncomplicated trauma, degenerative or resolving lesion, benign neoplasia, bone cyst (Figure 1.8)	Example: malignant neoplasia, fulminant osteomyelitis (Figure 1.9)
Well demarcated	Poorly demarcated
Short zone of transition	Long zone of transition
Absent or geographic osteolysis	Permeative osteolysis
Cortex may be displaced and thinned, but rarely broken	Cortex interrupted
Continuous solid or smooth periosteal reaction	Interrupted, irregular periosteal reaction
With or without surrounding sclerosis	No surrounding sclerosis
Static or slow rate of change	Rapid rate of change
If mixed signs are present the lesion should be categorised according to its most aggressive feature.	

1.9 Fractures – radiography, classification, assessment of healing

Causes of fractures

1. Trauma.
2. Pathological; spontaneous or following minor trauma to weakened bone
   a. Neoplasia.
   b. Bone cyst.
   c. Osteomyelitis.

7

SMALL ANIMAL RADIOLOGICAL DIFFERENTIAL DIAGNOSIS

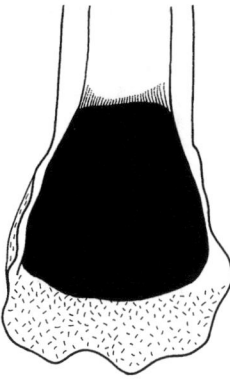

Figure 1.8 Non-aggressive osteolytic bone lesion, with geographic osteolysis, short zone of transition, intact overlying cortex and smooth periosteal reaction.

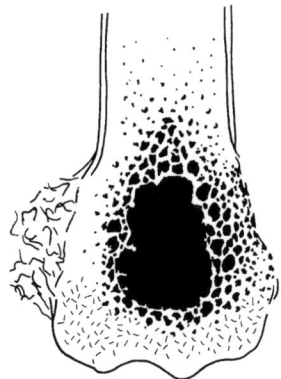

Figure 1.9 Aggressive bone lesion, with a mixed pattern of osteolysis, long zone of transition, cortical erosion and interrupted periosteal reaction.

    d. Diffuse osteopenia such as nutritional secondary hyperparathyroidism (usually folding fractures).
3. "Stress protection" – weakened bone at the end of an orthopaedic plate.
4. Defect in bone due to biopsy or surgery.

Radiography

1. Obtain at least two radiographs, including views at 90° to one another.
2. Include joints above and below to check for joint involvement and rotation of fragments.
3. In young animals examine growth plates for signs of injury.
4. Radiograph the opposite leg for assessment of true bone length if surgery is planned.
5. Use a horizontal beam if necessary (for example if pain, spinal instability or thoracic trauma prevent dorsal recumbency).
6. Increase exposure factors if soft tissue swelling is present.
7. Thoracic and abdominal studies are often required in cases of road accident or falls from high buildings (e.g. to detect pulmonary contusion, pneumothorax or bladder rupture).
8. If hairline fractures are suspected but not seen repeat the radiographs 7–10 days later (or use scintigraphy).
9. Stressed views may be needed to detect fracture (sub)luxations or collateral ligament damage (see 2.1).

Radiographic signs of fractures

1. Disruption of the normal contour of bone, of the cortex or of the trabecular pattern.
2. Radiolucent fracture lines can be mimicked by
   a. nutrient foramen
   b. overlying fascial plane fat
   c. skin defect or gas in fascial planes – open fracture
   d. normal growth plate or skull suture
   e. Mach line – dark lines appear along the edge of two overlapping bones due to an optical illusion
   f. grid line artefact (from damaged grid).

N.B. hairline or minimally displaced fractures radiating along the shaft from the main fracture site may be seen only if parallel to the X-ray beam; this may require additional views.

3. Increased radio-opacity of cortex and medulla if the fracture is folding or impacted or if fragments overlap in the plane of the X-ray beam.
4. Small free fragments of variable size can be mimicked by
   a. unusual centres of ossification
   b. inconstant sesamoids
   c. multipartite sesamoids

These are often bilateral. If in doubt, radiograph the opposite limb for comparison.

5. Ballistics, foreign material and gas – compound fractures.
6. Evidence of fracture healing – see below.
7. Muscle atrophy and disuse osteopenia.

Reasons for overlooking fractures include incorrect exposure/processing, non-displacement of fracture fragments, insufficient number of views, confusion with growth plates and fracture reduced by positioning.

1 SKELETAL SYSTEM – GENERAL

Classification of fractures

1. Closed/open or compound (risk of infection).
2. Simple (single fracture)/comminuted (three or more fragments)/multiple (fracture lines do not connect; same bone or different bones)/segmental (two or more separate fracture lines in a single bone).
3. Transverse/oblique/spiral/irregular.
4. Complete (entire bone width)/incomplete (one cortex only)
   a. greenstick fracture – convex side cortex
   b. torus fracture – concave side fracture.
5. Chip fracture (no or one articular surface involved)/slab fracture (two joint surfaces involved).
6. Articular/non-articular.
7. Avulsion (traction by soft tissue attachment).
8. Fatigue or stress fracture – one cortex only, from repeated minor trauma.
9. Impaction or compression fracture – shortening of bone due to stress along its length; especially occurs in the vertebrae.
10. Fracture (sub)luxation – fracture with associated soft tissue injury causing joint instability or displacement.
11. Salter-Harris fractures (Figure 1.10) – fractures involving unfused growth plates may lead to growth disturbances e.g. shortening or angulation of bone. Can occur surprisingly late in neutered cats as the growth plates remain open longer.

Assessment of fracture: at the time of injury

1. Location – which bone, which anatomical area of the bone?
2. Type of fracture – see above.
3. Displacement of fragments – distal relative to proximal fragment.
4. Underlying bone radio-opacity, for evidence of pathological fracture (Figure 1.11).
5. Involvement of joints – subsequent osteoarthritis possible.
6. Presence of foreign material.
7. Soft tissue injuries.
8. Injuries elsewhere in body.

Assessment of fracture: postoperative radiographs

1. Degree of reduction – at least 50% bone contact needed for healing (on orthogonal views).
2. Alignment
   a. side-to-side and cranial–caudal
   b. rotational alignment – include joints above and below.
3. Adequacy of implant type, size and placement.
4. Joints – congruency, lack of entry by implants.

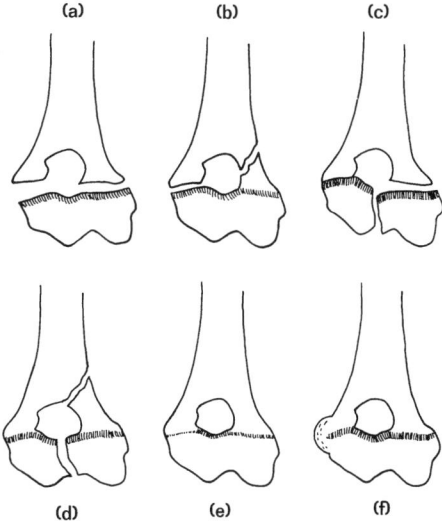

Figure 1.10 Salter-Harris classification of growth plate fractures. (a) Type 1: separation through the growth plate; (b) Type 2: a metaphyseal fragment remains attached to the epiphysis; (c) Type 3: fracture through the epiphysis into the growth plate; (d) Type 4: fracture through the epiphysis and metaphysis crossing the growth plate; (e) Type 5: crush injury to the growth plate (may not be radiographically visible, but leads to growth disturbance); (f) Type 6: bridging of the growth plate by periosteal new bone.

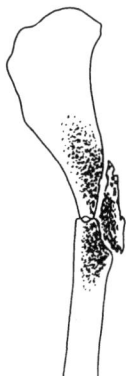

Figure 1.11 Pathological fracture – tibial fracture through an area of diffuse bone rarefaction caused by metastatic neoplasia.

SMALL ANIMAL RADIOLOGICAL DIFFERENTIAL DIAGNOSIS

5. Presence of cancellous bone grafts.
6. Soft tissues.

(Useful mnemonic for assessing postoperative radiographs: ABCDS: alignment, bone, cartilage, device, soft tissues).

Fracture healing

Two orthogonal views are needed to assess healing as the fracture may appear bridged on one view and not on another. Healing occurs more rapidly in young animals.

Primary bone healing

Direct bridging of the fracture by osseous tissue, re-establishing cortex and medulla without intermediate callus. Occurs with perfect reduction and stabilisation of the fracture site. Stages 1, 2 and 5.

Secondary bone healing

Unstructured bone laid down in soft tissue and subsequently remodelled. Stages 1–5 (Figure 1.12).

- Stage 1 (recent injury): sharp fracture ends; well-defined fragments; soft tissue swelling; disruption to skin and emphysema if the fracture is compound.
- Stage 2 (7–14 days): reducing soft tissue swelling; fracture line blurred due to hyperaemia and bone resorption; hairline fractures widened and more obvious; early, indistinct periosteal reaction especially in young animals.
- Stage 3 (2–3 weeks): abundant, unstructured bony callus forming (size depends on the type of fracture, location, use of limb, stability at site, vascularisation); partial bridging of fracture line; structurally strong.
- Stage 4 (3–8 weeks): continued filling-in of the fracture line; early remodelling of the callus.
- Stage 5 (8 weeks on): continued remodelling and reduction in size of callus; restoration of cortices and trabecular pattern; the limb may straighten slightly if malunion occurred originally.

Assessment of fracture: subsequent examinations

1. Use equivalent technique (reduce exposure factors if soft tissue is less due to reduction of swelling or muscle wastage).
2. Alignment of fragments.
3. Position and integrity of implants – migration, bending, cracking or fracture of implants may occur.
4. Stability of fracture site – evidence of instability following surgical repair includes migration of implants and radiolucent haloes around screws and pins (DDx infection, bone necrosis from high-speed drill).
5. Stage of fracture healing.
6. Evidence of infection – lysis especially around implants, unexpected periosteal reactions (DDx periosteal stripping), sequestrum formation, soft tissue swelling +/− emphysema.
7. Evidence of secondary joint disease.
8. Evidence of disuse – muscle wastage, osteopenia.

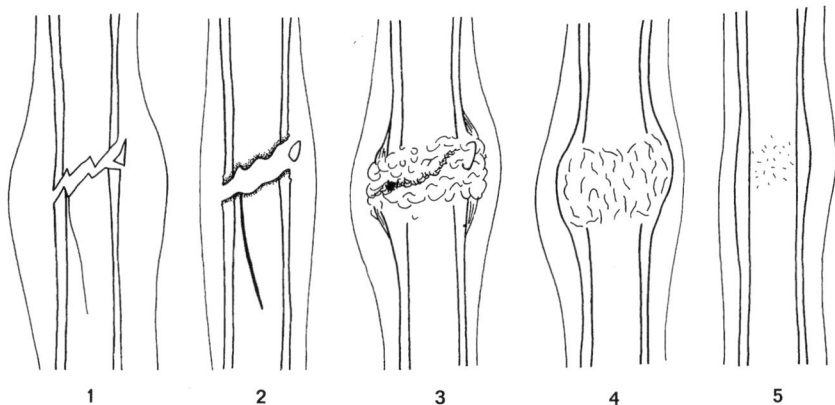

Figure 1.12 The five stages of fracture healing. Stage 1: sharp fragments, hairline fractures line easily overlooked, marked soft tissue swelling; Stage 2: fracture margins becoming blurred; hairline fractures more obvious; reduced soft tissue swelling; Stage 3: unstructured bony callus with partial bridging of fracture line; Stage 4: callus becoming more solid; early remodelling; Stage 5: continued remodelling results in reduction in callus size.

1 SKELETAL SYSTEM – GENERAL

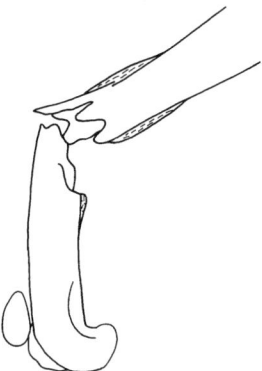

Figure 1.13 Atrophic non-union of a femoral fracture.

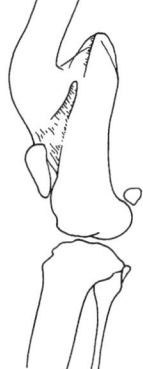

Figure 1.15 Malunion of a femoral fracture.

Complications of fracture healing

1. Delayed union – time taken to heal is longer than expected for type and location of fracture, but evidence of bone activity is present
   a. disuse
   b. instability
   c. poor reduction
   d. poor nutrition
   e. old age
   f. infection
   g. poor vascularity
   h. large intramedullary pin
   i. undetected underlying pathology.
2. Non-union – fracture healing has apparently ceased without uniting the fragments; bone ends smooth with sealed medullary cavity
   a. atrophic (dying-back) (Figure 1.13) – no callus, pointed bone ends; especially the radius and ulna in toy breeds of dog
   b. hypertrophic ("elephant's foot") (Figure 1.14) – new bone surrounds bone ends but does not cross the fracture line giving a bell-shaped appearance; fragment ends parallel.

   Both types may form a false joint in which the fragment ends are contoured – e.g. one is concave and the other is convex or pointed.
3. Malunion (Figure 1.15) – bones fuse with incorrect alignment.
4. Excessive callus formation
   a. movement at fracture site
   b. infection
   c. periosteal stripping
   d. incorporation of bone grafts.
5. Ossification of stripped periosteum – e.g. "rhino horn" callus caudal to femur. Not usually a clinical problem.
6. Osteomyelitis – leads to delayed or non-union.
7. "Fracture disease" – a clinical syndrome with joint stiffness and muscle wastage due to disease. Radiographs show osteopenia.
8. Neoplastic transformation – may be years later; especially if metallic implants present or healing was complex. Mechanism not known, but possibly chronic inflammation.
9. Metallosis – a sterile, chronic, proliferative osteomyelitis which may result from reaction to metallic implants especially if dissimilar metals have been combined; less common in domestic animals than in humans due to their shorter life span.

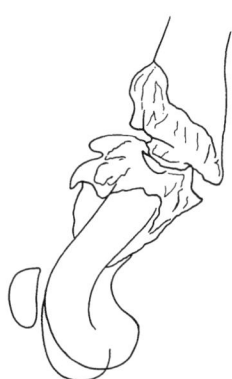

Figure 1.14 Hypertrophic non-union of a femoral fracture.

BONES

1.10 Altered shape of long bones

See also Section 1.15
1. Bowing of bone(s) (Figure 1.16)
   a. "Normal" in chondrodystrophic breeds (e.g. Basset Hound, Bulldog, Dachshund); especially radius and ulna. Long bones in affected breeds often also have prominent apophyses (enesthesiopathies – bony spurs within attachments of soft tissues).
   b. Growth plate trauma resulting in uneven growth.
   c. Radius – passive bowing due to shortening of ulna and secondary "bowstring" effect (see 3.5.4 and Figure 3.12).
   d. Chondrodysplasias (dyschondroplasias) are recognised in numerous breeds and in the Domestic Shorthaired cat (see 1.21.7). Failure of normal endochondral ossification leads to bowing of long bones, especially the radius and ulna, and epiphyseal changes resulting in arthritis.
   e. Rickets; bowing of long bones, especially the radius and ulna.
   f. Congenital hypothyroidism; bowing of long bones, especially the radius and ulna; seen especially in Boxers (see 1.21.9).
   g. Asymmetric bridging of a growth plate, resulting in uneven growth. For example, severe periosteal reaction in metaphyseal osteopathy (hypertrophic osteodystrophy), surgical staple left in too long.
   h. Tension from shortened soft tissues (e.g. quadriceps contracture).
   i. Altered stresses due to bone or joint disease elsewhere in the limb.
   j. Hemimelia (rare) – either radius or ulna is absent (usually radial agenesis), putting abnormal stress on the remaining bone.
2. Angulation of bone
   a. Traumatic folding (greenstick) fracture.
   b. Pathological fracture:
      - primary, secondary or pseudohyperparathyroidism (see 1.16.4 and Figure 1.21)
      - osteolytic neoplasia (primary, secondary, multiple myeloma) (see 1.18.1, 1.19.1 and Figure 1.24)
      - enchondromatosis (see 1.18.7)
      - bone cyst (see 1.18.8)
      - osteomyelitis (see 1.19.2 and Figures 1.27 and 1.28)
      - severe osteopenia (see 1.16)
      - osteogenesis imperfecta (see 1.16.13).
   c. Malunion.
3. Abnormally straight bone (e.g. radius, due to premature closure of the distal radial growth plate).
4. Expansion or irregular margination of bone
   a. Osteochondroma (single)/multiple cartilaginous exostoses (multiple) (see 1.15.2 and Figure 1.19).
   b. Enchondromatosis (see 1.18.7).
   c. Other expansile tumour (see 1.18.7 and Figure 1.25).
   d. Bone cyst (see 1.18.8).
   e. Late, remodelled metaphyseal osteopathy (see 1.23.3 and Figure 1.30).
   f. Disseminated idiopathic skeletal hyperostosis (DISH) – mainly spine but also extremital periarticular new bone and enesthesiopathies.
   g. Insertion tendinopathies:
      - "normal" in chondrodystrophic breeds
      - pathological (see Chapter 3).

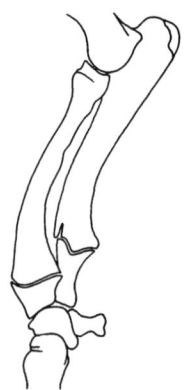

Figure 1.16 Bowing of the radius and ulna – shortening of the ulna due to a distal ulnar growth plate injury in an immature animal.

1.11 Dwarfism

1. Proportionate dwarfism
   a. Pituitary dwarfism; mainly German Shepherd dog, also reported in the Miniature Pinscher, Spitz and Covelian Bear dog. May be hypothyroid too (see below).
2. Disproportionate dwarfism

a. Chondrodysplasias (see 1.21.7).
b. Hypothyroidism; mainly in Boxer (see 1.21.9).
c. Rickets (see 1.22.8 and Figure 1.29).
d. Zinc-responsive chondrodysplasia in the Alaskan Malamute and possibly other northern breeds.
e. Cats – mucopolysaccharidosis Types VI and VII – especially cats with Siamese ancestry; rarely occurs in dogs but mucopolysaccharidosis Type VII is reported to cause dwarfism in mongrels.
f. Cats – mucolipidosis Type II (rare).
g. Cats – hypervitaminosis A in kittens.

1.12 Delayed ossification or growth plate closure

Delayed ossification is mainly recognised in epiphyses, carpal and tarsal bones. The various conditions listed below may be difficult to differentiate and chondrodysplasias are often initially misdiagnosed as rickets. However, rickets does not manifest until after weaning whereas other conditions begin to develop before weaning. The table summarises the radiographic changes that may be present.
1. Chondrodysplasias – effect on growth plate closure time variable.
2. Congenital hypothyroidism – especially Boxers.
3. Pituitary dwarfism – especially German Shepherd dogs.
4. Rickets.
5. Hypervitaminosis D – a massive intake in young animal causes retarded growth, bone deformity and osteopenia.
6. Copper deficiency.
7. Cats – mucopolysaccharidoses, especially in cats with Siamese ancestry; rarely affects dogs.
8. Cats – neutering (especially males) delays growth plate closure.

1.13 Increased radio-opacity within bone

It may be difficult to differentiate increased radio-opacity within a bone from increased radio-opacity due to superimposition of surrounding new bone. Both will produce an increased radio-opacity often referred to as *sclerosis*.
1. Technical factors causing artefactual increased radio-opacity
   a. Underexposure (too low a kV or mAs)
   b. Underdevelopment.
2. Normal
   a. Normal "metaphyseal condensation" in the metaphysis of skeletally immature animals; also termed "idiopathic osteodystrophy"
   b. Subchondral bone.
3. Neoplasia
   a. Primary malignant bone tumour of blastic type, although usually there is some evidence of osteolysis as well (see 1.19.1 and Figure 1.26)
   b. Bone metastases – may be sclerotic or osteolytic; atypical sites for primary tumours; often multiple in one bone or polyostotic (see 1.19.1).
   c. Cats – feline leukaemia (FeLV)-induced medullary osteosclerosis – rare; likely to be widespread in the skeleton.
4. Osteomyelitis – more likely to be a mixed lesion including osteolysis (see 1.19.2 and Figures 1.27 and 1.28). Haematogenous spread is the most common cause so there are likely to be multiple, possibly bilaterally symmetrical lesions.
   a. Bacterial
   b. Fungal
   c. Protozoal – leishmaniasis*. Periosteal and intramedullary bone proliferation in diaphyses and flat bones provoked by chronic osteomyelitis; mixed, aggressive bone lesions; also osteolytic joint lesions.

	Epiphyseal dysplasia	Wide growth plates	Late-closing growth plates	Osteopenia	Long bone bowing
Chondrodysplasia	Yes	Yes	Some	No	Yes
Hypothyroidism	Yes	Yes	Yes	No	Yes
Hypervitaminosis A (young cats)	Stunting due to degeneration of physes			Yes	Shortening
Pituitary dwarfism	Yes	Yes	Yes	No	No
Mucopolysaccharidosis	Yes	"Retarded growth"		Yes	No
Rickets	No	Yes	Yes	Yes	Yes

5. Panosteitis – usually in young adult male German Shepherd dogs, producing shifting lameness, which may be severe at times. Other large breeds of dog may also be affected. Lesions are seen in long bones (Figure 1.17) and several patterns of increased diaphyseal radio-opacity may occur
   a. Ill-defined medullary patches often near the nutrient foramen; main DDx osteomyelitis
   b. Coarse, sclerotic trabecular pattern
   c. Narrow transverse sclerotic lines as recovery occurs; DDx growth arrest lines
   d. Increased radio-opacity due to superimposed periosteal reaction.
6. Growth arrest lines – fine, transverse sclerotic lines due to periods of arrested and increased growth, of no clinical significance; DDx panosteitis.
7. Metaphyseal osteopathy (MO), also known as hypertrophic osteodystrophy (HOD) – affects young dogs, especially the distal radius and ulna; initially osteolytic metaphyseal bands +/− sclerotic borders; later superimposed periosteal new bone adds to increased radio-opacity (see 1.23.3 and Figure 1.30).
8. Fractures – if impaction of bone or overlapping of fragments occur a sclerotic band rather than a bone defect may be seen.
   a. Folding fractures:
      - "greenstick fractures" (single cortex) in young animals
      - osteopenia, especially nutritional secondary hyperparathyroidism

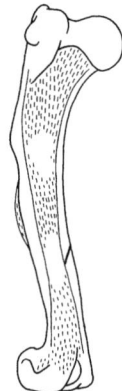

Figure 1.17 Panosteitis of the humerus: patches of increased medullary radio-opacity, coarse trabeculation and smooth periosteal reaction.

   b. Compression or impaction fractures – especially vertebrae
   c. Superimposition of overridden fragments seen on one radiographic projection, but shown to be displaced using orthogonal view
   d. Healing fracture.
9. Osteopenia – sparing of subchondral bone and bone along epiphyseal and metaphyseal margins of growth plates creates *apparent* sclerotic bands (see 1.16).
10. Skeletal immaturity – a sclerotic metaphyseal band is also seen in skeletally immature dogs as a normal finding ("metaphyseal condensation").
11. Lead poisoning – in rare cases thin sclerotic bands are seen in the metaphyses of long bones and vertebrae of young animals suffering lead poisoning; also causes osteopenia.
12. Bone infarcts (rare) – multiple, irregular sclerotic patches in medullary cavities of limb bones and cranial diploë; may be associated with osteosarcoma. Mainly affect smaller breeds (e.g. Shetland Sheepdog, Miniature Schnauzer). Cause unknown, possibly vascular disease leading to hypoxia.
13. Osteopetrosis (osteosclerosis fragilis, marble bones, chalk bones) – rare. Massive, diffuse increase in bone radio-opacity with coarsening of trabeculae, obliteration of medulla and thickening of cortices; bones are brittle and pathological fractures occur. May cause anaemia if medullary cavities are severely compromised.
   a. Congenital:
      - autosomal recessive gene, usually lethal
      - hereditary anaemia in the Basenji
   b. Acquired due to various causes:
      - chronic dietary excess of calcium
      - chronic vitamin D toxicity
      - myelofibrosis
      - idiopathic
      - cats – FeLV-induced medullary osteosclerosis.

1.14 Periosteal reactions

Periosteal reactions forming new bone may be localised or diffuse, depending upon the aetiology. Localised periosteal reactions appearing as bony masses are also described in Section 1.15.

1 SKELETAL SYSTEM - GENERAL

1. Trauma
   a. Direct blow to the cortex producing periosteal stimulation (a single episode or repetitive milder trauma)
   b. Periosteal tearing or elevation associated with fractures
   c. Subperiosteal haematoma – often caudal skull; also sometimes in dogs with coagulopathies (e.g. Dobermanns with von Willebrand's disease).
2. Infection (more likely to produce diffuse reaction in young animals in which the periosteum is loosely attached)
   a. Bacterial – usually associated with an open wound (trauma, surgery):
      - focal anaerobic osteomyelitis occurs following bite wounds, with a small central sequestrum surrounded by a raised, ring-like periosteal reaction
   b. Fungal – may be multifocal due to haematogenous spread; more often mixed osteolytic/proliferative lesion (see 1.19.2)
   c. Protozoal:
      - leishmaniasis* – a spectrum of periosteal reactions varying from smooth to irregular; also intramedullary sclerosis, mixed bone lesions and osteolytic joint disease
      - hepatozoonosis* – chronic myositis, debilitation and death, often with periosteal reactions varying from subtle to dramatic
   d. Cats – feline tuberculosis – various *Mycobacterium* spp. (rare). Also mixed lesions, discospondylitis and arthritis.
3. Neoplasia – early malignancy (primary bone, metastatic or soft tissue tumours before osteolysis becomes apparent). Follow-up radiography may help to distinguish neoplasia from infection or trauma.
4. Panosteitis – severe cases may show mild smooth or lamellated periosteal reactions on the diaphyses (see 1.13.5 and Figure 1.17). The diagnosis is usually obvious from the signalment and the presence of medullary lesions.
5. Metaphyseal osteopathy (hypertrophic osteodystrophy) – advanced cases show collars of periosteal new bone and paraperiosteal soft tissue mineralisation around the metaphyses which may obscure the characteristic mottled metaphyseal band (see 1.23.3 and Figure 1.30). Subsequent remodelling causes thickening of metaphyses. In severe cases the adjacent epiphysis may be bridged, resulting in an angular limb deformity.
6. Hypertrophic (pulmonary) osteopathy (HPO, Marie's disease. Figure 1.18) – florid periosteal new bone on the diaphyses of long bones, usually beginning distally in the limb and being bilaterally symmetrical. More severe on the abaxial margins of digits. Classically the new bone is in a palisade pattern, but it may also be smooth and solid, irregular or lamellated. The thorax and abdomen should be radiographed to look for underlying lesions (usually pulmonary masses). The diagnosis is usually obvious from the type and extent of the periosteal reaction and the presence of a primary lesion.
7. Craniomandibular osteopathy (mainly terriers, especially West Highland White Terrier) – florid periosteal new bone on the skull (see 4.10.1 and Figure 4.4). Masses of paraperiosteal new bone adjacent to distal ulnar metaphyses are occasionally seen.
8. Cats – hypervitaminosis A: focal periosteal new bone around vertebrae (mainly cervical/thoracic), joints (especially elbow and stifle), sternum and ribs. Usually young adult cats on raw liver diets; DDx mucopolysaccharidosis.
9. Cats – mucopolysaccharidoses: lysosomal storage diseases causing new bone on the spine which appears very similar to hypervitaminosis A; also dwarfism, facial deformity, pectus excavatum and hip dysplasia. Especially seen in cats with Siamese ancestry; DDx hypervitaminosis A. Rare in dogs.

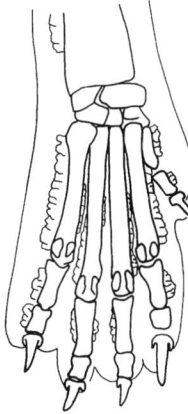

Figure 1.18 Hypertrophic pulmonary osteopathy – palisading periosteal new bone with overlying diffuse soft tissue swelling.

1.15 Bony masses (see also 1.10 and 1.14)

Differential diagnoses for bony masses include mixed osteoproductive/osteolytic lesions in which new bone predominates and obscures underlying lysis, and soft tissue mineralisation which is close to or superimposed over bone (e.g. calcinosis circumscripta) (see 12.2.2 and Figure 12.1).

1. Trauma
   a. Exuberant, localised periosteal reaction following direct injury
   b. Large fracture callus – due to movement, infection, periosteal stripping
   c. Hypertrophic non-union – bone defect at the fracture line should be evident
   d. "Rhino horn callus" from periosteal stripping caudal to the femur associated with femoral fracture.
2. Neoplasia
   a. Osteochondroma (single)/multiple cartilaginous exostoses (multiple). A skeletal dysplasia rather than a true neoplastic process. In dogs, seen when skeletally immature at osteochondral junctions e.g. long bone metaphyses (often bilateral), ribs and costochondral junctions, pelvis and vertebrae (Figure 1.19). Hereditary tendency; especially affects Yorkshire Terriers. Generally smooth, cauliflower-like or nodular projections with cortex and medulla continuous with underlying bone, but may appear more granular and aggressive during the active growth phase. Lesions in long bone may be more irregular than those elsewhere. Whilst still ossifying they may appear not to be attached to underlying bone, and may mimic calcinosis circumscripta (see 12.2.2 and Figure 12.1). Osteochondromata in ribs may mimic healing rib fractures. Growth of osteochondromata ceases at skeletal maturity, but malignant transformation may occur.
   Rare in cats, seen in older animals, possibly with a viral aetiology. Arise from the perichondrium of flat or irregular bones such as the skull and may continue to grow, becoming more aggressive.
   b. Osteoma (benign) – rare, usually skull; often affects younger dogs. Dense, bony mass without underlying osteolysis
   c. Ossifying fibroma – skull
   d. Multilobular tumour of bone – skull
   e. Predominantly osteoblastic primary malignant bone tumour – mainly metaphyses of long bones; also skull

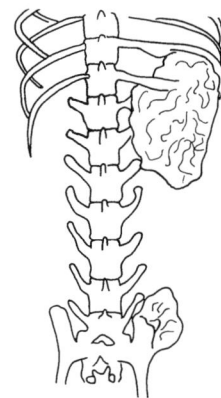

Figure 1.19 Multiple cartilaginous exostoses (dog) – expansile masses arising from a rib and the wing of the ilium.

   f. Parosteal osteosarcoma – rare; radiographically and pathologically distinct from other osteosarcomata. Slow-growing, sclerotic, smooth or lobulated, non-aggressive bony masses arising from periosteum or parosteal connective tissue with little or no underlying osteolysis; seen especially around the stifle.
3. Enthesiopathies
   a. Normal prominence of apophyses in chondrodystrophic breeds; bilaterally symmetrical (Figure 1.20)
   b. Enthesiopathies in individuals of other breeds suffering from chondrodysplasias; bilaterally symmetrical
   c. Enthesiopathies in specific tendon and ligament attachments (see Chapter 3)
   d. Disseminated skeletal hyperostosis (DISH) – spurs of new bone, mainly on the spine but also extremital periarticular new bone and enthesiopathies.
4. Proliferative joint diseases (see also 2.5)
   a. Severe osteoarthritis
   b. DISH
   c. Cats – hypervitaminosis A; especially the elbow and stifle.
5. Craniomandibular osteopathy – masses of periosteal new bone on the skull, mainly mandibles and temporal bones; rare limb changes (see 3.5, 4.10.1 and Figure 4.4).

1.16 Osteopenia

Osteopenia is a radiographic term meaning reduction in radiographic bone radio-opacity. This may be due to *osteoporosis* (reduced

1 SKELETAL SYSTEM – GENERAL

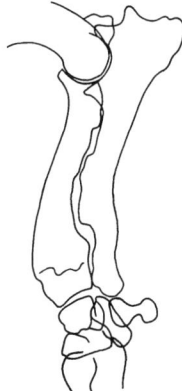

Figure 1.20 "Normal" radius and ulna of a chondrodystrophic dog showing bowing of the long bones, prominence of apophyses and bony proliferation in the interosseus space.

bone mass but normal ratio of organic matrix and inorganic salts) or *osteomalacia* (organic matrix present in excess due to failure of mineralisation), and these cannot be differentiated radiographically. This section lists differential diagnoses for diffuse osteopenia usually affecting the whole skeleton (or, in the case of disuse, a whole limb). More localised areas of osteopenia are described in section 1.18.

Osteopenia is most readily apparent in parts of the skeleton with high bone turnover such as trabeculated bone in the metaphyses and epiphyses of long bones, vertebrae and the skull. The radiographic signs of osteopenia are:

- a reduction in bone radio-opacity compared with soft tissues
- thinning of cortices, sometimes with a "double cortical line"
- relative sparing of subchondral bone leading to apparent sclerosis, especially in the endplates of the vertebrae and adjacent to physes
- coarse trabeculation due to resorption of smaller trabeculae
- pathological folding or compression fractures.

Most causes of osteopenia are metabolic diseases, and the aetiology may be complex. The condition is reversible if the cause is corrected. Osteopenia may also be mimicked by incorrect technical factors during radiography.

1. Technical factors causing artefactual osteopenia:
   a. overexposure (kV or mAs too high)
   b. overdevelopment
   c. fogging of the film (numerous causes).
2. Reduction in overlying soft tissue leading to relative overexposure, e.g. in limb with chronic disuse. Compare with the opposite limb if possible.
3. Disuse (limb) – paralysis, fracture or severe lameness; often most severe distal to a fracture and particularly affecting epiphyses and the cuboidal bones of the carpus and tarsus.
4. Hyperparathyroidism (osteitis fibrosa cystica, fibrous osteodystrophy). Dystrophic or metastatic calcification may occur secondarily in soft tissues, such as the kidneys, gastric rugae and major blood vessels
   a. Nutritional secondary hyperparathyroidism (juvenile osteoporosis, Butcher's dog disease; Figure 1.21) – especially young animals due to high skeletal activity. Seen after weaning in animals on a high meat diet that is low in calcium and high in phosphorus. Clinical signs of lameness, lordosis and para/tetraplegia due to folding fractures occur. More common in cats than in dogs
   b. Renal secondary hyperparathyroidism (renal rickets, renal osteodystrophy) – chronic renal failure in young animals with renal dysplasia or in older animals with chronic renal disease; mainly affects the skull, causing "rubber jaw" (see 4.9.4 and Figure 4.3), but other skeletal changes may also be seen (as above)
   c. Primary hyperparathyroidism – rare; parathyroid gland hyperplasia or neoplasia
   d. Pseudohyperparathyroidism; hypercalcaemia of malignancy – various neoplastic causes, especially lymphosarcoma and anal sac adenocarcinoma; also mammary adenocarcinoma, myeloma, gastric squamous cell carcinoma, thyroid adenocarcinoma, testicular interstitial cell tumours
   e. Other causes of secondary hyperparathyroidism include pregnancy and lactation, vitamin D deficiency, acidosis, osteomalacic anticonvulsant therapy.
5. Corticosteroid excess
   a. Hyperadrenocorticism – Cushing's disease
   b. Iatrogenic – long-term corticosteroid administration.

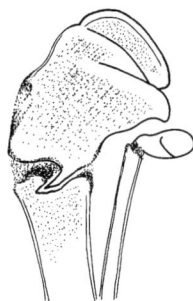

Figure 1.21 Nutritional secondary hyperparathyroidism – folding fractures in an osteopenic tibia and fibula.

6. Senility – especially in aged cats.
7. Chronic protein deprivation or loss
   a. Starvation
   b. Liver disease
   c. Malabsorption.
8. Hyperthyroidism.
9. Diabetes mellitus.
10. Panosteitis – not a true osteopenia but residual changes include paucity of trabeculae in long bones, giving a "hollow" appearance, although the cortices are of normal thickness and radio-opacity.
11. Rickets – probably via associated nutritional secondary hyperparathyroidism (see 1.22.8 and Figure 1.29).
12. Multiple myeloma (plasma cell myeloma) – genuine osteopenia; also apparent osteopenia due to confluence of areas of osteolysis (see 1.18.1 and Figure 1.24).
13. Osteogenesis imperfecta – a rare inherited collagen defect resulting in multiple pathological fractures; may occur with dentinogenesis imperfecta, in which teeth also fracture. Seen in young animals so the main DDx is nutritional secondary hyperparathyroidism.
14. Lead poisoning in immature animals; sclerotic metaphyseal lines are also seen.
15. Hypervitaminosis D – a massive intake in a young animal can produce osteopenia with bone deformity and retarded growth, but the main changes are soft tissue calcification.
16. Prolonged high-dose anticonvulsant therapy – primidone, phenytoin and phenobarbitone in humans; however, effects in animals are not proven; due to liver damage and effect on vitamin D production.
17. Cats – hypervitaminosis A: osteopenia due to disuse and concomitant nutritional secondary hyperparathyroidism; however, the proliferative spine and joint changes predominate.
18. Cats – mucopolysaccharidosis and mucolipidosis: likewise; may occur rarely in dogs.

1.17 Coarse trabecular pattern

1. Osteopenia – osteopenia is most apparent in areas of trabecular bone because here bone turnover is highest. Small trabeculae are resorbed first, leaving a coarse trabecular pattern due to the remaining larger trabeculae. For causes see Section 1.16.
2. Panosteitis – coarse, sclerotic trabeculae may be seen in large or small patches, or arising from the endosteal surface of the cortices (see 1.13.5 and Figure 1.17). In a dog of suggestive age and breed, this finding is usually considered pathognomonic for the disease.
3. Multiple myeloma (plasma cell myeloma) – the disease may produce multiple, confluent osteolytic lesions and osteopenia which together can create an apparent coarse trabecular pattern (see 1.18.1 and Figure 1.24).
4. Osteopetrosis (see 1.13.13).

1.18 Osteolytic lesions

1. Neoplasia (see 1.19.1 and Figure 1.26)
   a. Primary malignant bone tumour of osteolytic type (especially in cats), although usually there is also some evidence of new bone production
   b. Bone metastases – may be osteolytic or sclerotic; usually in atypical sites

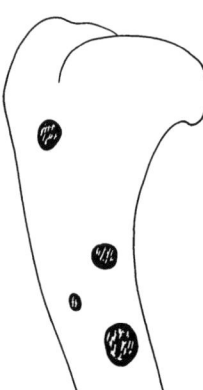

Figure 1.22 Bone metastases – multiple osteolytic lesions, in atypical sites for primary neoplasia.

1 SKELETAL SYSTEM – GENERAL

for primary tumours; often multiple in one bone or polyostotic (Figure 1.22). Lymphosarcoma in bone is usually osteolytic

c. Malignant soft tissue tumour invading bone – usually soft tissue swelling and cortical destruction are obvious (Figure 1.23). If near a joint more than one bone may be affected (see 2.4.6 and Figure 2.3)

d. Multiple myeloma (plasma cell myeloma Figure 1.24) – discrete, "punched out" osteolytic areas of variable size and lacking any sclerotic margin; usually multiple/confluent/polyostotic, less often solitary. Where lesions are confluent the affected bone has a polycystic or marbled appearance or may appear osteopenic with coarse trabeculation. Mainly affects pelvis, spine, ribs, long bones. Pathological fractures are common.

2. Infection (see 1.19.2 and Figures 1.27 and 1.28)
   a. Bacterial:
      - osteolytic halo around infected teeth due to periapical granuloma; DDx renal secondary hyperparathyroidism (see 4.9.4 and Figure 4.3)
      - around sequestra
      - around metallic implants; DDx movement, bone necrosis due to heat from high-speed drill
      - at fracture sites, especially following an open wound
      - haematogenous osteomyelitis, especially in metaphyses (see 1.23.4 and Figure 1.31; DDx metaphyseal osteopathy (hypertrophic osteodystrophy)

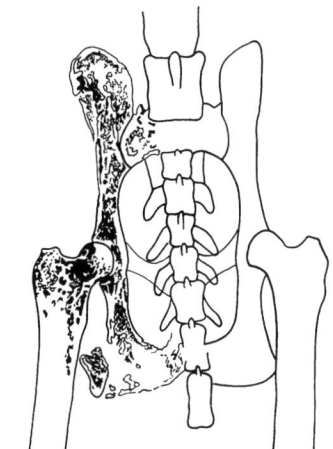

Figure 1.24 Multiple myeloma (cat) – extensive osteolysis affecting multiple bones, with a pathological fracture of the ischiatic tuberosity.

   b. Fungal* – usually spread by the haematogenous route and therefore likely to be multiple lesions
   c. Protozoal – leishmaniasis* – may cause severe osteolytic arthritis.

3. Trauma
   a. Superimposition of skin defect or gas in open wound
   b. Fracture line before full bridging
   c. Osteolytic halo around surgical implants caused by infection, movement or bone necrosis due to the use of a high-speed drill
   d. Stress protection – a localised area of osteopenia and bone weakness at the end of a bone plate.

4. Pressure atrophy – a smoothly bordered area of superficial bone loss due to pressure from an adjacent mass (e.g. rib tumour, mass between digits).

5. Fibrous dysplasia – rare fibro-osseous defect of bone thought to be developmental in origin as mainly seen in young animals; mono- or polyostotic osteolytic lesions which may undergo pathological fracture.

6. Osteolytic lesions at specific locations
   a. Metaphyseal osteopathy (see 1.23.3 and Figure 1.30)
   b. Metaphyseal osteomyelitis (see 1.23.4 and Figure 1.31)
   c. Retained cartilaginous cores (see 1.23.2, 3.5.3 and Figure 3.11) – not truly osteolytic but areas of non-ossification of cartilage

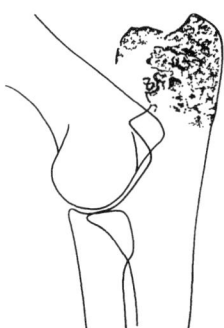

Figure 1.23 Malignant soft tissue tumour invading bone. Osteolysis predominates.

d. Avascular necrosis of the femoral head (Legg–Calvé–Perthe's disease) – young dogs of terrier breeds – may affect both hips (see 3.9.3 and Figure 3.22)
e. Intra-osseous epidermoid cysts – rare in bone; usually osteolytic; distal phalanges and vertebrae
f. Cats – feline femoral neck "metaphyseal osteopathy" (see 3.9.10).

The following lesions are likely to be *expansile*, that is, they are osteolytic lesions arising within bones which displace the cortex outwards and cause thinning rather than frank lysis of the cortex (Figure 1.25). Pathological fracture may occur. They are usually benign, or of low-grade malignancy.

7. Neoplasia
   a. Giant cell tumour (osteoclastoma) – a rare tumour, usually seen in the epiphyses and metaphyses of long bones, especially the distal ulna. Expansile, osteolytic lesion with multiloculated, septate appearance and variable transition to normal bone. May look identical to bone cyst but the patients are usually older
   b. Rarely, other non-osteogenic malignancies may appear expansile
   c. Enchondroma (single)/enchondromatosis (multiple) – synonyms osseous chondromatosis, dyschondroplasia, Ollier's disease. Rare; larger breeds. A benign but debilitating condition in which foci of physeal cartilage are displaced through the metaphyses into the diaphyses, causing weakening of the bone due to expansile, non-ossified lesions; animals usually present whilst immature due to pathological fractures
   d. Osteochondroma/multiple cartilaginous exostoses – may appear expansile because the cortex is continuous with underlying bone (see 1.15.2 and Figure 1.19).
8. Benign bone cysts – rare, mainly in young dogs of large breeds, male predominance, often distal radius or ulna. Expansile, often septate, osteolytic lesions which may appear identical to giant cell tumours although affected dogs are generally younger and the lesion is likely to be confined to the metaphysis, not crossing the growth plate, although it may migrate along the diaphysis with skeletal maturity. Usually single (unicameral, mono-ostotic), occasionally multiple (polyostotic).
9. Aneurysmal bone cysts appear similar but are due to vascular anomalies such as arteriovenous fistulae or vascular defects resulting from trauma or neoplasia; usually older animals.
10. Fibro-osseous dysplasia (see 1.18.5) – may be expansile.
11. Bone abscess – rare.

1.19 Mixed osteolytic/osteogenic lesions

As bone can respond to disease or injury only by loss or production of new bone, diseases of different aetiology can appear very similar radiographically. One of the main challenges for the radiologist is to distinguish between neoplasia and infection, although it may be impossible to do this with certainty and a biopsy, follow-up radiographs or other tests may be required. There may be an equal combination of bone destruction and new bone production and the mixed nature of the lesion may be obvious; in other cases one or other process may predominate.

1. Neoplasia
   a. Primary malignant bone tumour – 80% are osteosarcoma; also chondrosarcoma, fibrosarcoma and tumours arising from soft tissue elements such as haemangiosarcoma, liposarcoma. It is impossible to differentiate histological types radiographically. In dogs, osteosarcoma usually arises in long bone metaphyses in larger breeds (especially the proximal humerus and distal radius), although any bone including the axial skeleton may be affected

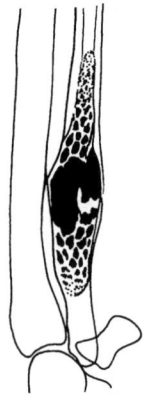

Figure 1.25 Expansile bone lesion – giant cell tumour of the distal ulna. Although malignant, the lesion does not appear particularly aggressive.

by malignancy). The lesions are usually mixed and aggressive with a long transition zone to normal bone, although some lesions may appear almost entirely osteolytic (osteoclastic type) or sclerotic (osteoblastic type). New bone production varies from minimal to florid, and in the case of osteosarcoma includes tumour bone as well as reactive bone (Figure 1.26). Lung metastases are common and pathological fracture may occur. Primary malignant bone tumours are usually confined to single bones and rarely cross joints. In small dog breeds and in cats, the tumours may be less aggressive and less likely to metastasise

b. Bone metastases – mixed, fairly aggressive lesions although lysis or sclerosis may predominate strongly; usually in atypical sites for primary tumours, such as diaphyses; often multiple in one bone or polyostotic. Rarer than in humans; usually from primary tumours of epithelial type such as mammary or prostate. The main DDx is osteomyelitis, especially where fungal diseases are endemic; sclerotic lesions may mimic panosteitis although the patient with metastases is likely to be older

c. Malignant soft tissue tumour invading bone – osteolysis usually predominates although there may be some bony reaction or pre-existing osteoarthritis. If arising near a joint more than one bone may be affected (see 2.4.6 and Figure 2.3)

d. Neoplastic transformation at the site of a previous fracture – rare, but well recognised in humans and animals. Usually several years after internal fixation – postulated causes include the presence of a metallic implant or chronic, low-grade infection. Radiographic signs are of an active and aggressive lesion superimposed over obvious previous fracture; DDx chronic infection

e. Benign bone tumours may occasionally show lysis as well as a bony mass (osteoma, osteochondroma), or bone reaction as well as lysis (enchondroma).

2. Infection
   a. Bacterial:
      - solitary lesions in older animals are usually associated with a known wound, surgery or extension from soft tissue infection. A mixed, aggressive lesion, but more likely to show a surrounding sclerotic zone (walling-off) than is neoplasia (Figure 1.27). Sequestrum/involucrum formation is an occasional finding (Figure 1.28). Pathological fractures are less common than with neoplasia
      - Multiple lesions are seen with haematogenous osteomyelitis, which is more common in young animals. Aggressive osteolytic lesions result, especially in metaphyses, due to sluggish blood flow (long bones, vertebrae, ribs) with surrounding sclerosis and/or

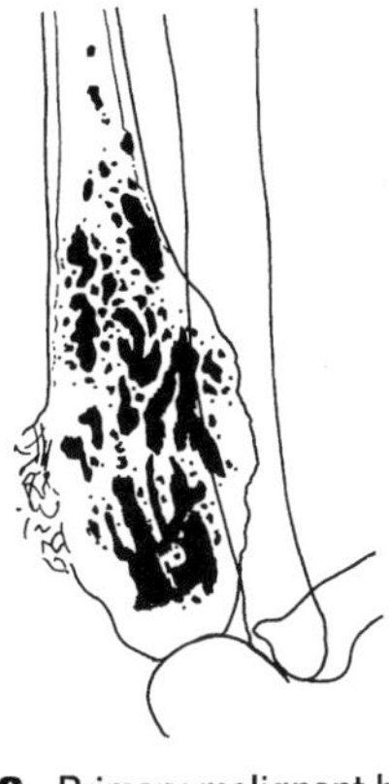

Figure 1.26 Primary malignant bone tumour – osteosarcoma of the distal radius. Note the more aggressive appearance than the lesion shown in Figure 1.25.

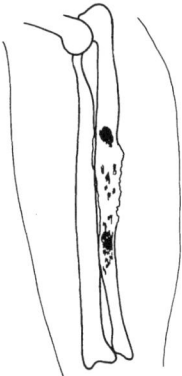

Figure 1.27 Acute osteomyelitis in the ulna of a cat, following a dog bite – a mixed, aggressive lesion with marked surrounding soft tissue swelling. The two focal radiolucent areas are the result of injury caused by the canine teeth of the attacking animal.

periosteal reaction; pathological fracture may occur. DDx metaphyseal osteopathy (hypertrophic osteodystrophy) in young dogs (see 1.23.3, 1.23.4 and Figures 1.30 and 1.31)

b. Fungal – usually spread haematogenously, producing single or multiple lesions, again often metaphyseal. Usually aggressive, mixed osteolytic/proliferative bone lesions. Main DDx is metastatic neoplasia, but with fungal infection the patient is more likely to be systemically ill; also consider bacterial osteomyelitis
- coccidioidomycosis* – fever and depression with respiratory, skin, ocular and skeletal lesions. As many as 90% of the bone lesions are in the appendicular skeleton, mainly in the distal ends of long bones
- blastomycosis* – affects mainly large breed, young male dogs, causing a spectrum of syndromes as above. Bone involvement occurs in 30% of dogs, with lesions usually solitary and distal to the elbow or stifle
- aspergillosis* – as well as destructive rhinitis, other aggressive bone lesions and pneumonia have been reported in the German Shepherd dog and immunocompromised patients, in areas where other fungal diseases are not endemic (e.g. the UK)
- histoplasmosis* – various systemic illnesses (mainly gastrointestinal in the dog); rarely causes osteolytic or mixed bone lesions
- cryptococcosis* – usually part of a more generalised disease process, especially in immunosuppressed patients

c. Protozoal – leishmaniasis* – may cause multifocal, mixed, aggressive bone lesions although the most common presentation is osteolytic joint disease

d. Cats – feline tuberculosis – various *Mycobacterium* species (rare). Skin and lung lesions predominate but occasionally aggressive mixed bone lesions are seen; also periosteal reactions, discospondylitis and osteoarthritis.

3. Trauma
a. Healing fracture – partial bridging of the fracture line with resorption of damaged bone
b. Osteomyelitis at a fracture site
c. Late neoplastic transformation at a fracture site.

4. Metaphyseal osteopathy – lesions in metaphyses only; DDx metaphyseal osteomyelitis (hypertrophic osteodystrophy) (see 1.23.3, 1.23.4 and Figures 1.30 and 1.31).

5. Multifocal idiopathic pyogranulomatous bone disease – sterile, polyostotic bone disease thought to be part of the group of histiocytic diseases.

6. Canine leucocyte adhesion deficiency (CLAD) (see 1.23.7).

Differentiating malignant bone neoplasia from osteomyelitis

- The degree and extent of osteolysis is usually greater in malignancy; the cortex is more likely to be breached.
- Pathological fracture is therefore more likely with neoplasia.
- Periosteal new bone formation is much more irregular in neoplasia, with a tendency to form spicules, often radiating out from the centre of the lesion; with osteomyelitis the new bone tends to be more solid.
- A Codman's triangle of new bone at one end of the lesion is more likely to be associated with neoplasia.
- Sequestrum formation may occur with osteomyelitis but not neoplasia.
- Most primary malignant bone tumours affect only a single bone and rarely cross joints.

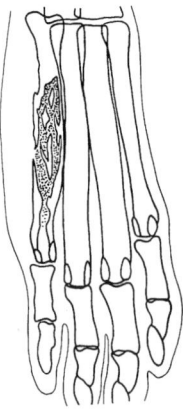

Figure 1.28 Chronic osteomyelitis and sequestrum formation in the metatarsus of a cat, following a cat bite. This lesion is less aggressive in nature than that shown in Figure 1.27 and appears partly walled off.

- The thorax should be radiographed to check for lung metastases if there is a suspicion of neoplasia. Abdominal ultrasonography may also be helpful.

1.20 Multifocal diseases

Multifocal diseases may produce more than one lesion in the same bone (mono-ostotic), or may affect multiple bones (polyostotic). For multifocal joint diseases see 2.7.

Multiple lesions of increased radio-opacity (see 1.13)

1. Panosteitis.
2. Sclerotic bone metastases.
3. Haematogenous osteomyelitis, especially fungal.
4. Bone infarcts – rare.
5. Osteopetrosis – rare.

Multiple lesions of reduced radio-opacity (see 1.18)

6. Osteolytic bone metastases.
7. Plasma cell myeloma (multiple myeloma).
8. Enchondromatosis.
9. Lymphosarcoma – may occasionally produce multiple or polyostotic osteolytic bone lesions.
10. Multiple bone cysts (more often single).
11. Metaphyseal osteopathy (hypertrophic osteodystrophy) – early cases show a radiolucent metaphyseal band (see 1.23.3 and Figure 1.30).
12. Metaphyseal osteomyelitis (see 1.23.4 and Figure 1.31).
13. Disuse osteopenia – seen especially in epiphyses and small bones (see 1.16).

Multiple lesions of mixed radio-opacity (see 1.19)

14. Bone metastases.
15. Haematogenous osteomyelitis
    a. Fungal*
    b. Bacterial, especially in young animals
    c. Protozoal – leishmaniasis*
16. Multifocal idiopathic pyogranulomatous bone disease.

Multiple mineralised or bony masses

17. Multiple cartilaginous exostoses (multiple osteochondromata) (see 1.15.2).
18. Calcinosis circumscripta – usually single, occasionally multiple; in soft tissues close to but not attached to bone (see 12 2.2 and Figure 12.1).
19. Synovial osteochondromatosis – masses around joints (see 2.8.18).
20. Cats – hypervitaminosis A: masses around joints – cats on raw liver diet; mainly spinal new bone but may also see exostoses near the limb joints, especially the elbow.

1.21 Lesions affecting epiphyses

See also Chapter 2 for joint diseases and Chapter 5 for vertebral epiphyseal lesions.

Lesions usually affecting single or few epiphyses

1. Fractures (see 1.9 and Figure 1.10) – usually Salter-Harris growth plate fractures in skeletally immature animals; Types III and IV cross the epiphysis causing disruption to the articular surface with variable displacement of the fragment. In skeletally mature animals the most common epiphyseal fracture is the lateral humeral condylar fracture seen especially in Spaniel breeds (see 3.4.14 and Figure 3.9).
2. Remodelling of epiphyses due to altered stresses following angular limb deformities and traumatic subluxations, e.g. of the distal radial epiphysis following radiocarpal subluxation as a result of premature closure of the distal ulnar growth plate. May be bilateral in giant breeds.
3. Disuse osteopenia (see 1.16) – due to fracture or paralysis of a limb. The osteopenia usually affects the distal limb most severely with loss of bone radio-opacity especially in epiphyses and cuboidal bones; for example, non-union of radial/ulnar fractures in toy breeds of dog with severe osteopenia in the carpus and distal limb epiphyses. Disuse osteopenia is reversible if the cause is corrected.
4. Giant cell tumour (osteoclastoma) (see 1.18.7).
5. Irregularity or osteolysis of the articular surface of an epiphysis (see 2.4–2.6)
    a. Osteochondrosis – may be bilateral or in other joints
    b. Septic arthritis – in multiple joints if of haematogenous origin
    c. Chronic osteoarthritis – may affect more than one joint, depending on the underlying cause
    d. Soft tissue tumour near joint

e. Avascular necrosis of the femoral head (Legg–Calvé–Perthe's disease) – young dogs of terrier breeds, especially West Highland White Terrier. May affect both hips (see 3.9.3 and Figure 3.22).

Lesions usually affecting numerous epiphyses

These include diseases that result in epiphyseal dysplasia or dysgenesis, often together with other widespread skeletal defects such as delayed growth plate closure, long bone curvature and dwarfism.

6. Normal skeletal immaturity – endochondral ossification occurs from the centre of epiphyses and apophyses and in the young animal the bone surface may appear ragged and irregular due to normal, incomplete ossification. Compare with other animals of similar age.
7. Chondrodysplasias (dyschondroplasias) recognised in numerous breeds (e.g. Alaskan Malamute, Australian Shepherd dog**, Beagle, Bedlington Terrier**, Cocker Spaniel, Dachshund, Dobermann**, English Pointer, English Springer Spaniel**, French Bulldog, German Shorthaired Pointer, Irish Red Setter, Japanese Akita, Labrador Retriever**, Miniature Poodle, Newfoundland, Norwegian Elkhound, Pyrenean Mountain dog, Saint Bernard, Samoyed**, Scottish Deerhound, Scottish Terrier, Shetland Sheepdog, Swedish Lapphund**); may have ocular defects as well

    Cats – Domestic Shorthair. Inherited abnormalities of endochondral ossification which produce generalised stippling and fragmentation of epiphyses leading to secondary osteoarthritis. Clinically may mimic rickets but may be seen before weaning and in related animals on different diets; radiographically rickets does not show epiphyseal changes, just physeal widening and long bone bowing.
8. Multiple epiphyseal dysplasia ("stippled epiphyses") – similar epiphyseal changes without other skeletal abnormalities are recognised in the Beagle and Poodle.
9. Congenital hypothyroidism – especially the Boxer. A congenital disease resulting in disproportionate dwarfism; DDx chondrodysplasia. Affected dogs suffer from epiphyseal dysgenesis leading to secondary osteoarthritis, delayed growth plate closure and shortened, bowed limbs. Facial and spinal changes are also seen (see 5.3.10).
10. Pituitary dwarfism – some cases show epiphyseal dysplasia, although this may be due to concurrent hypothyroidism.
11. Mucopolysaccharidosis Types VI and VII – especially seen in cats with Siamese ancestry; facial and spinal lesions with varying degrees of epiphyseal dysplasia and secondary osteoarthritis, especially in the shoulders and hips. Rare in dogs, although mucopolysaccharidosis Type I (Plott Hound) and II (Pointers) are reported – epiphyseal dysplasia and periarticular bony proliferations.
12. Cats – mucolipidosis Type II – rare; less severe epiphyseal lesions reported.

1.22 Lesions affecting physes

Loss of physeal line

1. Poor positioning so the growth plate is not parallel to the X-ray beam.
2. Premature closure of the growth plate due to trauma
    a. Salter-Harris Type V crushing injury – probably responsible for "idiopathic" premature closure of the distal ulnar growth plate in giant breeds; may be bilateral
    b. Bridging of the margin of a growth plate due to superimposed periosteal new bone – Salter-Harris Type VI injury.

Widening of physeal lines – single

3. Salter-Harris Type I fracture with displacement.
4. Infection (physitis) – although haematogenous osteomyelitis more often occurs in metaphyses due to sluggish blood flow in these areas. Vertebral physitis is recognised – younger dogs, caudal lumbar physes; may also be associated with portosystemic shunts.

Widening of physeal lines – generalised

Affected animals are often stunted and may also have epiphyseal dysplasia and secondary osteoarthritis. Physeal lesions are often most severe in the distal radius and ulna due to the normally rapid growth rate at these sites.

1 SKELETAL SYSTEM – GENERAL

5. Chondrodysplasias – variable effects on growth plates with widening, ragged margination and delayed closure in some affected animals. Often initially misdiagnosed as rickets (see 1.21.7).
6. Congenital hypothyroidism – wide and irregular growth plates with delayed closure, especially in the spine (see 5.3.10). Affects the Boxer particularly.
7. Pituitary dwarfism – some cases may show wide and irregular growth plates with delayed closure, perhaps due to concomitant hypothyroidism.
8. Rickets (juvenile osteomalacia).
   a. Rare, dietary deficiency of calcium or Vitamin D (Figure 1.29); seen after weaning. Growth plates are wide transversely and longitudinally due to failure of ossification at the metaphyseal border; metaphyses flare or mushroom laterally and show beaked margins due to continued periosteal bone growth. Long bones may be demineralised (concomitant nutritional secondary hyperparathyroidism) and bowed. Unlike hereditary chondrodysplasias there is no effect on the epiphyses
   b. Hypovitaminosis D due to failure to absorb or metabolise vitamin D (e.g. extrahepatic biliary atresia or common bile duct obstruction in young animals).
9. Infection – haematogenous physitis may affect more than one growth plate.

Masses arising at physes

10. Osteochondroma (single)/multiple cartilaginous exostoses (multiple) – arise at osteochondral junctions in young dogs and are often seen protruding from the site of previous growth plates (see 1.15.2 and Figure 1.19).

1.23 Lesions affecting metaphyses

1. Neoplasia
   a. Primary malignant bone tumours (e.g. osteosarcoma) – long bone metaphyses are a strong predilection site, especially the proximal humerus and distal radius in giant dog breeds (see 1.19.1 and Figure 1.26)
   b. Osteochondroma (single)/multiple cartilaginous exostoses (multiple) – in young dogs, arise at osteochondral junctions and therefore often protrude from the metaphyseal area in older animals (see 1.15.2 and Figure 1.19)
   c. Enchondromatosis – persistent segments of physeal cartilage are displaced through metaphyses into diaphyses producing multiple, expansile, osteolytic lesions which may undergo pathological fracture (see 1.18.7).
2. Retained cartilaginous cores – retention of physeal cartilage in metaphyses due to incomplete endochondral ossification, producing conical or "candle flame"-shaped radiolucent areas with fine sclerotic margins in the distal ulnar metaphyses (occasionally the distal radius or femur). Giant breeds. Often bilateral; may co-exist with retarded growth or premature closure of the distal ulnar growth plate but a causal relationship is not certain (see 3.5.3 and Figure 3.11).
3. Metaphyseal osteopathy (hypertrophic osteodystrophy, skeletal scurvy, Moller–Barlow's disease) – affects young, rapidly growing dogs of larger breeds on a high plane of nutrition; self-limiting. Pain, heat and swelling at metaphyses, the patient is usually febrile and ill. Radiography shows a radiolucent band +/– narrow sclerotic margins, or a mottled band, crossing metaphyses parallel to but not involving the growth plate (Figure 1.30a). Later, subperiosteal haemorrhages provoke collars of mineralisation and paraperiosteal new bone which may become large and deforming. The distal radius and ulna are most severely affected (Figure 1.30b). DDx

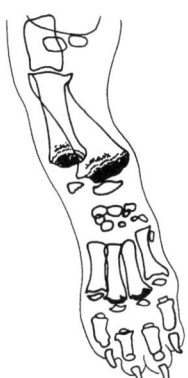

Figure 1.29 Rickets – forearm of a young puppy, showing lesions especially in the distal radial and ulnar growth plates.

25

SMALL ANIMAL RADIOLOGICAL DIFFERENTIAL DIAGNOSIS

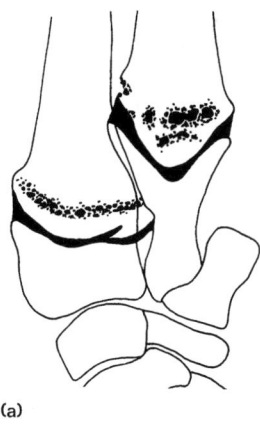

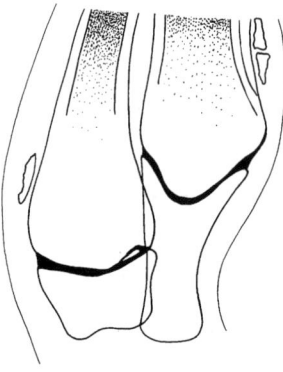

Figure 1.30 (a) Early metaphyseal osteopathy – a mottled band or line of radiolucency in the metaphysis parallel to the growth plate. (b) Late metaphyseal osteopathy – the metaphyses are surrounded by successive layers of periosteal and paraperiosteal new bone, the deeper layers becoming remodelled into the cortex. Superimposition of new bone creates a sclerotic appearance.

   a. Bacterial – metaphyseal osteomyelitis (Figure 1.31) is an unusual condition in young dogs with aggressive, osteolytic metaphyseal lesions which may undergo pathological fracture; definitive diagnosis requires blood culture; DDx metaphyseal osteopathy (hypertrophic osteodystrophy)
   b. Fungal* – aggressive, usually mixed lesions.
5. Bone cysts – often metaphyseal (see 1.18.8).
6. Chondrodysplasias, rickets and other growth abnormalities (see 1.12) – often metaphyses are widened due to abnormal endochondral ossification at the growth plate.
7. CLAD – an inherited disease in the Irish Red Setter causing osteolytic or mixed osteolytic/proliferative lesions in metaphyses, especially the distal radius and ulna, and skull changes similar to craniomandibular osteopathy; clinical signs include gingivitis, lameness, mandibular swelling and lymphadenopathy.
8. Craniomandibular osteopathy – rarely, additional masses of paraperiosteal new bone appear adjacent to distal ulnar metaphyses; may mimic metaphyseal osteopathy (hypertrophic osteodystrophy) (see 4.10.1 and Figure 4.4).
9. Lead poisoning – rarely see radiographic lesions; thin, transverse sclerotic bands in metaphyses.
10. Cats – feline femoral neck "metaphyseal osteopathy" (see 3.9.10).

metaphyseal osteomyelitis, normal "cutback zone" in large dogs (areas of ill-defined cortical irregularity due to remodelling of bone), unusual forms of craniomandibular osteopathy (CMO), canine leucocyte adhesion disorder (CLAD), lead poisoning (if the band appears mainly sclerotic).
4. Infection – usually produces metaphyseal lesions if the infection is spread haematogenously, especially in young animals; likely to be multifocal and often bilaterally symmetrical.

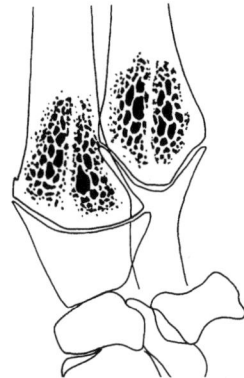

Figure 1.31 Metaphyseal osteomyelitis. The osteolysis is more diffuse and aggressive than with metaphyseal osteopathy.

1 SKELETAL SYSTEM – GENERAL

1.24 Lesions affecting diaphyses

Conditions that are mainly seen in diaphyses are listed in this section, although some of these lesions may also produce changes in other parts of the skeleton.

Thinning of cortices

1. Osteopenia – various causes (see 1.16). Results in reduced bone radio-opacity, coarse trabecular pattern and folding fractures.
2. Expansile lesion within medullary cavity – e.g. bone cyst, giant cell tumour, enchondroma (see 1.18.7–11 and Figure 1.25). The cortex is displaced outwards and is smoothly thinned but not often interrupted.
3. Osteolytic lesions (e.g. neoplasia, osteomyelitis). The cortex is irregularly thinned and often interrupted.
4. Pressure atrophy – a smoothly bordered area of superficial bone loss due to pressure from an adjacent mass (e.g. rib tumour, mass between digits).
5. Convex side of a bowed long bone.
6. Atrophic non-union of a fracture.

Thickening of cortices

7. Remodelling periosteal reaction – numerous causes (see 1.14).
8. Hypertrophic osteopathy (Maries' disease – see 1.14.6 and Figure 1.18) – a specific type of periosteal reaction.
9. Healing fracture.
10. Chronic osteomyelitis.
11. Leishmaniasis* – although osteolytic joint disease is more common there is also a pattern of periosteal and intramedullary bone proliferation in diaphyses and flat bones provoked by chronic osteomyelitis.
12. Concave side of bowed long bone, in response to increased load.
13. Congenital hypothyroidism – especially Boxers; shortened, bowed radius and ulna with thickened cortices and increased medullary radio-opacity.
14. Osteopetrosis.

Interruption of cortices

15. Trauma.
16. Neoplasia.
17. Osteomyelitis.
18. Large expansile lesion.
19. Biopsy site.

Radiolucent lines in diaphyses

20. Artefacts
    a. Overlying skin defect
    b. Overlying fat or gas in fascial planes
    c. Mach effect from other superimposed bones.
21. Nutrient foramen – location usually known anatomically; compare with the opposite limb if in doubt.
22. Fissure fractures.

Sclerotic lines in diaphyses (see 1.13)

23. Growth arrest lines.
24. Panosteitis.
25. Fractures – if impaction of bone or overlapping of fragments occur a sclerotic band rather than a bone defect may be seen
    a. Folding fractures:
       - "greenstick fractures" (single cortex) in young animals
       - osteopenia, especially due to nutritional secondary hyperparathyroidism
    b. Compression or impaction fractures – especially vertebrae
    c. Superimposition of overridden fragments seen on one radiographic projection, but shown to be displaced using the orthogonal view
    d. Healing fracture.

Osteolytic areas in diaphyses (see 1.18)

26. Neoplasia
    a. Bone metastases – may be predominantly osteolytic; often multiple in one bone or polyostotic. Metastases in bone are usually in atypical locations for primary bone tumours, and especially in the diaphyses. They may be osteolytic or sclerotic and are less often mixed lesions. Little surrounding reaction results. Any primary tumour may metastasise to bone but mammary tumours are over-represented
    b. Plasma cell myeloma (multiple myeloma) – usually multiple, discrete osteolytic lesions affecting more than one bone
    c. Malignant soft tissue tumour invading bone – osteolysis predominates
    d. Osteolytic primary bone tumour extending into the diaphysis or in an atypical location (usually they are metaphyseal).

27. Infection – mixed lesions are more common than purely osteolytic lesions.
28. Bone cysts – discrete, expansile lesions; rare.
29. Enchondromatosis – discrete, expansile lesion; rare.

Sclerotic areas in diaphyses (see 1.13)

30. Neoplasia
    a. Bone metastases – may be predominantly sclerotic; often multiple in one bone or polyostotic
    b. Osteoproductive primary bone tumour extending into the diaphysis or in an atypical location (usually they are metaphyseal)
    c. Lymphosarcoma – may rarely cause medullary sclerosis
    d. Cats – FeLV-induced medullary osteosclerosis – rare; likely to be widespread in the skeleton.
31. Osteomyelitis – haematogenous osteomyelitis may produce ill-defined patches of sclerosis.
32. Panosteitis.
33. Healing fractures.
34. Bone infarcts.
35. Osteopetrosis – affects the whole skeleton but is most obvious radiographically in the diaphyses.

Mixed osteolytic/osteogenic lesions (see 1.19)

36. Neoplasia
    a. Bone metastases – may be mixed lesions, although they are often predominantly osteolytic or sclerotic; often multiple in one bone or polyostotic
    b. Malignant soft tissue tumour invading bone
    c. Neoplastic transformation at the site of a previous fracture
    d. Mixed primary bone tumour in an atypical location (usually they are metaphyseal).
37. Infection.
38. Trauma.
    a. Healing fracture
    b. Infected fracture
    c. Neoplastic transformation at the site of a previous fracture.

Altered shape of diaphyses

See Section 1.10.

FURTHER READING

General

Kramer, M., Gerwing, M., Hach, V. and Schimke, E. (1997) Sonography of the musculoskeletal system in dogs and cats. *Veterinary Radiology and Ultrasound* **38** 139–149.

Samii, V.F., Nyland, T.G., Werner, L.L. and Baker, T.W. (1999) Ultrasound guided fine needle aspiration biopsy of bone lesions. *Veterinary Radiology and Ultrasound* **40** 82–86.

Papageorges M. and Sande R.D. (1990) The Mach phenomenon *Veterinary Radiology* **32** 191–195.

Papageorges, M. (1991) How the Mach phenomenon and shape affect the radiographic appearance of skeletal structures. *Veterinary Radiology* **32** 191–195.

Weinstein, J.M., Mongil, C.M. and Smith, G.K. (1995) Orthopedic conditions of the Rottweiler – Part I. *Compendium of Continuing Education for the Practicing Veterinarian (Small Animal)* **17** 813–830.

Weinstein, J.M., Mongil, C.M., Rhodes, W.H. and Smith, G.K. (1995) Orthopedic conditions of the Rottweiler – Part II. *Compendium of Continuing Education for the Practicing Veterinarian (Small Animal)* **17** 925–938.

Normal anatomy, normal variants and artefacts

Fagin, B.D., Aronson, E. and Gutzmer, M.A. (1992) Closure of the iliac crest ossification centre of dogs. *Journal of the American Veterinary Medical Association* **200** 1709.

Root, M.V., Johnston, S.D. and Olson, P.N. (1997) The effect of prepubertal and postpubertal gonadectomy on radial physeal closure in male and female domestic cats. *Veterinary Radiology and Ultrasound* **38** 42–47.

Congenital and developmental diseases; diseases of young animals

Campbell, B.G., Wootton, J.A.M., Krook, L., DeMarco, J. and Minor, R.R. (1997) Clinical signs and diagnosis of osteogenesis imperfecta in three dogs. *Journal of the American Veterinary Medical Association* **211** 183–187.

Konde, L.J., Thrall, M.A., Gasper, P., Dial, S.M., McBiles, K., Colgan, S. and Haskins, M. (1987) Radiographically visualized skeletal changes associated with mucopolysaccharidosis VI in cats. *Veterinary Radiology* **28** 223–228.

Muir, P., Dubielzig, R.R. and Johnson, K.A (1996) Panosteitis. Compendium of Continuing Education for the Practicing Veterinarian (Small Animal) **18** 29–33.

Muir, P., Dubielzig, R.R., Johnson, K.A. and Shelton, D.G. (1996) Hypertrophic osteodystrophy and calvarial hyperostosis. *Compendium of Continuing Education for the Practicing Veterinarian (Small Animal)* **18** 143–151.

Scott, H. (1998) Non-traumatic causes of lameness in the forelimb of the growing dog. *In Practice* **20** 539–554.

Scott, H. (1999) Non-traumatic causes of lameness in the hindlimb of the growing dog. *In Practice* **21** 176–188.

Trowald-Wigh, G., Ekman, S., Hansson, K., Hedhammar, A. and Hard af Segerstad, C. (2000) Clinical, radiological and pathological features of 12 Irish Setters with canine leucocyte adhesion deficiency. *Journal of Small Animal Practice* **41** 211–217.

Metabolic bone disease (some overlap with above)

Allan, G.S., Huxtable, C.R.R., Howlett, C.R., Baxter, R.C., Duff, B. and Farrow, B.R.H. (1978) Pituitary dwarfism in German Shepherd dogs. *Journal of Small Animal Practice* **19** 711–729.

Buckley, J.C. (1984) Pathophysiologic considerations of osteopenia. *Compendium of Continuing Education for the Practicing Veterinarian (Small Animal)* **6** 552–562.

Dennis, R. (1989) Radiology of metabolic bone disease. *Vet Ann* **29** 195–206.

Johnson, K.A., Church, D.B., Barton, R.J. and Wood, A.K.W. (1988) Vitamin D-dependent rickets in a Saint Bernard dog. *Journal of Small Animal Practice* **29** 657–666.

Konde, L.J., Thrall, M.A., Gasper, P., Dial, S.M., McBiles, K., Colgan, S. and Haskins, M. (1987) Radiographically visualized skeletal changes associated with mucopolysaccharidosis VI in cats. *Veterinary Radiology* **28** 223–228.

Kramers, P., Flueckiger, M.A., Rahn, B.A. and Cordey, J. (1988) Osteopetrosis in cats. *Journal of Small Animal Practice* **29** 153–164.

Lamb, C.R. (1990) The double cortical line: a sign of osteopenia. *Journal of Small Animal Practice* **31** 189–192.

Saunders, H.M. and Jezyk, P.K. (1991) The radiographic appearance of canine congenital hypothyroidism: skeletal changes with delayed treatment. *Veterinary Radiology* **32** 171–177.

Tomsa, K., Glaus, T., Hauser, B., Flueckiger, M., Arnold, P., Wess, G. and Reusch, C. (1999) Nutritional secondary hyperparathyroidism in six cats. *Journal of Small Animal Practice* **40** 533–539.

Infective and inflammatory conditions

Canfield, P.J., Malik, R., Davis, P.E. and Martin, P. (1994) Multifocal idiopathic pyogranulomatous bone disease in a dog. *Journal of Small Animal Practice* **35** 370–373.

Dunn, J.K., Dennis, R. and Houlton, J.E.F. (1992) Successful treatment of two cases of metaphyseal osteomyelitis in the dog. *Journal of Small Animal Practice* **33** 85–89.

Turrel, J.M. and Pool, R.R. (1982) Bone lesions in four dogs with visceral leishmaniasis. *Veterinary Radiology* **23** 243–249.

Neoplasia

Blackwood, L. (1999) Bone tumours in small animals. *In Practice* **21** 31–37.

Dubielzig, R.R., Biery, D.N. and Brodey, R.S. (1981) Bone sarcomas associated with multifocal medullary bone infarction in dogs. *Journal of the American Veterinary Medical Association* **179** 64–68.

Gibbs C., Denny, H.R. and Kelly, D.F. (1984) The radiological features of osteosarcoma of the appendicular skeleton of dogs: a review of 74 cases. *Journal of Small Animal Practice* **25** 177–192.

Gibbs, C., Denny, H.R. and Lucke, V.M. (1985) The radiological features of non-osteogenic malignant tumours of bone in the appendicular skeleton of the dog: a review of 34 cases. *Journal of Small Animal Practice* **26** 537–553.

Jacobson, L.S. and Kirberger, R.M. (1996) Canine multiple cartilaginous exostoses: unusual manifestations and a review of the literature. *Journal of the American Animal Hospital Association* **32** 45–51.

Lamb C.R., Berg, J. and Schelling, S.H. (1993) Radiographic diagnosis of an expansile bone lesion in a dog. *Journal of Small Animal Practice* **34** 239–241.

Matis, U., Krauser, K., Schwartz-Porsche, D. and Putzer-Brenig, A.v. (1989) Multiple enchondromatosis in the dog. *Veterinary and Comparative Orthopaedics and Traumatology* **4** 144–151.

Russel, R.G. and Walker, M. (1983) Metastatic and invasive tumors of bone in dogs and cats. *Veterinary Clinics of North America* **13** 163–180.

Schrader, S.C., Burk, R.L. and Lin, S. (1983) Bone cysts in two dogs and a review of similar cystic bone lesions in the dog. *Journal of the American Veterinary Medical Association* **182** 490–495.

Turrel, J.M. and Pool, R.R. (1982) Primary bone tumors in the cat: a retrospective study of 15 cats and a literature review. *Veterinary Radiology* **23** 152–166.

Wrigley, R.H. (2000) Malignant versus nonmalignant bone disease. *Veterinary Clinics of North America; Small Animal Practice* **30** 315–348.

Trauma

Anderson, M.A., Dee, L.G. and Dee, J.F. (1995) Fractures and dislocations of the racing greyhound – Part I. *Compendium of Continuing Education for the Practicing Veterinarian (Small Animal)* **17** 779–786.

Anderson, M.A., Dee, L.G. and Dee, J.F. (1995) Fractures and dislocations of the racing greyhound – Part II. *Compendium of Continuing Education for the Practicing Veterinarian (Small Animal)* **17** 899–909.

Sande, R. (1999) Radiography of orthopaedic trauma and fracture repair. *Veterinary Clinics of North America; Small Animal Practice* **29** 1247–1260.

Miscellaneous

Canfield P.J., Malik R., Davis, P.E. and Martin P. (1994) Multifocal idiopathic pyogranulomatous bone disease in a dog. *Journal of Small Animal Practice* **35** 370–373.

Kramer, M., Gerwing, M., Hach, V. and Schimke, E. (1997) Sonography of the musculoskeletal system in dogs and cats. *Veterinary Radiology and Ultrasound* **38** 139–149.

2

Joints

2.1 Radiography of joints: technique and interpretation
2.2 Soft tissue changes around joints
2.3 Altered width of joint space
2.4 Osteolytic joint disease
2.5 Proliferative joint disease
2.6 Mixed osteolytic/proliferative joint disease
2.7 Conditions that may affect more than one joint
2.8 Mineralised bodies in or near joints

2.1 Radiography of joints: technique and interpretation

Technique

Lesions in joints may be radiographically subtle, and so attention to good radiographic technique is essential.
1. High-definition film/screen combination; no grid is necessary except for the upper limb joints in large dogs; optimum processing technique.
2. Accurate positioning and centring with a small object/film distance to minimise geometric distortion.
3. Straight radiographs in two planes are usually required (i.e. orthogonal views) with oblique views as necessary.
4. Use of stressed views (traction, rotation, sheer, hyperextension/flexion and fulcrum-assisted) and weight-bearing or simulated weight-bearing views for the detection of subluxation and altered joint width – great care with radiation safety is needed if the patient is manually restrained. The vacuum phenomenon may occur with traction views of the shoulder and spine (see 2.2.12).
5. Close collimation to enhance radiographic definition and safety.
6. Correct exposure factors to allow examination of soft tissue as well as bone.
7. Beware of hair coat debris creating artefactual shadows.
8. Radiograph the opposite joint for comparison if necessary.

Arthrography (negative, positive, double contrast)

INDICATIONS
Detection of the extent or rupture of joint capsule; examination of the bicipital tendon sheath (shoulder joint); assessment of cartilage thickness and flap formation; detection of synovial masses and intra-articular filling defects; to see if a mineralised body is intra-articular. Most often performed in the shoulder joint.

PREPARATION
General anaesthesia; sterile preparation of the injection site; survey radiographs.

TECHNIQUE (SHOULDER)
Insert a 20–22 g short-bevel needle 1 cm distal to the acromion and direct it caudally, distally and medially into the joint space. Joint fluid may flow freely or require aspiration; obtain a sample for laboratory analysis.
- Positive-contrast arthrogram – use 2–7ml isotonic iodinated contrast medium (e.g. a non-ionic medium such as isohexol) depending on the patient size, withdraw the needle and apply pressure to the injection site; manipulate the joint gently to ensure even contrast medium distribution; take mediolateral, caudocranial and cranioproximal–craniodistal (skyline) radiographs. Use lower volumes for assessment of the joint space only and higher volumes for the biceps tendon sheath.
- Negative-contrast arthrogram – use air.

SMALL ANIMAL RADIOLOGICAL DIFFERENTIAL DIAGNOSIS

- Double-contrast arthrogram – use a small volume of positive contrast medium followed by air.

TECHNICAL ERRORS ON ARTHROGRAPHY

Contrast medium not entering the joint space; insufficient or too much contrast medium used.

INTERPRETATION OF ARTHROGRAMS

1. Reduce the viewer area to mask glare and increase the visibility of lesions.
2. Use a spotlight, dimmer and magnifying glass as necessary.
3. Compare with the contralateral joint and use radiographic atlases and bone specimens.
4. Consider patient signalment and associated clinical and laboratory findings.
5. Assess number of joints affected (e.g. single – trauma or neoplasia; bilateral – osteochondrosis, bilateral trauma; multiple – systemic or immune-mediated disease).
6. Assess joint space alignment and congruity.
7. Assess joint space width (changes only seen if gross or if weight-bearing views obtained).
8. Assess articular surface contour – remodelling, erosion.
9. Assess subchondral bone opacity – sclerosis, erosion, cyst formation, osteopenia
10. Assess joint space opacity – gas, fat, mineralisation, foreign material.
11. Assess osteoarthritis (see 2.5).
12. Assess soft tissue changes (may be more obvious radiographically than clinically):
    a. increased soft tissue – concept of "synovial mass", as synovial tissue and synovial fluid cannot be differentiated on plain radiographs
    b. reduced soft tissue – muscle wastage due to disuse (especially in the thighs).
13. Other articular and periarticular changes:
    a. intra- and periarticular mineralisation (see 2.8)
    b. joint "mice"
    c. intra-articular fat pads reduced by synovial effusion; fascial planes and sesamoids displaced by effusions and soft tissue swelling
    d. periarticular chip and avulsion fractures
    e. periarticular osteolysis
    f. periarticular new bone other than due to osteoarthritis.

2.2 Soft tissue changes around joints

Soft tissue swelling (with or without bony changes)

Differentiation between joint effusion and surrounding soft tissue swelling may not be possible except in the stifle joint, but both are often present. A joint effusion will compress or displace any intra-articular fat and adjacent fascial planes and is limited in extent by the joint capsule; the effusion may be visible only when the radiograph is examined using a spotlight. Periarticular swelling may be more extensive and will obliterate fascial planes.

1. Joint effusion/soft tissue swelling (Figure 2.1)
   a. External trauma
   b. Strain or rupture of an intra-articular structure such as a cruciate ligament
   c. Early osteochondrosis confined to cartilage
   d. Early septic arthritis
   e. Systemic lupus erythematosus (SLE) – usually multiple joints
   f. Ehrlichiosis*
   g. Lyme disease* (*Borrelia burgdorferi* infection)
   h. Polyarthritis/polymyositis syndrome, especially spaniel breeds
   i. Polyarthritis/meningitis syndrome – Weimaraner, German Shorthaired Pointer, Boxer, Bernese Mountain dog, Japanese Akita, also cats

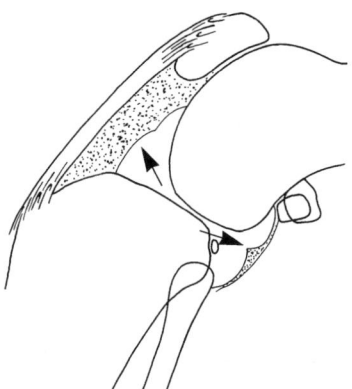

Figure 2.1 Joint effusion – stifle. The effusion is seen as a soft tissue radio-opacity compressing the patellar fat pad and displacing fascial planes caudally (arrows).

j. Heritable polyarthritis of the adolescent Japanese Akita
k. Polyarteritis nodosa – "stiff Beagle disease"
l. Drug-induced polyarthritis, especially certain antibiotics
m. Immune-mediated vaccine reactions
n. Idiopathic polyarthritis
o. Chinese Shar Pei Fever syndrome – short-lived episodes of acute pyrexia and lameness with mono/pauciarticular joint pain and swelling of the hocks and carpi; occasionally enthesiopathies.
2. Recent haemarthrosis.
3. Joint capsule thickening.
4. Periarticular oedema, haematoma, cellulitis, abscess, fibrosis.
5. Soft tissue tumour.
6. Synovial cysts – herniation of joint capsule, bursa or tendon sheath.
7. Soft tissue callus – large dogs, especially elbows.
8. Villonodular synovitis (VNS) – often bone erosion at the chondrosynovial junction too.
9. Cats – various erosive and non-erosive feline polyarthritides; the latter showing soft tissue swelling only.

Gas in joints

10. Fat mistaken for gas.
11. Post-arthrocentesis.
12. Vacuum phenomenon – seen in humans in joints under traction, when gas (mainly nitrogen) diffuses out from extracellular fluid. In dogs, reported only in the shoulder, intervertebral disc spaces and intersternebral spaces and only in the presence of joint disease e.g. osteochondrosis, disc disease
13. Open wound communicating with the joint
14. Infection with gas-producing bacteria.

2.3 Altered width of joint space

Decreased joint space width

1. Artefactual – X-ray beam not centred over the joint space.
2. Articular cartilage erosion due to degenerative joint disease.
3. Articular cartilage erosion due to rheumatoid disease; usually multiple joints.
4. Periarticular fibrosis.
5. Advanced septic arthritis with erosion of articular cartilage and collapse of subchondral bone.

Increased joint space width

6. Traction during radiography.
7. Skeletal immaturity and incomplete epiphyseal ossification.
8. Joint effusion.
9. Recent haemarthrosis.
10. Subluxation.
11. Intra-articular soft tissue mass.
12. Intra-articular pathology causing subchondral osteolysis (e.g. osteochondrosis, septic arthritis, soft tissue tumour, rheumatoid arthritis).
13. Various epiphyseal dysplasias (see 1.21.7–12).

Asymmetric joint space width

14. Normal variant in some joints, dependent on positioning (e.g. caudocranial views of the shoulder and stifle)
15. Congenital subluxation/dysplasia.
16. Collateral ligament rupture (Figure 2.2) – stressed views may be required to demonstrate subluxation.
17. Asymmetric narrowing or widening of the joint space due to other pathology – see above.

2.4 Osteolytic joint disease

1. Apparent osteolysis due to incomplete ossification in the young animal.
2. Apparent osteolysis due to abnormalities of ossification (see epiphyseal dysplasias, 1.21.7–12).
3. Osteochondrosis (OC) – focal subchondral lucencies at specific locations, mainly the shoulder, elbow, stifle and hock in young, medium and large breed dogs, male preponderance; often bilateral; also joint effusion +/– mineralised cartilage flap, fragmentation of subchondral bone, joint mice, subchondral sclerosis, secondary osteoarthritis (see 3.2.4, 3.4.4–7, 3.11.4, 3.13.1 and Figures 3.1, 3.4–3.6, 3.23, 3.29).
4. Legg–Calvé–Perthe's disease (avascular necrosis of the femoral head) – patchy osteolysis and collapse of femoral head in young, small breed dogs; often bilateral (see 3.9.3 and Figure 3.22).
5. Septic arthritis – usually involves all bones comprising a joint, including the articular surfaces. Multiple joints may be affected if the infection has been spread haematogenously. Main DDx soft tissue tumour (if in an older animal with solitary joint involvement).

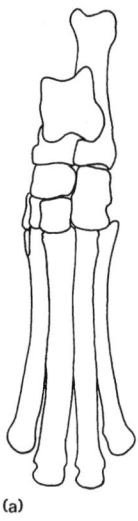

(a)

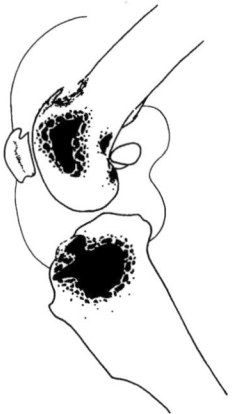

Figure 2.3 Soft tissue tumour around the stifle joint – osteolysis in several bones, joint effusion and surrounding soft tissue swelling.

7. Rheumatoid arthritis (Figure 2.4) – immune-mediated, erosive, symmetrical polyarthritis; progressive and deforming; usually in small to medium middle-aged dogs and rare in cats; many joints may be affected but there is a predilection for the carpus and hock. Radiographic changes include joint effusion and soft tissue swelling, changes in joint space width, subchondral osteolysis and cyst formation, osteolysis at sites of soft tissue attachment, severe osteoarthritis, periarticular calcification and eventual luxation or ankylosis.

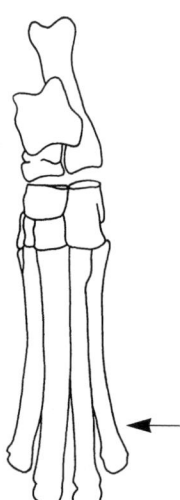

(b)

Figure 2.2 Lateral collateral ligament rupture of the tarsus. (a) The unstressed dorsoplantar view appears normal; (b) subluxation of the intertarsal joint space caused by laterally applied stress.

6. Soft tissue tumour (Figure 2.3) – if at or near a joint will usually affect more than one bone, mainly causing multiple areas of punched-out osteolysis; articular surfaces may be spared with lysis predominantly at sites of soft tissue attachment. DDx septic arthritis; severe osteoarthritis with superimposition of irregular new bone mimicking osteolysis
   a. Synovial sarcoma
   b. Other periarticular soft tissue tumours.

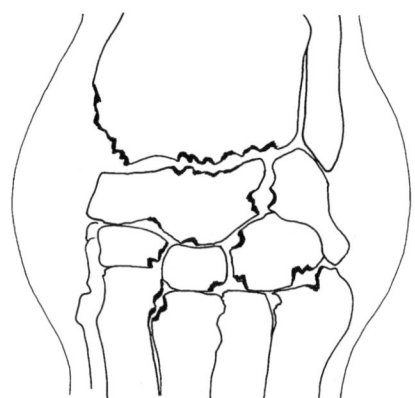

Figure 2.4 Rheumatoid arthritis affecting the carpus – widening of joint spaces (they may also be narrowed), subchondral osteolysis and surrounding soft tissue swelling.

8. Osteopenia (e.g. disuse, metabolic) – epiphyses and carpal/tarsal bones are especially affected (see 1.16).
9. Chronic haemarthrosis – usually also with secondary osteoarthritis.
10. Villonodular synovitis (VNS) – intracapsular, nodular synovial hyperplasia thought to be due to trauma. Smooth, cyst-like areas of osteolysis at the chondrosynovial junction; intra-articular mass can be shown by arthrography or ultrasound.
11. Leishmaniasis* – 30% of affected dogs develop locomotor problems including severe osteolytic joint disease which may affect multiple joints. Main DDx septic arthritis, rheumatoid arthritis.
12. *Mycoplasma* polyarthritis – immunosuppressed or debilitated animals; also *M. spumans* polyarthritis in young greyhounds.
13. Subchondral cysts associated with osteoarthritis – occasional finding.
14. Cats – feline metastatic digital carcinoma – multiple digits/feet, primary lesion in lung. DDx paronychia (see 3.7.9, 3.7.11 and Figure 3.16).
15. Cats – feline tuberculosis – various *Mycobacteria*; occasionally affects the skeletal system – osteolytic joint disease; also periostitis, osteoarthritis and mixed bone lesions.

2.5 Proliferative joint disease

The term *osteoarthritis* implies the presence of an inflammatory component to the disease process whereas *osteoarthrosis* is generally used to imply a non-inflammatory condition. However, the two conditions may exist together and cannot be differentiated radiographically, and so the terms are often used synonymously. In some cases, new bone proliferation may be accompanied by marked remodelling of underlying bone.

1. Osteoarthritis secondary to elbow and hip dysplasia (see 3.4.4–7, 3.4.16, 3.9.2 and Figures 3.4–3.6, 3.10, 3.19).
2. Osteoarthritis secondary to damaged articular soft tissues (e.g. strained or ruptured cranial cruciate ligament. Figure 2.5)
3. Osteoarthritis secondary to osteochondrosis – typical breeds and joints, may be bilateral (3.2.4, 3.4.4–7, 3.11.4, 3.13.1 and Figures 3.1, 3.4–3.6, 3.23, 3.29).
4. Osteoarthritis secondary to generalised skeletal chondrodysplasias (see 1.21.7–12).
5. Osteoarthritis secondary to trauma or other abnormal stresses (e.g. angular limb deformities).
6. Osteoarthritis secondary to repeated haemarthroses (may also see osteolysis).
7. Enthesiopathies at specific locations, although these may not be clinically significant (e.g. enthesiopathy of the short radial collateral ligament in the greyhound. See 3.6.10 and Figure 3.14).
8. Neoplasia – single joints, large bony masses
   a. Osteoma – rare in small animals
   b. Parosteal osteosarcoma – mainly proliferative, unlike other osteosarcomas.
9. Disseminated idiopathic skeletal hyperostosis (DISH) – large dogs, mainly spondylotic lesions in the spine but may also affect extremital joints causing osteoarthritis, enthesiopathies and prominence of tuberosities and trochanters.
10. Synovial osteochondroma – calcified intra-articular and periarticular bodies +/– osteoarthritis (see 2.8.18).
11. Systemic lupus erythematosus (SLE) – very mild osteoarthritis may occur in chronic cases.
12. Cats – hypervitaminosis A: raw liver diet; mainly spinal new bone but may also see exostoses near the limb joints, especially the elbow
13. Cats – mucopolysaccharidoses – inherited epiphyseal dysplasia; mainly spinal changes similar to hypervitaminosis A but also osteoarthritis secondary to epiphyseal dysplasia. Rare in dogs.

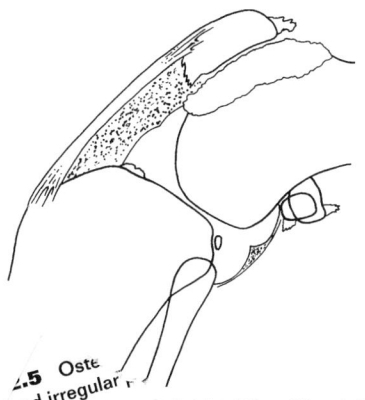

Fig 2.5 Osteoarthritis of the stifle – joint effusion and irregular periarticular osteophytes.

2.6 Mixed osteolytic/proliferative joint disease

1. Soft tissue neoplasia – osteolysis usually predominates but there may be some periosteal reaction or the tumour may be superimposed over pre-existing osteoarthritis as patients are usually older (see 2.4.6 and Figure 2.3).
2. Rheumatoid arthritis – osteolytic or mixed joint lesions affecting small joints especially (see 2.4.7 and Figure 2.4).
3. Legg–Calvé–Perthe's disease (avascular necrosis of the femoral head) with secondary osteoarthritis – hip only (see 3.9.3 and Figure 3.22).
4. Septic arthritis – bacterial or fungal; if haematogenous spread has occurred multiple joints may be affected and the animal is likely to be systemically ill.
5. Chronic/repeated haemarthroses – animals with bleeding disorders, often multiple joints.
6. Leishmaniasis* – mainly osteolytic.
7. Villonodular synovitis (see 2.4.10).
8. Cats – feline non-infectious erosive polyarthritis.
9. Cats – feline tuberculosis.
10. Cats – periosteal proliferative polyarthritis (Reiter's disease); especially carpi and tarsi. Rare in dogs.

2.7 Conditions that may affect more than one joint

For further details of conditions which affect specific joints, see Chapter 3.

1. Elbow and hip dysplasia – often bilateral (see 3.4.4–7, 3.9.2 and Figures 3.4–3.6, 3.19).
2. Osteochondrosis – primary lesions and secondary osteoarthritis; mainly shoulder, elbow, stifle and hock in larger breed dogs. Often bilateral and may affect more than one pair of joints (see 3.2.4, 3.4.4–7, 3.11.4, 3.13.1 and Figures 3.1, 3.4–3.6, 3.23, 3.29).
3. Primary osteoarthritis – an ageing change, but less common in small animals than in humans; mainly the shoulder and elbow; often bilateral or multiple joints affected.
4. Stifle osteoarthritis secondary to cruciate ligament disease or patellar subluxation; often bilateral (see 3.11.16 and Figure 2.5).
5. Rheumatoid arthritis – osteolytic or mixed joint lesions affecting small joints especially (see 2.4.7 and Figure 2.4).
6. SLE – usually mild soft tissue swelling only.
7. Haematogenous bacterial or fungal septic arthritis – mixed osteolytic/proliferative changes.
8. Leishmaniasis* – mainly osteolytic joint disease.
9. Chronic/repeated haemarthroses – animals with bleeding disorders.
10. DISH – large dogs, mainly spondylotic lesions in the spine but may also affect extremital joints causing osteoarthritis, enthesiopathies and prominence of tuberosities and trochanters.
11. Skeletal dysplasias – e.g. chondrodysplasias, pituitary dwarfism and congenital hypothyroidism; multiple joints affected (see 1.21.7–12).
12. Rocky Mountain spotted fever* (*Rickettsia rickettsii* infection).
13. Ehrlichiosis*.
14. Lyme disease * (*Borrelia burgdorferi* infection) – usually a shifting monoarticular or pauciarticular condition rather than a true polyarthritis.
15. Polyarthritis/polymyositis syndrome, especially spaniel breeds.
16. Polyarthritis/meningitis syndrome – Weimaraner, German Shorthaired Pointer, Boxer, Bernese Mountain dog, Japanese Akita, also cats.
17. Heritable polyarthritis of the adolescent Japanese Akita.
18. *Mycoplasma* polyarthritis – immunosuppressed or debilitated animals; also *M. spumans* polyarthritis in young greyhounds.
19. Chinese Shar Pei fever syndrome – short-lived episodes of acute pyrexia and lameness with mono/pauciarticular joint pain and swelling of hocks and carpi; occasionally enthesiopathies.
20. Polyarteritis nodosa – "stiff Beagle disease".
21. Drug-induced polyarthritis, especially due to certain antibiotics.
22. Immune-mediated vaccine reactions.
23. Cats – feline non-infectious erosive and non-erosive polyarthritides.
24. Cats – feline calicivirus.
25. Cats – periosteal proliferative polyarthritis (Reiter's disease); especially carpi and tarsi. Rare in dogs.
26. Cats – hypervitaminosis A: raw liver diet; mainly spinal new bone but joints, esee exostoses near the limb
27. Cats – mucopolysaccharidoses – inherited epiphyseal d

changes similar to hypervitaminosis A but also osteoarthritis secondary to epiphyseal dysplasia. Rare in dogs.
28. Cats – feline tuberculosis.

2.8 Mineralised bodies in or near joints

Normal anatomical structures

1. Small sesamoid in tendon of abductor pollicis longus et indicus proprius muscle, medial aspect of carpus.
2. Sesamoids of metacarpo/tarsophalangeal joints (one dorsal, two palmar/plantar).
3. Patella.
4. Fabellae in heads of gastrocnemius muscle – caudal aspect of distal femur; medial much larger than lateral in cats.
5. Popliteal sesamoid – caudal aspect of stifle or proximal tibia; may be absent in small dogs.
6. Epiphyseal, apophyseal and small bone centres of ossification in young animals.
7. Cats – clavicles.

Normal variants – occasional findings of no clinical significance

These are likely to be bilateral, so if there is doubt as to their significance, radiograph the other leg.

8. Accessory centres of ossification – usually larger dogs; examples are caudal glenoid rim, anconeus, dorsal aspect of wing of ilium (often remains unfused), craniodorsal margin of acetabulum.
9. Occasional sesamoids – e.g. sesamoid craniolateral to elbow (in humeroradial ligament, lateral collateral ligament, supinator or ulnaris lateralis).
10. Bipartite or multipartite sesamoids – e.g. palmar metacarpophalangeal sesamoids II and VII in Rottweilers; medial fabella of stifle (see 3.7.4, 3.11.2 and Figure 3.15); DDx traumatic fragmentation.
11. Rudimentary clavicles in some dogs.
12. Multiple centres of ossification at the base of the os penis.
13. Stifle meniscal calcification or ossification – especially old cats (may also be associated with lameness in some animals).

Structures likely to be clinically significant

See also Chapter 3 for details of specific joints

14. Osteochondrosis (OC) – mineralised cartilage flaps and osteochondral fragments (joint mice).
15. Fractures:
    a. avulsion fractures
    b. chip fractures
    c. fractured osteophytes from pre-existing osteoarthritis.
16. Calcifying tendinopathy.
17. Meniscal calcification or ossification (stifle, see 3.11.18).
18. Synovial osteochondromatosis (chondrometaplasia) – primary, or secondary to joint disease; osteochondral nodules in synovial tissue of joint, bursa or tendon sheath; main DDx in the cat is hypervitaminosis A and in the dog is parosteal osteosarcoma.
19. Calcinosis circumscripta – usually young German Shepherd dogs; masses of amorphous calcified material in soft tissues over limb prominences; also in the neck and tongue; self-limiting (see 12.2.2 and Figure 12.1).
20. Severe arthritis – dystrophic calcification of soft tissues around joint; other arthritic changes seen too
    a. Steroid arthropathy following intra-articular steroid injection
    b. Rheumatoid arthritis
    c. Infectious arthritis
    d. Severe degenerative osteoarthritis.
21. Myositis ossificans – heterotopic bone formation in muscle
    a. Primary idiopathic
    b. Secondary to trauma.
22. Chondrocalcinosis/pseudogout (calcium pyrophosphate deposition disease CPDD) – rare, unknown aetiology; older animals.

FURTHER READING

General

Carrig, C.B. (1997) Diagnostic imaging of osteoarthritis. *Veterinary Clinics of North America; Small Animal Practice* **27** 777–814.

Farrow, C.S. (1982) Stress radiography: applications in small animal practice. *Journal of the American Veterinary Medical Association* **181** 777–784.

Morgan, J.P., Wind, A. and Davidson, A.P. (1999) Bone dysplasias in the Labrador retriever: a radiographic study. *Journal of the American Animal Hospital Association* **35** 332–340.

Techniques and normal anatomy

Muhumuza, L., Morgan, J.P., Miyabayashi, T. and Atilola, A.O. (1988) Positive-contrast arthrography – a study of the humeral joints in normal beagle dogs. *Veterinary Radiology* **29** 157–161.

Congenital and developmental diseases; diseases of young animals

Various authors (1998) Osteochondrosis. *Veterinary Clinics of North America; Small Animal Practice* **28** number 1.

Infective and inflammatory conditions

Bennett, D. and Taylor, D.J. (1988) Bacterial infective arthritis in the dog. *Journal of Small Animal Practice* **29** 207–230.

Bennett, D. (1988) Immune based erosive inflammatory joint disease of the dog: canine rheumatoid arthritis. I Clinical, radiological and laboratory investigations. *Journal of Small Animal Practice* **28** 779–797.

Bennett, D. and Nash, A.S. (1988) Feline immune-based polyarthritis: a study of thirty-one cases. *Journal of Small Animal Practice* **29** 501–523.

Ettinger, S.J. and Feldman, E.C. (1995) *Textbook of Veterinary Internal Medicine* 4th ed., Philadelphia: W.B. Saunders.

Gunn-Moore, D.A., Jenkins, P.A. and Lucke, V.M. (1996) Feline tuberculosis: a literature review and discussion of 19 cases caused by an unusual mycobacterial variant. *Veterinary Record* **138** 53–58.

Hanson, J.A. (1998) Radiographic diagnosis – canine carpal villonodular synovitis. *Veterinary Radiology and Ultrasound* **39** 15–17.

Marti, J.M. (1997) Bilateral pigmented villonodular synovitis in a dog. *Journal of Small Animal Practice* **38** 256–260.

May, C., Hammill, J. and Bennett, D. (1992), Chinese Shar Pei fever syndrome: a preliminary report. *Veterinary Record* **131** 586–587.

Owens, J.M., Ackerman, N. and Nyland, T. (1978) Roentgenology of arthritis. *Veterinary Clinics of North America* **8** 453–464.

Neoplasia

Whitelock, R.G., Dyce, J., Houlton, J.E.F. and Jeffries, A.R. (1997) *Veterinary and Comparative Orthopaedics and Traumatology* **10** 146–152.

Thamm, D.H., Mauldin, E.A., Edinger, D.T. and Lustgarten, C. (2000) Primary osteosarcoma of the synovium in a dog. *Journal of the American Animal Hospital Association* **36** 326–331.

Trauma

Owens, J.M., Ackerman, N. and Nyland, T. (1978) Roentgenology of joint trauma. *Veterinary Clinics of North America; Small Animal Practice* **8** 419–451.

Miscellaneous conditions

Allan, G.S. (2000) Radiographic features of feline joint diseases. *Veterinary Clinics of North America; Small Animal Practice* **30** 281–302.

de Haan, J.J. and Andreasen, C.B. (1992) Calcium crystal-associated arthropathy (pseudogout) in a dog. *Journal of the American Veterinary Medical Association* **200** 943–946.

Kramer, M., Gerwing, M., Hach, V. and Schimke, E. (1997) Sonography of the musculoskeletal system in dogs and cats. *Veterinary Radiology and Ultrasound* **38** 139–149.

Mahoney P.N. and Lamb C.R. (1996) Articular, periarticular and juxtaarticular calcified bodies in the dog and cat: a radiological review. *Veterinary Radiology and Ultrasound* **37** 3–19.

Prymak, C. and Goldschmidt, M.H. (1991) Synovial cysts in five dogs and one cat. *Journal of the American Animal Hospital Association* **27** 151–154.

Short, R.P. and Jardine, J.E. (1993) Calcium pyrophosphate deposition disease in a Fox Terrier. *Journal of the American Animal Hospital Association* **29** 363–366.

Stead, A.C., Else, R.W. and Stead, M.C.P. (1995) Synovial cysts in cats. *Journal of Small Animal Practice* **36** 450–454.

Weber, W.J., Berry, C.R. and Kramer, R.W. (1995) Vacuum phenomenon in twelve dogs. *Veterinary Radiology and Ultrasound* **36** 493–498.

3

Appendicular skeleton

3.1   Scapula
3.2   Shoulder
3.3   Humerus
3.4   Elbow
3.5   Radius and ulna (antebrachium, forearm)
3.6   Carpus
3.7   Metacarpus, metatarsus and phalanges

3.8   Pelvis
3.9   Hip (coxofemoral joint)
3.10 Femur
3.11 Stifle
3.12 Tibia and fibula
3.13 Tarsus (hock)

This chapter describes conditions that are most commonly associated with specific bones or joints. Lack of inclusion of a condition under an anatomical area may not mean that it cannot occur there, simply that this area is not a predilection site; for example synovial sarcomas most often arise around the elbow and stifle, although they may arise near any synovial joint. Conditions that may occur in any joint (e.g. infectious arthritis) are described in Chapter 2.

For each anatomical area, the conditions are listed in the following order:
- artefacts and normal anatomical variants
- congenital/developmental
- metabolic
- infective
- inflammatory
- neoplastic
- traumatic
- degenerative
- miscellaneous conditions.

Conditions that most closely resemble each other radiographically are indicated by DDx (differential diagnosis). Conditions involving joints are listed under the relevant bone but described more fully under the appropriate joint.

Joint trauma tends to affect the weakest area, hence physeal fractures occur in skeletally immature animals and ligamentous damage in older animals; young dogs rarely suffer from ligament trauma.

In many cases, where there is doubt as to the presence of genuine pathology, always consider radiographing the opposite limb for comparison.

3.1 Scapula

Views: mediolateral (ML), caudocranial (CdCr), distoproximal (DiPr) – dorsal recumbency with the affected limb pulled caudally so the scapula is vertical and the shoulder joint is flexed to 90°.
1. Ossification centre of the scapular tuberosity (supraglenoid tubercle), fuses to the body of the scapula by 4–7 months; DDx fracture.
2. Chondrosarcoma – flat bones are predisposed (scapula, pelvis, cranium, ribs).
3. Scapular fractures – usually young medium to large breeds of dog and after major trauma; often concurrent thoracic injuries
   a. Scapular body – non-articular
   b. Scapular spine – non-articular
   c. Scapular neck – non-articular
   d. Scapular tuberosity (supraglenoid tubercle) – avulsed by biceps tendon; articular; DDx separate centre of ossification
   e. Other glenoid fractures; articular.

3.2 Shoulder

Views: ML, ML with pronation and/or supination, CdCr, flexed cranioproximal-craniodistal oblique (CrPr-CrDiO), arthrography (see 2.1).
1. Clavicles – clearly seen in cats; smaller and less mineralised in dogs but rudimentary structures are sometimes visible, especially on the CdCr view of the shoulder; bilaterally symmetrical.

39

2. Caudal circumflex humeral artery seen end-on caudal to the joint surrounded by fat; DDx poorly mineralised joint mouse.
3. Separate ossification centre of glenoid – small, crescentic mineralised opacity adjacent to the caudal rim of the glenoid; may fuse to the scapula or persist throughout life; incidental finding but DDx osteochondrosis of glenoid (see 3.2.5).
4. Osteochondrosis (OC) of the humeral head (Figure 3.1); also called osteochondrosis dissecans (OCD) if there is evidence of cartilage flap formation – young dogs mainly 5–7 months old of larger breeds, with a male preponderance; often bilateral. Radiographic signs include flattening or concavity of the caudal third of the humeral articular surface +/− subchondral lucency or sclerosis, overlying mineralised cartilage flap, joint mice usually in the caudal joint pouch but also in the biceps tendon sheath or the subscapular joint pouch (CdCr view); mild secondary osteoarthritis. The presence of the vacuum phenomenon (see 2.2.12) is highly suggestive of an OC lesion. Arthrography is helpful in demonstrating irregularity of the articular cartilage layer and non-mineralised cartilage flap formation.
5. OC of the glenoid rim – unusual. Separate mineralised fragment adjacent to articular rim; DDx separate centre of ossification, but usually larger.

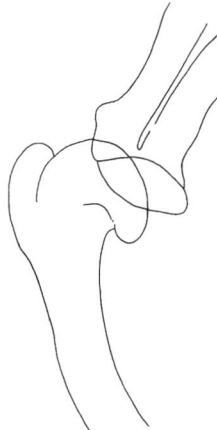

Figure 3.2 Congenital shoulder luxation or remodelling following trauma at a very early age. The glenoid of the scapula and the humeral head are both deformed with loss of congruity of the joint space; superimposition of the two bones on the ML view implies luxation in the sagittal plane.

6. Congenital shoulder luxation or subluxation (Figure 3.2) – rare, mainly miniature and toy breeds of dog; may be bilateral. The humerus is normally displaced medially due to underdevelopment of the medial labrum of the scapular glenoid but spontaneous reduction may occur on positioning for radiography. Radiographic signs include a flattened, underdeveloped glenoid with progressive remodelling of articular surfaces leading to osteoarthritis; DDx trauma at an early age.
7. Traumatic shoulder luxation – uncommon, unilateral. The humerus is usually displaced medially or laterally, occasionally cranially or caudally. With sagittal displacement ML radiographs show a slight overlap of the scapula and humerus with loss of the joint space; on CdCr radiographs the luxation is obvious unless spontaneous reduction has occurred; DDx normal medial widening of the shoulder joint space on a CdCr view, especially if poorly positioned and particularly in smaller dog breeds. Check also for associated chip fractures.
8. Fractures involving the shoulder joint
    a. Scapular tuberosity (supraglenoid tubercle) – Salter-Harris type I growth plate fracture in a skeletally immature animal or bone fracture in a mature animal. May be avulsed by biceps tendon. DDx separate centre of ossification

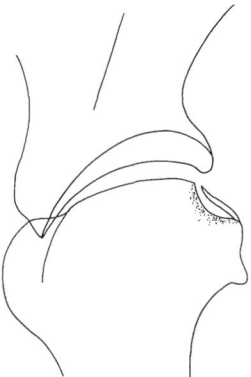

Figure 3.1 Shoulder osteochondrosis with secondary osteoarthritis – subchondral bone erosion affecting the caudal part of the humeral head, an overlying mineralised cartilage flap and an osteophyte on the caudal articular margin of the humerus.

b. Other articular glenoid fractures
   c. Salter–Harris type I fracture of the proximal humeral epiphysis in young animals – rare.
9. Shoulder osteoarthritis – usually osteophytes on the caudal glenoid rim and caudal articular margin of the humeral head. Joint mice may be visible in the caudal joint pouch, and may become very large in old dogs. Some may develop into synovial osteochondromata
   a. Primary – ageing change; often clinically insignificant
   b. Secondary – e.g. following osteochondrosis.
10. Calcifying tendinopathy (Figure 3.3) – usually supraspinatus and biceps brachii tendons; changes in the infraspinatus and coracobrachialis tendons are also reported. Mainly medium to large, middle-aged dogs, especially Rottweilers; aetiology unknown. Mild/chronic/intermittent lameness or clinically silent. May be bilateral. Radiographic signs include small areas of mineralisation in the region of the affected tendon; DDx rudimentary clavicles or joint mice in the biceps tendon sheath. The CrPr–CrDiO view and arthrography are helpful in identifying the tendon of origin. Bicipital calcifying tendinopathy may be associated with tenosynovitis (see 3.2.11). Ultrasonography of the tendons may be helpful in showing fibre disruption, areas of mineralisation and joint capsule or tendon sheath effusion.
11. Bicipital tenosynovitis and bursitis – signalment as in 3.2.10. Radiographs may be normal or may show ill-defined sclerosis and new bone in the intertubercular groove, enthesiophytes on the supraglenoid tubercle and mild osteoarthritis. Arthrography may show reduced or irregular filling of the biceps tendon sheath. Ultrasonography may be used to demonstrate fluid distension of the bursa and tendon sheath and changes within the tendon itself.

3.3 Humerus

Views: ML, CdCr or craniocaudal (CrCd).
1. Panosteitis – the humerus is a predilection site (see 1.13.5 and Figure 1.17).
2. Metaphyseal osteopathy (hypertrophic osteodystrophy) – proximal and distal humeral metaphyses are minor sites; the most obvious lesions are usually in the distal radius and ulna (see 1.23.3 and Figure 1.30).
3. Primary malignant bone tumours (most commonly osteosarcoma) – the proximal humeral metaphysis is a predilection site (see 1.19.1 and Figure 1.26); the distal humerus is very rarely affected.
4. Humeral fractures
   a. Distal two-thirds of diaphysis – most common area; usually spiral or oblique and may be comminuted, following the musculospiral groove; transient radial paralysis is commonly associated
   b. Proximal third of diaphysis – usually a transverse fracture near the deltoid tuberosity
   c. Salter–Harris type I fracture of the proximal humeral growth plate in skeletally immature animals
   d. Distal epiphysis – (see 3.4.14 and Figure 3.9):
      • lateral humeral condylar fracture
      • Y-fracture affecting both medial and lateral parts of the condyle
      • medial humeral condylar fracture.

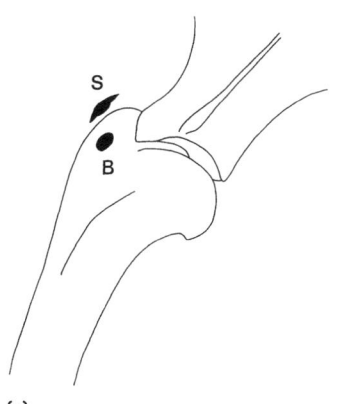
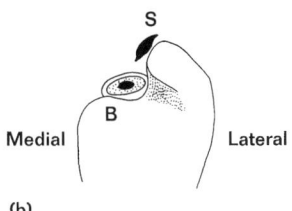

Figure 3.3 Calcifying tendinopathy of the shoulder joint. (a) ML view; (b) CrPr–CrDiO view (right shoulder). Calcification is seen as a radio-opaque area radiographically, although shown here in black. B = In biceps brachii tendon; S = in supraspinatus tendon.

3.4 Elbow

Views: flexed, extended and neutral ML, CrCd or CdCr, craniolateral–caudomedial oblique (CrL–CdMO), craniomedial–caudolateral oblique (CrM–CdLO), arthrography.

1. Ossification centres visible in the elbow – medial and lateral parts of the distal humeral condyle, medial humeral epicondyle, anconeus, olecranon, proximal radial epiphysis; occasional small separate centre of ossification in the lateral humeral epicondyle seen on the CrCd view.
2. Elbow sesamoids – mineralised elbow sesamoids are commonly seen in both dogs (mainly larger breeds) and cats; small, smooth, round bodies craniolateral to the radial head; usually bilateral. Mainly in the supinator muscle but also reported in the annular ligament and lateral collateral ligament. DDx joint mice, chip fractures.
3. Absence of the supratrochlear foramen of the distal humerus – occasionally noted in small, chondrodystrophic breeds of dog.
4. Fragmentation of the medial coronoid process of ulna (FCP; Figure 3.4) – part of the elbow dysplasia complex seen in young dogs of medium and large breeds especially the Labrador Retriever, Golden Retriever, Bernese Mountain dog, Rottweiler, Newfoundland; male preponderance; often bilateral. Predisposed to by elbow incongruity with widening of the humeroradial joint space, which puts increased pressure on the medial coronoid process. The diagnosis of FCP and of humeral condylar OC is often made by identification of secondary osteoarthritis in an appropriate patient rather than by visualisation of a primary lesion (see 3.4.16 and Figure 3.10 for description); a specific diagnosis may not be possible without arthrotomy, arthroscopy or high resolution CT or MR imaging. The primary radiographic findings are flattening, rounding or fragmentation of the process on the ML and Cr15°L– CdMO (15° supinated ML) views; the CrCd view shows not the process itself but a more medial projection of bone, which may be remodelled. "Kissing" subchondral lesions may also be seen on the opposing articular surface of the humeral condyle; DDx humeral osteochondrosis.
5. OC of the medial part of the distal humeral condyle (Figure 3.5) – also part of the elbow dysplasia complex with signalment as above. The primary lesion is best seen on the CrCd view as subchondral bone flattening or irregularity, subchondral sclerosis, +/– overlying mineralised cartilage flap; severe lesions may also be visible on the ML view; DDx "kissing" lesion created by a fragmented medial coronoid process.
6. Ununited anconeal process (UAP. Figure 3.6) – also part of the elbow dysplasia complex, although mainly in the German Shepherd dog, Irish Wolfhound, Great Dane, Gordon Setter and Basset Hound; predisposed to by elbow incongruity with a short ulna or long radius putting pres-

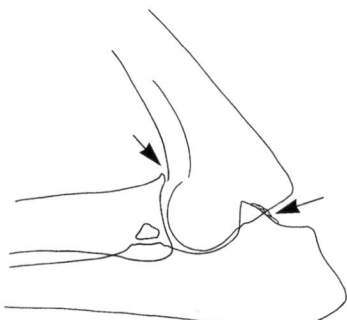

Figure 3.4 Fragmented medial coronoid process with early secondary osteoarthritis. A small bone fragment is seen lying adjacent to the medial coronoid region of the ulna, which is flattened. Small osteophytes are present on the radial head and anconeal process (arrowed).

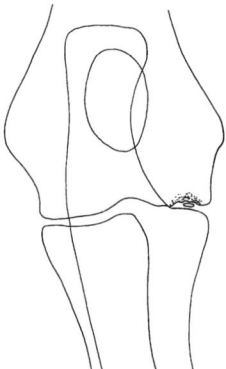

Figure 3.5 Humeral condylar OC (CrCd view of the right elbow). A shallow subchondral defect is seen in the medial part of the humeral condyle, with an overlying small, mineralised fragment.

3 APPENDICULAR SKELETON

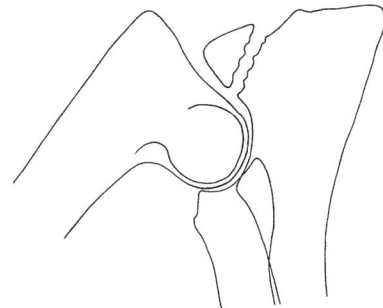

Figure 3.6 Ununited anconeal process – a large, triangular bone fragment is clearly seen, separated from the adjacent ulna.

sure on the anconeus, but may also be due to trauma; some cases are bilateral. The separate centre of ossification for the anconeus usually fuses to the ulna between 4 and 5 months and persistence of a radiolucent cleavage line beyond this time indicates separation. The flexed ML view is diagnostic, showing a substantial triangular bone fragment either adjacent to the ulna or displaced proximally; chronic cases show remodelling of the fragment and/or osteoarthritis.

7. Elbow incongruity – seen in the various breeds predisposed to elbow dysplasia, but especially in the Bernese Mountain dog. Poor congruity between the humerus, radius and ulna puts increased pressure on the medial coronoid process or the anconeus and may lead to fragmentation or separation of these processes respectively. Usually the humeroradial joint space is widened distal to the joint; this is best assessed on a CrCd view as it is quite position-sensitive. May be seen alone, or with FCP, OC, UAP +/- osteoarthritis.
8. Medial epicondylar spurs (flexor tendon enthesiopathy. Figure 3.7) – usually larger breeds of dog; may be bilateral; aetiology and significance not known: in some dogs it is an incidental radiographic finding. The ML radiograph shows a distally projecting bony spur on the caudal aspect of the medial humeral epicondyle or, less commonly, mineralisation in adjacent soft tissues.
9. "Ununited medial epicondyle" – unusual; aetiology not known but may be part of the elbow dysplasia complex as similar breeds are affected, mainly young Labradors; may be bilateral. Single or multiple mineralised fragments of varying size and shape are seen at several locations near the medial epicondyle on the ML or CrCd view, sometimes with an adjacent bone defect. Secondary osteoarthritis may be very minor. Some cases are radiographically similar to flexor enthesiopathies and these may be different manifestations of the same condition.

International Elbow Working Group (IEWG) grading system for elbow dysplasia

The IEWG recommends the following grading system for elbow dysplasia screening based on the degree of secondary osteoarthritis:
- Grade 0 – normal elbow, no osteoarthritis or primary lesion
- Grade 1 – mild osteoarthritis with osteophytes <2 mm
- Grade 2 – moderate osteoarthritis with osteophytes 2–5 mm
- Grade 3 – severe osteoarthritis with osteophytes >5 mm.

Primary lesions described include malformed or fragmented medial coronoid process, ununited anconeal process, osteochondrosis of the humeral condyle, incongruity of the articular surfaces and mineralisation in deep tendons caudal to the medial epicondyle. Grading schemes in different countries vary in their grading of primary lesions.

10. Elbow subluxation
    a. Severe elbow incongruity
    b. Secondary to relative shortening of ulna or radius, usually due to traumatic lesions at the distal growth

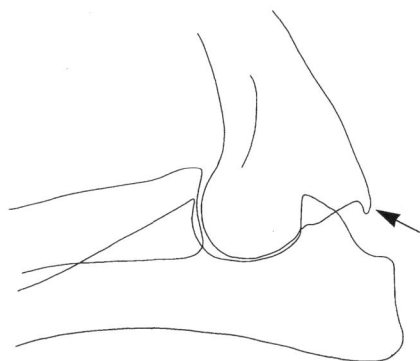

Figure 3.7 Medial epicondylar spur. A small, distally projecting osteophyte arises from the caudal aspect of the medial humeral epicondyle (arrowed).

plates (see 3.5.4–7). Shortening of the ulna causes widening of the humeroulnar space distally and increased pressure on the anconeal process; shortening of the radius causes widening of the humeroradial space and of the humeroulnar space proximally, resulting in increased pressure on the medial coronoid process of the ulna

c. Distractio cubiti/dysostosis enchondralis (see 3.5.5)
d. Congenital elbow (sub)luxation – several types; mainly small breeds of dogs (e.g. Pekinese), but also cats; often bilateral. Deformity is recognised at an early age
- the most common type is lateral displacement of the radial head with a normal humeroulnar articulation; the radius is elongated and the radial head is rounded and remodelled (Figure 3.8)
- the second most common type is lateral displacement and 90° medial rotation of the ulna with a normal humeroradial articulation; the semilunar notch of the ulna faces medially and is seen in profile on a CrCd projection of the elbow.

11. Patella cubiti – a rare fusion defect through the semilunar notch of the ulna such that the olecranon and proximal ulnar metaphysis are separated from the rest of the ulna and distracted by the triceps; so called because the fragment of bone is patella-shaped. May be bilateral. DDx avulsion fracture through the proximal ulnar growth plate or semilunar notch.

12. Cats – hypervitaminosis A; usually due to excessive ingestion of raw liver, leading to bony exostoses mainly on the spine, but the elbow is also a predilection site.

13. Synovial sarcoma (occasionally other soft tissue tumours) – the elbow is a predilection site (see 2.4.6 and Figure 2.3); mainly larger breeds of dog; DDx severe osteoarthritis where superimposition of new bone may mimic osteolysis, septic arthritis. The diagnosis may be difficult in cases where tumour is superimposed over pre-existing osteo-

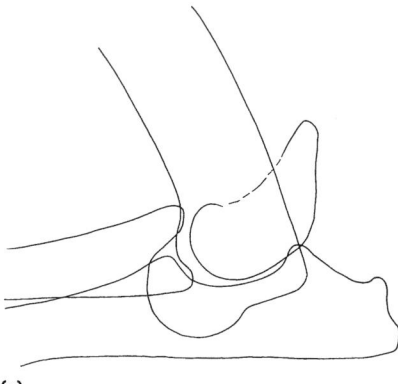

(a)

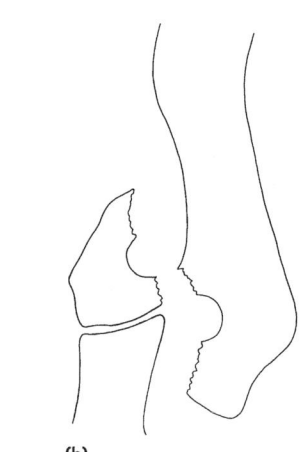

(b)

Figure 3.9 Lateral humeral condylar fracture. (a) On the ML view the medial and lateral parts of the humeral condyle are no longer superimposed; (b) on the CrCd view (right elbow) the displaced fracture is clearly seen (the ulna has been omitted on this view for clarity). The radius remains articulating with the lateral condylar fragment, and these bones override the humeral shaft.

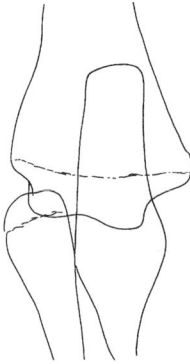

Figure 3.8 Congenital lateral luxation of the radial head (CrCd view of the right elbow). The radial head is markedly remodelled and no longer contoured to the humeral condyle.

3 APPENDICULAR SKELETON

arthritis. In the case of a tumour, a soft tissue mass may be palpable or radiographically visible adjacent to the joint.
14. Fractures involving the elbow joint
    a. Lateral humeral condylar fracture (Figure 3.9) – usually Spaniels and Spaniel crosses; often minor trauma only; may be bilateral. Young dogs or adults; in the latter thought to be predisposed to by incomplete ossification between the medial and lateral parts of the humeral condyle together with the increased loading of the lateral part of the condyle by its articulation with the radius and its weak attachment to the humeral shaft. Best seen on the CrCd view, but overriding of the fragments is also seen on the ML view
    b. "Y" fractures of the humeral condyle – also Spaniels; the fracture line runs proximally between the medial and lateral parts of the condyle into the supracondylar foramen and then separate fracture lines emerge through the medial and lateral humeral cortices. Best seen on the CrCd view
    c. Medial humeral condylar fractures – uncommon
    d. Salter-Harris type I fracture of the distal humeral epiphysis in skeletally immature animals – uncommon
    e. Olecranon fractures – through the proximal ulnar physis (non-articular) or into the semilunar notch (articular), both with distraction by triceps muscle; DDx patella cubiti (see 3.4.11)
    f. Monteggia fracture – uncommon; a proximal ulnar fracture (articular or non-articular) with cranial luxation of the radius and distal ulnar fragment.
15. Traumatic elbow luxation – usually due to a road-traffic accident or suspension by the limb from a fence. ML radiographs may be almost normal but the CrCd view shows dislocation of radius/ulna from humerus clearly; small chip fractures may also be seen.
16. Elbow osteoarthritis – new bone mainly on the anconeus and radial head (seen on the ML view; Figure 3.10a) and medial and lateral humeral epicondyles (seen on the CrCd view; Figure 3.10b). The lameness may be quite severe with mild radiographic changes
    a. Primary – ageing change; radiographic findings are usually minor

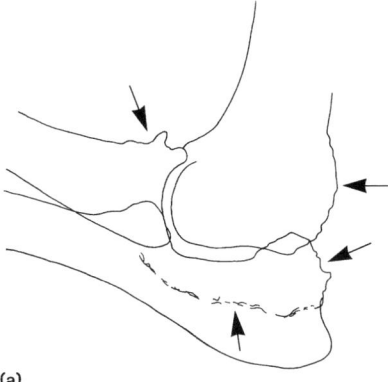

(a)

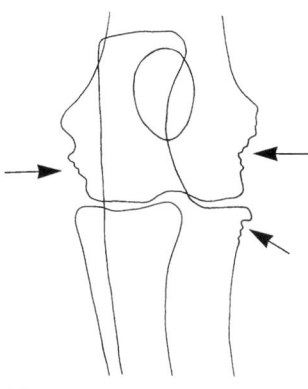

(b)

Figure 3.10 Elbow osteoarthritis. (a) ML and (b) CrCd views (right elbow) showing periarticular new bone (arrowed).

b. Secondary – usually due to elbow dysplasia; radiographic findings may be severe.

3.5 Radius and ulna (antebrachium, forearm)

Views: ML, CrCd.
1. Late closure of the radial growth plates in neutered cats (males – distal only; females – both proximal and distal); leads to an overall longer radius than in entire cats.
2. Hemimelia – one of the paired bones is congenitally absent, usually the radius; rare; usually unilateral. Limb deformity and disability are evident from birth. Possibly heritable as seen in several sibling cats.
3. Retained cartilaginous core, distal ulnar metaphysis (Figure 3.11) – common,

SMALL ANIMAL RADIOLOGICAL DIFFERENTIAL DIAGNOSIS

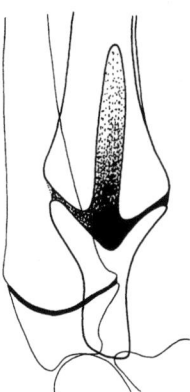

Figure 3.11 Retained cartilaginous core in the distal ulnar metaphysis, seen as a conical radiolucent area extending proximally from the growth plate.

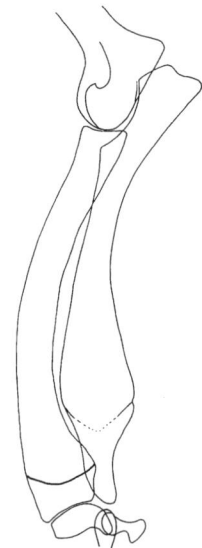

Figure 3.12 Premature closure of the distal ulnar growth plate. Relative shortening of the ulna leading to cranial bowing of the antebrachium and often elbow and carpal subluxation.

often bilateral, ossification defect in giant dog breeds in which a central core of distal growth plate cartilage is slow to ossify, forming a "candle-flame"-shaped lucency with faintly sclerotic borders. Implicated in growth disturbances but may be a coincidental finding as often also seen in normal dogs.
4. Premature closure of the distal ulnar growth plate ("radius curvus" syndrome. Figure 3.12) – a common growth disturbance in young dogs of giant breeds; often bilateral. The cause is usually not identified so deemed idiopathic, but proposed mechanisms include:
   a. Salter-Harris type V crush injury of the distal ulnar growth plate – susceptible to such injury due to its deep conical shape, which prevents lateral movement. May also occur unilaterally in other breeds
   b. metaphyseal osteochondrosis/retained cartilaginous core.

Radiographs should include the whole forearm including the elbow and carpus, and show shortening of the ulna and distraction of the lateral styloid process from the carpus, craniomedial bowing of the radius and ulna with thickening of cortices on the concave aspect, carpal subluxation and remodelling of the distal radius, carpal valgus and supination of the foot, and secondary elbow subluxation, usually of the distal aspect of the humeroulnar articulation (Figure 3.12).
5. Distractio cubiti/dysostosis enchondralis – asynchronous growth of the radius and ulna in chondrodystrophic breeds (e.g. Bassett Hound), leading to elbow incongruity and pain; widening of the distal aspect of the humeroulnar articulation. Usually present with elbow lameness at about 12 months of age; may be bilateral.
6. Premature closure of the distal radial growth plate – trauma at or near the growth plate causes reduction in growth of the radius with shortening of the bone and subluxation of the elbow; widening of the humeroradial articulation +/− increased width of the humeroulnar space proximally. Angular limb deformity is usually minor and the main clinical problem is elbow pain
   a. Symmetric closure – radius short and unusually straight, ulna may also be slightly short, elbow subluxation
   b. Asymmetric closure – distal radius remodelled
      • lateral aspect (more common) – mimics premature closure of the distal ulnar growth plate with bowing of the radius and ulna and carpal valgus
      • medial aspect – carpal varus.
7. Premature closure of the proximal radial growth plate – rare; presumed to be due to trauma; radiographic signs as for 3.5.6a but the proximal radius may be obviously remodelled. Only 30% of the

radial growth occurs proximally therefore radial shortening is less severe than that following distal growth plate trauma.
8. Osteochondrodysplasias – various types of hereditary dwarfism are recognised in a number of dog breeds and in cats (see 1.21.7). Pathological and radiographic lesions are often most severe in the distal ulna and radius due to the high rate of growth at this site. The main abnormality is delayed growth at the distal ulnar growth plate leading to shortening and bowing of the forearm. Some conditions may also resemble rickets radiographically (see 3.5.12). The hindlimbs are less severely affected and may be normal.
9. Congenital hypothyroidism – causes dwarfism with radiographic changes similar to hereditary osteochondrodysplasias (see 1.21.9).
10. Metaphyseal osteopathy (hypertrophic osteodystrophy) – young, rapidly growing dogs of larger breeds; lesions usually most severe in the distal ulnar and radial metaphyses (see 1.23.3 and Figure 1.30). Severe periosteal and paraperiosteal new bone may occasionally bridge growth plates, leading to angular limb deformities.
11. Panosteitis – the radius and ulna are predilection sites (see 1.13.5 and Figure 1.17).
12. Rickets (juvenile osteomalacia) – young animals after weaning; lesions usually most severe in the distal ulnar and radial growth plates (see 1.22.8 and Figure 1.29).
13. Hypertrophic (pulmonary) osteopathy (HPO, Marie's disease) – the radius and ulna may be affected by palisading periosteal new bone, although the distal limb is likely to be affected first (see 1.14.6 and Figure 1.18).
14. Craniomandibular osteopathy (CMO) – rarely, paraperiosteal new bone may be seen surrounding the distal ulna and radius, mimicking metaphyseal osteopathy, sometimes in the absence of the typical skull lesions although in dogs of appropriate breed and age (see 4.10.1 and Figure 4.4).
15. Canine leucocyte adhesion disorder (CLAD) – a hereditary, fatal disease in Irish Red Setters causing lesions similar to metaphyseal osteopathy and craniomandibular osteopathy.
16. Primary malignant bone tumours (most commonly osteosarcoma) – the distal radial metaphysis is the main predilection site, especially in large and giant dog breeds such as Great Dane, Irish Wolfhound (see 1.19.1 and Figure 1.26).
17. Giant cell tumour (osteoclastoma) – the distal ulnar metaphysis is a predilection site; DDx solitary bone cyst (see 1.18.7 and Figure 1.25).
18. Solitary bone cyst – the distal ulnar metaphysis is a predilection site; DDx giant cell tumour (see 1.18.8).
19. Forearm fractures
    a. Transverse fracture of the radius and ulna is very common; usually distal one-third
    b. Fracture of one bone occurs only occasionally due to direct trauma.
20. Radial/ulnar fracture delayed union or non-union – common in toy breeds of dog due to failure to use the injured limb; radiographs show atrophic non-union and disuse osteopenia (see 1.9 and 1.16).

3.6 Carpus

Views: ML, flexed ML, dorsopalmar (DPa), dorsolateral–palmaromedial oblique (DL–PaMO), dorsomedial–palmarolateral oblique (DM–PaLO), stressed and weight-bearing views.

The carpus is a complex joint and small lesions may easily be overlooked; oblique radiographs and similar radiographs of the normal leg for comparison are helpful in interpretation.

1. Normal sesamoid in the insertion of abductor pollicis longus muscle on proximal MC I, seen on a DPa radiograph medial to the radial carpal bone; DDx old chip fracture.
2. Antebrachiocarpal subluxations – secondary to growth disturbances in the forearm and angular limb deformities; most commonly premature closure of the distal ulnar growth plate with cranial bowing of the radius leading to articulation of the distal radius with the dorsoproximal margin of the radial carpal bone and remodelling of the distal radial epiphysis.
3. Cats – osteodystrophy of the Scottish Fold cat; changes more severe in the hindlimbs (see 3.7.6).
4. Rheumatoid arthritis – the carpus and tarsus are predilection sites; often bilateral (see 2.4.7 and Figure 2.4).
5. Cats – various feline polyarthritides; the carpus and tarsus are predilection sites.

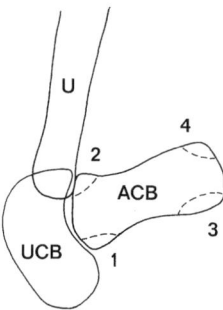

Figure 3.13 Diagrammatic representation of Types 1–4 accessory carpal bone fractures (ML view). U = ulna; UCB = ulnar carpal bone; ACB = accessory carpal bone.

6. Chinese Shar Pei fever syndrome/familial renal amyloidosis of Chinese Shar Pei dogs – mainly the tarsus, but the carpus is occasionally affected – (see 3.13.6).
7. Carpal fractures
    a. Accessory carpal bone fractures (Figure 3.13) – especially Greyhounds and other athletic dogs; mainly the right carpus due to loading when running anti-clockwise; best seen on a ML radiograph. Five types are described:
        • Type 1 – accessoroulnar ligament avulsion from the base of the bone
        • Type 2 – avulsion of ligaments attaching to the radius and ulna, on the proximal border of the bone
        • Type 3 – avulsion of the origin of the accessorometacarpal ligaments
        • Type 4 – avulsion of the tendon of insertion of flexor carpi ulnaris muscle
        • Type 5 – comminuted

    Types 1, 2 +/– 5 are articular and may lead to osteoarthritis of the accessoroulnar joint
    b. Radial carpal bone fractures – may occur without known trauma; Boxers are over-represented; may be bilateral; possibly due to a fusion defect of the three centres of ossification in the bone. Usually sagittal or oblique sagittal fractures which are best seen on DPa projections.
8. Carpal luxations and subluxations
    a. Carpal overextension injuries/palmar ligament rupture – due to jumping from a height; also arise insidiously in Shetland Sheepdogs and Collies; may be bilateral. Unstressed ML radiographs may appear normal but with

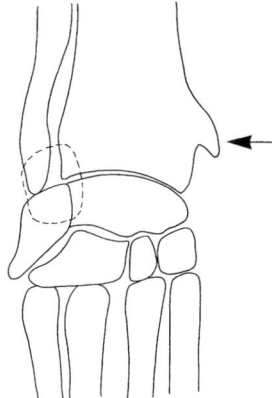

Figure 3.14 Enthesiopathy of the short radial collateral ligament (arrow). Small spurs may be seen in Greyhounds; larger masses of new bone may be associated with carpal osteoarthritis in other large breeds of dog.

    pressure from the palmar aspect or weight-bearing radiographs overextension may be seen at any of the three carpal joints. Chronic cases show secondary osteoarthritis
    b. Antebrachiocarpal joint (sub)luxation – the carpus is usually displaced in a palmar direction; +/– ligament damage and avulsion fractures
    c. Radial carpal bone luxation – an uncommon injury which appears to be due to antebrachial joint hyperextension and rotation combined with rupture of the short radial collateral ligament and dorsal joint capsule; the radial carpal bone is displaced palmarly or palmaroproximally.
9. Collateral ligament trauma
    a. Rupture of the collateral ligaments – medially and laterally stressed DPa radiographs are needed to confirm the injury
    b. Avulsion fractures of the origins of the oblique and straight short radial collateral ligaments – especially Greyhounds; best seen on a DPa projection. Chronic cases may show dystrophic mineralisation and enthesiopathy (see 3.6.11).
10. Enthesiopathy of the short radial collateral ligament (Figure 3.14) – Greyhounds, although does not necessarily cause lameness.
11. Carpal osteoarthritis and enthesiopathy – common in older dogs, especially of larger breeds; radiographic changes may

be much less severe than the clinical signs suggest. Often a focal, firm soft tissue swelling medial to the carpus with underlying enthesiophytes on the medial aspect of the distal radius and proximal second metacarpal bone.

3.7 Metacarpus, metatarsus and phalanges

Views: ML, dorsopalmar/dorsoplantar (DPa/DPl), dorsolateral – palmaromedial oblique (DL – PaMO), dorsomedial – palmarolateral oblique (DM – PaLO), ML with digits separated using ties.

1. Artefacts created by radio-opaque dirt on the foot, especially between the pads.
2. Radio-opaque foreign bodies embedded in the pads (e.g. wire, glass).
3. Variation in the appearance of digit I (dew claw), especially in dogs that have undergone removal of this digit as puppies.
4. "Sesamoid disease" (Figure 3.15) – especially young Rottweilers; fragmentation of the palmar metacarpal sesamoids (metatarsal less commonly), mainly sesamoids 2 and 7 (axial sesamoids of digits 2 and 5); unknown cause but possibly abnormal endochondral ossification; lameness variable or absent so check for other causes. DDx congenital bipartite or multipartite sesamoids; fractures.
5. Congenital polydactyly – e.g. six-toed cats; may be hereditary.
6. Cats – osteodystrophy of the Scottish Fold cat (chondro-osseous dysplasia): an inherited condition in which both homozygotes and heterozygotes are affected;

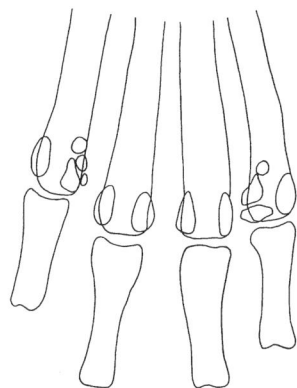

Figure 3.15 Fragmentation of the palmar metacarpophalangeal sesamoids, typically sesamoids 2 and 7.

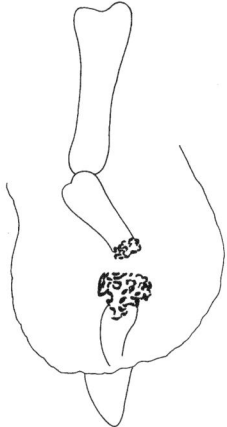

Figure 3.16 Paronychia or digital neoplasia – osteolysis of adjacent articular surfaces of P2 and P3 with surrounding soft tissue swelling.

osseous deformities are most obvious in the distal appendicular skeleton especially in the hindlimbs; inconsistently shortened and thickened metapodial bones, splayed phalanges, exostoses and ankylosing polyarthropathy affecting the tarsus, carpus and digits; occasionally osteolysis and a more aggressive radiographic appearance.

7. Hypertrophic (pulmonary) osteopathy (HPO, Marie's disease) – affects the distal limbs initially, with new bone most obvious on the abaxial margins of metapodial bones and phalanges (see 1.14.6 and Figure 1.18).
8. Calcinosis circumscripta – may affect the lower limbs including the pads; (see 12.2.2 and Figure 12.1).
9. Paronychia (nail bed infection) and osteomyelitis of P3 – an osteolytic or mixed osteolytic/proliferative lesion affecting P2–3 joint or P3; paronychia may affect multiple toes. DDx malignant neoplasia; intra-osseous epidermoid cysts (see 3.7.11, 3.7.12 and Figure 3.16).
10. Malignant neoplasia of the metacarpal and metatarsal bones (e.g. osteosarcoma) (Figure 3.16) – an occasional occurrence.
11. Malignant neoplasia of the digits – osteolytic or mixed osteolytic/proliferative lesions. DDx paronychia; osteomyelitis; intra-osseous epidermoid cysts
    a. Squamous cell carcinoma of nail bed – mostly large breed dogs and unpigmented areas; primarily osteolytic

b. Malignant melanoma – mainly pigmented areas
   c. Cats – polyostotic digital metastases from pulmonary carcinoma; often several feet affected.
12. Intraosseous epidermoid cysts – reported to affect P3 in dogs although more common in the skin; cause unknown, but secondary to trauma in humans when arising in phalanges. DDx paronychia; osteomyelitis; malignant neoplasia.
13. Metacarpal and metatarsal fractures
    a. A common traumatic injury, especially in the forelimb; often multiple, displaced
    b. MT III stress fracture of right hindlimb occasionally seen in racing Greyhounds; minimally displaced as supported by adjacent metatarsal bones.
14. Interphalangeal subluxations – racing Greyhounds, especially digit V of the left forefoot. May reduce spontaneously leaving only soft tissue swelling
    a. Distal interphalangeal joint – "knocked-up" or "sprung" toe; dorsal elastic ligament remains intact
    b. Proximal interphalangeal joint.
15. Sesamoid fractures – usually palmar metacarpal sesamoids II and VII; especially the right forefoot in racing Greyhounds. Recent injuries show sharp fracture lines; fragments remodel with time. DDx congenital bipartite or multipartite bones; sesamoid disease in Rottweilers.

3.8 Pelvis

Views: ventrodorsal (VD), laterolateral (LL), oblique lateral to reduce superimposition of the two hemipelves.
1. Ossification centres (Figure 3.17)
   a. Crescentic centre of ossification dorsal to the wing of the ilium – fusion time to the ilium is highly variable and it may remain incompletely ossified throughout life
   b. The four pelvic bones (ilium, ischium, pubis and acetabular bones) fuse at the acetabulum at about 12 weeks
   c. Centres of ossification of the ischiatic tuberosities
   d. Occasionally a triangular centre of ossification is seen in the caudal part of the pelvic symphysis, apex directed cranially
   e. The caudal margin of the ischium often appears roughened during ossification, especially in large dogs.
2. Neoplasia
   a. Osteochondroma – especially the wing of the ilium, young dogs (see 1.15.2 and Figure 1.19)
   b. Chondrosarcoma – flat bones are predisposed to chondrosarcoma although other primary malignant tumours (e.g. osteosarcoma, fibrosarcoma) may also occur in the pelvis.
   c. Multiple myeloma (plasma cell myeloma) – the pelvis is a predilection site (see 1.18.1 and Figure 1.24).
3. Pelvic fractures (Figure 3.18) – common traumatic injuries; usually multiple and displaced. Complications include concurrent lower urinary tract injury, sacrocaudal luxations and subsequent pelvic malunion leading to obstipation and dystocia.
4. Sacroiliac separation – a common injury, especially in cats (Figure 3.18); alone or associated with pelvic fractures. If bilateral, or if associated with ipsilateral pelvic fractures, cranial displacement of part of the pelvis may occur. DDx the normal radiolucency of the sacroiliac joint seen on a slightly oblique ventrodorsal radiograph.

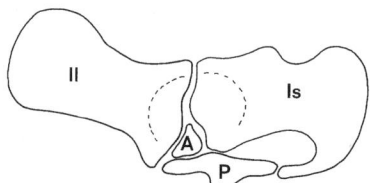

Figure 3.17 Main ossification centres of the pelvis (LL view). Il = ilium; Is = ischium; P = pubis; A = acetabular bone.

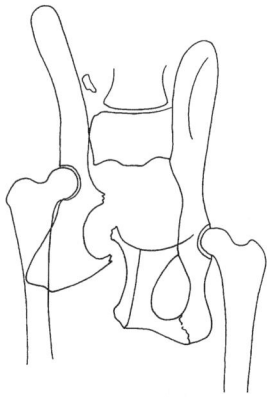

Figure 3.18 Pelvic fractures and unilateral sacroiliac separation in a cat.

3 APPENDICULAR SKELETON

3.9 Hip (coxofemoral joint)

Views: extended VD, flexed (frog-legged) ventrodorsal, ML, dorsal acetabular rim view (DAR), distraction ventrodorsal view (PennHIP).

1. Accessory ossification centre of the craniodorsal margin of the acetabular rim – an occasional finding and may remain unfused; DDx osteochondrosis of the dorsal acetabular edge (see 3.9.4).
2. Hip dysplasia (Figure 3.19) – a developmental and partly inherited condition of hip joint laxity leading to bony deformity and secondary degenerative changes; clinical signs are usually limited to larger breeds of dog (especially prevalent in the German Shepherd dog and Labrador Retriever) but radiographic changes may also be observed in small breeds and in cats. Radiographic screening programmes exist in a number of countries. The main radiographic signs include femoral head subluxation, shallow conformation of acetabulum, flattening of the cranial acetabular edge, new bone around the acetabular margins and femoral neck, recontouring of the femoral head and muscle wastage in severe cases. Symmetrical VD radiographs are required since lateral tilting of the pelvis may result in apparent subluxation of the hip joint closer to the table. The extended VD projection is standard; some screening programmes also require a flexed VD radiograph. The degree of subluxation and the depth of the acetabulum together are evaluated by measuring the Norberg angle (Figure 3.20).

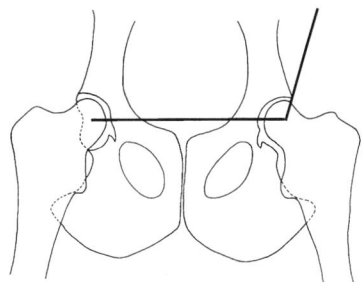

Figure 3.20 Method for measuring the Norberg angle. The base line joins the centres of the femoral heads and then for each hip joint a second line is taken from the femoral head centre to the junction between the cranial and dorsal acetabular edges. In normal hips the angle between the lines is 105° or greater. Reduction in the Norberg angle denotes femoral head subluxation and/or a shallow acetabulum, in proportion to the degree of dysplasia present.

PennHIP scheme

Distraction index (DI) is a quantitative measurement of hip laxity, calculated by comparing the position of the femoral head centre without and with traction applied to the hip joints using a fulcrum between the femora (Figure 3.21). A DI of 0 shows a fully congruent and non-lax joint; DI of 1 indicates luxation. DI is a good predictor of subsequent hip osteoarthritis as hips with a DI less than 0.3 rarely develop secondary change.

Dorsal acetabular rim view (DAR)

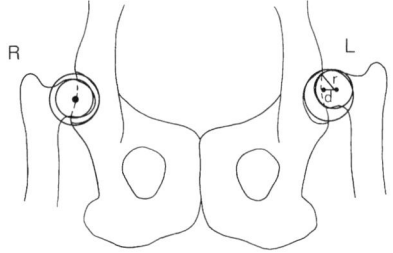

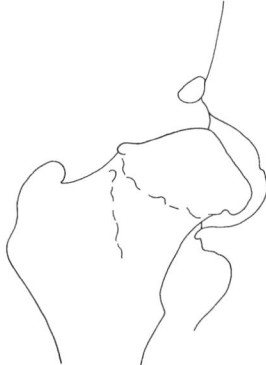

Figure 3.19 Severe hip dysplasia and secondary osteoarthritis. The femoral head is subluxated and remodelled and the acetabulum is shallow and irregular. New bone is present in the acetabular fossa, around the margins of the acetabulum, encircling the femoral neck and running vertically along the metaphyseal area (a "Morgan line").

Figure 3.21 Calculation of the distraction index. The right hip remains fully congruent with traction and the centre of the femoral head does not move; DI = 0. The left hip becomes subluxated with traction and the femoral head centre moves outwards; DI = distance moved (d) divided by the radius of the femoral head, r. (With permission from the Journal of the American Veterinary Medical Association.)

For assessing dogs for suitability for triple pelvic osteotomy. The dog is positioned in sternal recumbency with flexion of the lumbosacral and hip joints resulting in steep angulation of the pelvis. The roof of the acetabulum is projected tangentially and its slope can be measured.

3. Legg–Calvé–Perthe's disease (Perthe's disease (Figure 3.22); avascular necrosis of the femoral head) – adolescent dogs of small breeds, especially terriers; mostly unilateral but occasionally bilateral. Ischaemic necrosis of the femoral head with repair by fibrovascular tissue; probable autosomal recessive inheritance in some breeds (e.g. West Highland White Terrier). Radiographic signs include uneven radio-opacity of the femoral head leading to femoral head collapse, widening and irregularity of the joint space, varus deformity of the femoral neck, secondary osteoarthritis and muscle wastage. DDx intracapsular hip trauma, severe hip dysplasia (but atypical breeds), femoral head osteochondrosis.
4. Osteochondrosis (OC) – the hip joint is a highly unusual location
    a. Femoral head – reported in Pekinese and Border Collie; focal subchondral osteolysis +/– mineralised flap formation. DDx Perthe's disease, although appears more focal
    b. Dorsal acetabular rim – DDx accessory ossification centre (see 3.9.1).
5. Mucopolysaccharidoses/mucolipidoses – may produce hip dysplasia, especially in cats.

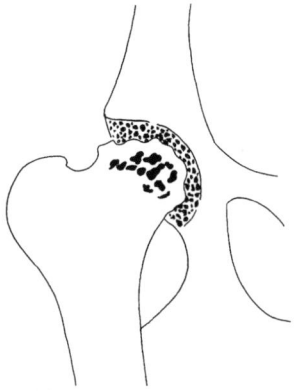

Figure 3.22 Advanced Perthe's disease. The femoral head shows a moth-eaten radio-opacity due to osteolysis, and has collapsed, resulting in a wide and irregular joint space.

6. Dislocation of the hip – a common traumatic injury in skeletally mature dogs and cats; the femoral head usually displaces craniodorsally. Both lateral and VD radiographs are required to confirm the direction of displacement. Small avulsion fractures from the insertion of the teres ligament onto the femoral head may be seen. Check for other pelvic fractures, sacroiliac separation and lower urinary tract damage. Chronic, unreduced hip dislocation results in new bone on the pelvis and false joint formation.
7. Fractures involving the hip joint
    a. Femoral neck fractures – intracapsular or extracapsular
    b. Proximal femoral growth plate fractures – Salter-Harris type I or II ("slipped epiphysis")
    c. Acetabular fractures – the femoral head displaces medially; secondary hip osteoarthritis is likely.

Types a and b fracture are common in young animals and may require both extended and flexed VD radiographs for diagnosis because the fracture may be reduced on one view. In skeletally immature animals the only femoral head blood supply is via the joint capsule, so untreated intracapsular neck fractures or growth plate fractures will probably result in avascular necrosis of the femoral head and non-union. In skeletally mature animals, blood supply exists via the medullary cavity.

8. Calcifying tendinopathy
    a. Middle gluteal muscle (less commonly deep and superficial gluteal muscles) – one or more rounded, mineralised bodies near the major trochanter of the femur, commonly seen on ventrodorsal hip radiographs of larger dogs; clinically insignificant
    b. Iliopsoas – a similar finding near the lesser trochanter
    c. Biceps femoris – near the ischiatic tuberosity.
9. Epiphysiolysis – separation of the proximal femoral epiphysis through the growth plate after no or minor trauma; recognised as a distinct syndrome in humans and pigs and possibly also occurs in dogs.
10. Cats – proximal femoral metaphyseal osteopathy; bone necrosis of the femoral neck of unknown aetiology leading to pathological fracture; unilateral or bilateral; male cats under 2 years old. DDx previous femoral neck fracture.

3.10 Femur

Views: ML, CrCd.
1. Growth arrest lines – fine, transverse, sclerotic lines in the medullary cavity of larger dogs; no clinical significance. DDx panosteitis.
2. Panosteitis – the femur is a predilection site (see 1.13.5 and Figure 1.17).
3. Metaphyseal osteopathy (hypertrophic osteodystrophy) – the proximal and distal femoral metaphyses are a minor site; the most obvious lesions are usually in the distal radius and ulna (see 1.23.3 and Figure 1.30).
4. Hypertrophic (pulmonary) osteopathy (HPO, Marie's disease) – the femur is a minor site (see 1.14.6 and Figure 1.18).
5. Neoplasia
   a. Primary malignant bone tumours (most commonly osteosarcoma) – the proximal femoral metaphysis is an occasional site, the distal metaphysis is affected more commonly although the incidence is less than in the forelimb
   b. Parosteal osteosarcoma – the distal femur is a predilection site (see 1.15.2)
   c. Infiltrative lipoma of thigh – swelling of thigh and displacement of muscle bellies by fat radio-opacity; rarely see femoral osteolysis or new bone formation.
6. Femoral fractures
   a. Diaphysis – common, often comminuted
   b. Proximal femur – (see 3.9.7)
   c. Distal femur – (see 3.11.12).

3.11 Stifle

Views: ML in various degrees of flexion, CrCd or CdCr, stressed views, flexed CrPr–CrDiO to skyline the trochlear groove.
1. Popliteal sesamoid not mineralised – an occasional finding, especially in small dogs.
2. Fabella variants
   a. Cats – the medial fabella is normally smaller than the lateral fabella
   b. Non-ossification of the medial fabella – an occasional finding
   c. Bipartite or multipartite fabellae – two or more smooth, rounded fragments; DDx old fabella fracture (no change over time if a developmental variant).
3. Patella variants
   a. Cats – normal tapering, pointed distal pole of patella, not to be confused with new bone
   b. Bipartite or multipartite patella – two or more smooth, rounded fragments probably with some distraction; DDx old patella fracture (no soft tissue swelling or change with time if developmental).
4. OC of the distal femur (Figure 3.23) – similar breed, age and sex predisposition as other manifestations of OC; may be bilateral; less common than forelimb OC
   a. Lateral femoral condyle (medial aspect) most common
   b. Medial femoral condyle
   c. Lateral trochlear ridge – rare; DDx normal rough appearance of immature bone until about 4 months of age

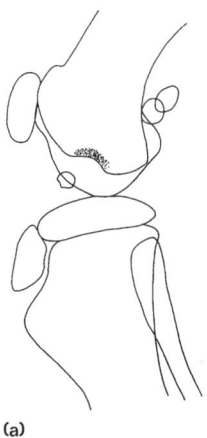

(a)

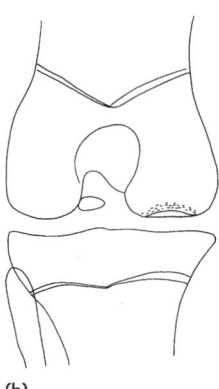

(b)

Figure 3.23 Stifle osteochondrosis affecting the medial femoral condyle. (a) ML view; (b) CrCd view (right stifle). A subchondral erosion is seen on the medial femoral condyle and a free mineralised body is present in the joint space. A joint effusion would also be present.

SMALL ANIMAL RADIOLOGICAL DIFFERENTIAL DIAGNOSIS

Radiographic signs of stifle OC are similar to those of shoulder OC and include stifle joint effusion (see 2.2.1, Figure 2.1); roughening or flattening of subchondral bone and underlying radiolucency, overlying mineralised cartilage flap, joint mice in various locations including the supratrochlear pouch, minor osteoarthritis.

5. Medial patellar luxation (Figure 3.24) – usually toy breeds of dog; unusual and may be incidental in cats, although there is a genetic predisposition in the Devon Rex cat; unilateral or bilateral. Usually secondary to underlying congenital/developmental malalignment of the quadriceps mechanism with femoral head and neck retroversion leading to outward rotation of the stifle (genu varum or bow-legged conformation). Radiographs may be normal in mild cases, but radiographic signs include medial displacement of the patella (although this may reduce on positioning for a CrCd view), lateral bowing and external rotation of the distal third of the femur, mediolateral tilting of the femorotibial joint, medial displacement and remodelling of the tibial tuberosity, medial bowing and internal rotation of the proximal tibia, shallow trochlear groove with hypoplastic medial ridge and hypoplastic medial femoral condyle (seen on a CrPr–CrDiO view) and secondary osteoarthritis.
6. Lateral patellar luxation – less common; usually large breeds of dog
    a. Due to trauma causing reduction in growth of the lateral aspect of the distal femur or proximal tibia
    b. Secondary to hip deformity (increased anteversion) leading to inward rotation of the stifle (genu valgum or knock-kneed conformation).
7. Premature closure of the distal femoral growth plate – usually the lateral aspect, leading to genu valgum and lateral patellar luxation; may be associated with hip dysplasia.
8. Premature closure of the proximal tibial growth plate (tibial plateau deformans; Figure 3.25) – usually young adult dogs; various breeds including the Rough Collie and West Highland White Terrier; thought to be due to Salter-Harris type I or V injury to the growth plate. In severe cases leads to inability to extend the stifle (resulting in a crouching hindlimb stance) with or without bow-legged conformation; affected dogs usually present due to secondary rupture of the cranial cruciate ligament. Radiographic signs include remodelling of the tibial plateau, a caudodistal slope to the femorotibial joint space, caudal bowing of the fibula, secondary joint effusion and osteoarthritis due to cruciate ligament damage.
9. Cats – hypervitaminosis A: raw liver diet; the stifle may be a predilection site after the spine and elbow; DDx synovial osteochondromatosis (see 3.11.17).
10. Idiopathic effusive arthritis/juvenile gonitis – especially the Boxer and Rottweiler, 1–3 years old; may be bi-

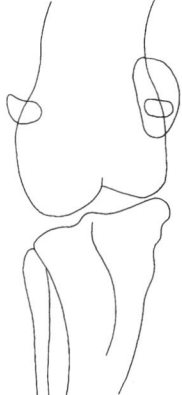

Figure 3.24 Medial patellar luxation (CrCd view of the right stifle). The patella is displaced medially and rotated about its long axis; the distal femur and proximal tibia are bowed and the femorotibial joint space lies obliquely.

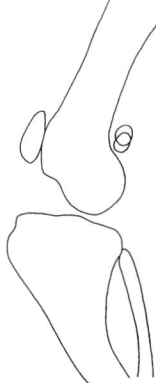

Figure 3.25 Premature closure of the proximal tibial growth plate (tibial plateau deformans). The proximal tibial articular surface slopes caudodistally and the fibula is bowed.

lateral; idiopathic arthropathy leading to rupture of the cranial cruciate ligament (see 3.11.13).
11. Synovial sarcoma (occasionally other soft tissue tumours) – the stifle is a predilection site (see 2.4.6, Figure 2.3); mainly larger breeds of dog. DDx severe osteoarthritis where superimposition of new bone may mimic osteolysis, septic arthritis. The cardinal radiographic sign may be displacement of the patella by a soft tissue mass.
12. Fractures involving the stifle joint
    a. Distal femoral supracondylar fractures – Salter-Harris type I or II fractures of the distal femoral growth plate in skeletally immature animals; the femoral condyles usually rotate caudally; may heal as a malunion
    b. Avulsion of the tibial tuberosity (Figure 3.26) – Salter-Harris type I fracture of the tibial tuberosity growth plate
        - extrinsic; due to external trauma
        - intrinsic; with no or minor trauma; especially the Greyhound and English or Staffordshire Bull Terrier, may be bilateral; osteochondrosis of the growth plate found in one litter

Radiographic signs include proximal displacement or rotation of the tibial tuberosity, +/– multiple small, mineralised fragments, soft tissue swelling. DDx normal wide growth plate (compare with the opposite leg unless there are bilateral clinical signs)

    c. Proximal tibial growth plate fractures – Salter-Harris type I or II; the tibial tuberosity may remain attached or may separate; the tibial shaft is usually displaced cranially; may heal as a malunion (see 3.11.8)
    d. Fractured patella – usually due to a direct blow; if transverse, the fragments will distract. With a chronic lesion with fragment remodelling the DDx is bipartite or multipartite patella
    e. Fractured fabellae – spontaneous fracture of the lateral fabella is reported in dogs. With a chronic lesion with fragment remodelling the DDx is bipartite or multipartite fabella
13. Cruciate ligament damage
    a. Strained or ruptured cranial cruciate ligament – acute trauma or chronic strain, especially in large dogs with straight hindlimb conformation; often bilateral. Radiographic signs include joint effusion, secondary osteoarthritis (see 2.5.2, 3.11.16 and Figure 2.5), joint mice and dystrophic mineralisation in the region of the ligament, remodelling of the tibial plateau at the site of attachment of the ligament and cranial displacement of the tibia on the femur in severe cases. Tibial compression radiography has been described as being a highly sensitive test – with the stifle flexed at 90°, the hock is maximally flexed, causing cranial displacement of the tibia and distal displacement of the popliteal sesamoid in cases of cranial cruciate ligament damage
    b. Avulsion of the insertion of the cranial cruciate ligament onto the tibial

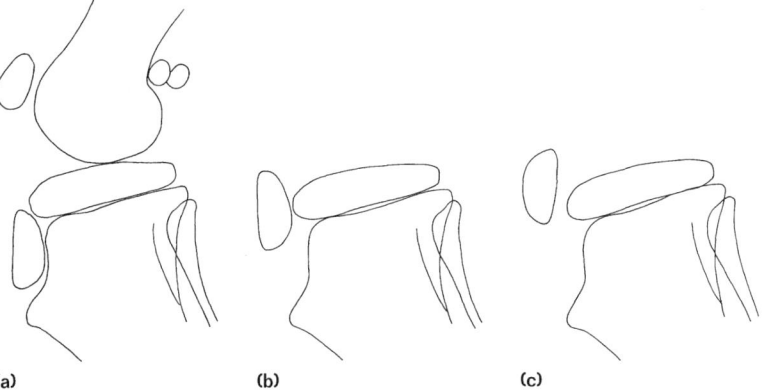

Figure 3.26 Avulsion of the tibial tuberosity. (a) Normal unfused tibial tuberosity; (b) separation and proximal displacement; (c) rotation of the fragment 180° in a clockwise direction.

SMALL ANIMAL RADIOLOGICAL DIFFERENTIAL DIAGNOSIS

plateau – dogs under 2 years old, in which the ligament is stronger than the bone. Radiographic signs include joint effusion and a small, mineralised fragment in the centre of the joint. DDx osteochondrosis, secondary osteoarthritis

c. Partial avulsion of the origin of the cranial cruciate ligament – rare; small, mineralised fragment in the intercondylar region of the distal femur and swelling of intracapsular soft tissues caudal to the patellar fat pad

d. Avulsion of the origin or insertion of the caudal cruciate ligament – often associated with multiple stifle injuries, and isolated injury is uncommon.

Radiographic signs include joint effusion, caudal displacement of the tibia, mineralised fragment(s) in the caudal part of the femoral intercondylar fossa or caudal to the tibial plateau and secondary osteoarthritis.

14. Tendon avulsions

a. Avulsion of the origin of the long digital extensor muscle (Figure 3.27) – usually skeletally immature dogs of larger breeds; may be no known trauma. Radiographic signs include a mineralised fragment adjacent or near to the extensor fossa of the distal femur, in the centre of the joint on the mediolateral radiograph but shown to be lateral on the craniocaudal view; also a radiolucent bone defect in the extensor fossa

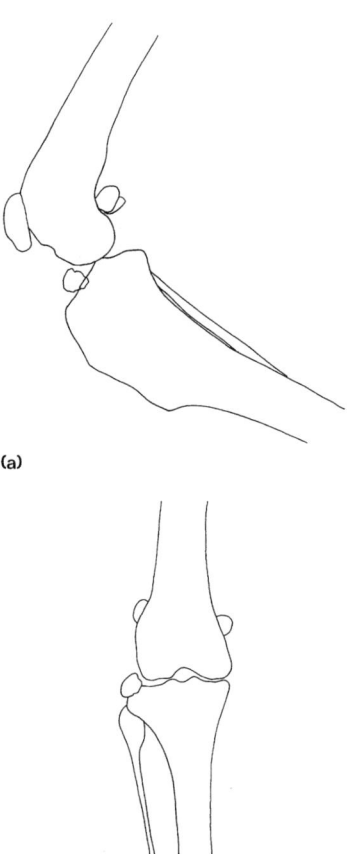

Figure 3.27 Avulsion of the tendon of origin of the long digital extensor muscle from its origin in the extensor fossa; a mineralised fragment is seen in the craniolateral aspect of the femorotibial joint space. (a) ML view; (b) CrCd view (right stifle).

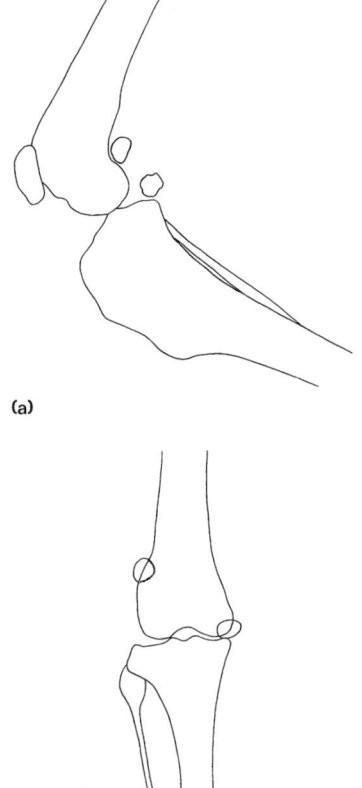

Figure 3.28 Avulsion of the medial head of gastrocnemius muscle resulting in distal displacement of the medial fabella. (a) ML view; (b) CrCd view (right stifle).

b. Avulsion of one or both heads of the gastrocnemius (Figure 3.28) – less common than distal injury to the Achilles tendon; may be bilateral; may be no known trauma; results in a plantigrade stance and hock hyperflexion. Radiographic signs include distal displacement of the associated fabella accentuated by hock flexion, new bone on the distal femoral supracondylar tuberosities where the tendons arise, new bone around the associated fabella, dystrophic mineralisation in surrounding soft tissues
c. Avulsion of the origin of the popliteal muscle – due to trauma, and may be associated with rupture of the cranial cruciate ligament; the CrCd radiograph may show an avulsed bone fragment and radiolucent bone defect on the lateral aspect of the lateral femoral condyle with distal displacement of the popliteal sesamoid. DDx rupture of the popliteal tendon, or when tibial compression radiography is performed in cases of damaged cranial cruciate ligament.
15. Other stifle ligamentous and soft tissue trauma
   a. Collateral ligament rupture – medial/lateral stressed CrCd radiographs needed
   b. Avulsion or rupture of the straight patellar ligament – proximal displacement of the patella exacerbated by stifle flexion, soft tissue swelling cranial to the infrapatellar fat pad
   c. Dislocation of the stifle – rupture of cruciate and collateral ligaments; more common in cats; the tibia is usually displaced cranially.
16. Stifle osteoarthritis – a very common degenerative condition especially in larger dogs; often bilateral; usually secondary to cranial cruciate ligament disease but also associated with osteochondrosis, patellar luxation, trauma etc. Radiographic signs include joint effusion which effaces the infrapatellar fat pad and displaces fascial planes caudal to the femorotibial joint, periarticular new bone at various sites – both poles of the patella, along the trochlear ridges of the distal femur, on the femoral epicondyles, around the fabellae and popliteal sesamoid and around the articular margins of the tibial plateau (see 2.2.1, 2.5.2 and Figures 2.1, 2.5); chronic cases may show multiple small, radiolucent, subchondral cysts in the intercondylar fossa on the CrCd/CdCr view.
17. Synovial osteochondromatosis/synovial chondrometaplasia – an uncommon condition; the stifle is a predilection site, especially in cats and larger dogs (see 2.8.18); DDx in cats, hypervitaminosis A.
18. Meniscal calcification or ossification – rare, dogs or cats; idiopathic or secondary to trauma (often associated with ruptured cranial cruciate ligament); small, mineralised body in the cranial horn of the medial (more common) or lateral meniscus.
19. Calcifying tendinopathy
   a. Quadriceps
   b. Gastrocnemius.
20. Mineralised bodies in or near the stifle joint (see 2.8)
   a. Normal sesamoids
   b. Fragmented sesamoids
   c. Osteochondrosis
   d. Cruciate ligament damage
      • dystrophic mineralisation of damaged tendon
      • avulsion fragments.
   e. Osteoarthritis – fractured osteophytes/enthesiophytes
   f. Fracture fragments
   g. Avulsion of the long digital extensor, gastrocnemius or popliteal muscles
   h. Meniscal calcification or ossification
   i. Synovial osteochondromatosis
   j. Pseudogout
   k. cats – hypervitaminosis A.

3.12 Tibia and fibula

Views: ML, CrCd.
1. Osteochondrodysplasias – various types of hereditary dwarfism in dogs and cats (see 1.21.7). The distal tibia is the second most common site for lesions after the distal radius and ulna, although often the hindlimbs are less severely affected than the forelimbs.
2. Metaphyseal osteopathy (hypertrophic osteodystrophy) – lesions may be seen in the proximal and distal tibial metaphyses, although less severe than in the distal radius and ulna (see 1.23.3 and Figure 1.30).
3. Panosteitis – the tibia may be affected (see 1.13.5 and Figure 1.17).
4. Rickets (juvenile osteomalacia) – the distal tibial growth plate is the second most severely affected site after the distal

radius and ulna (see 1.22.8 and Figure 1.29).
5. Hypertrophic (pulmonary) osteopathy (HPO, Marie's disease) – the tibia and/or fibula may be affected by palisading periosteal new bone, although the distal portion of the limb is likely to be affected first.
6. Primary malignant bone tumours (most commonly osteosarcoma) – the proximal and distal tibial metaphyses are predilection sites, although less commonly affected than the humerus and radius.
7. Tibial and fibular fractures
   a. Proximal tibia – (see 3.11.12).
   b. Diaphyseal – in the tibia may spiral or create incomplete fissure fractures.
   c. Distal tibia – (see 3.13.7).

3.13 Tarsus (hock)

Views: ML, flexed ML, dorsoplantar (DPl), flexed dorsoplantar, dorsolateral–plantaromedial oblique (DL–PlMO), dorsomedial–plantarolateral oblique (DM–PlLO), stressed and weight-bearing views. Like the carpus, the tarsus is a complex joint and bone specimens or comparable views of the normal limb may be helpful in interpretation.
1. OC of the tibiotarsal joint – similar breed and age predisposition as other manifestations of OC but apparently no sex predisposition; Labrador, Rottweiler, English and Staffordshire Bull terrier over-represented; may be bilateral; less common than forelimb OC.
   a. Medial trochlear ridge of talus (tibial tarsal bone; Figure 3.29) – by far the commonest site. Radiographic signs include joint effusion and periarticular soft tissue swelling, flattening and fragmentation of the ridge with widening of tibiotarsal joint space medially, joint mice and marked secondary osteoarthritis; variably visible on the DPI, extended and flexed ML views (may be better seen on ML views if the plantar aspect of the ridge is affected).
   b. Lateral trochlear ridge of talus – uncommon and harder to diagnose; Rottweiler possibly predisposed. Oblique views and flexed DPl are helpful projections.
   c. Fragmentation of the medial malleolus of the tibia – uncommon; possibly part of the OC complex and may be associated with medial trochlear ridge OC; Rottweiler predisposed.

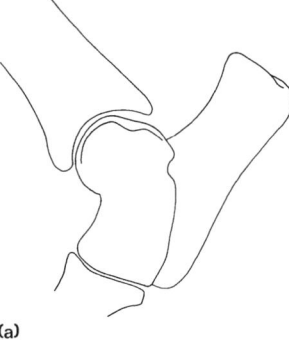

(a)

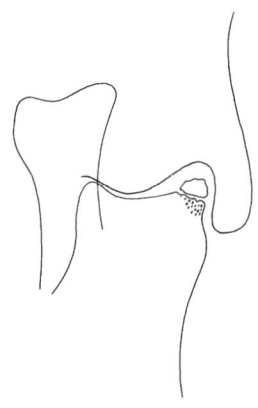

(b)

Figure 3.29 Osteochondrosis of the medial trochlear ridge of the talus; right hock. The ML view (a) shows flattening of one of the bony ridges; the DPI view (b) identifies this as the medial ridge and shows subchondral radiolucency and overlying fragmentation with widening of the joint space.

2. Premature closure of the distal tibial growth plate – Rough Collie predisposed; usually the lateral aspect of the growth plate more is severely affected, leading to tarsal valgus (cow-hocked conformation).
3. Cats – osteodystrophy of the Scottish Fold cat; the tarsi and hind paws are most severely affected (see 3.7.6).
4. Rheumatoid arthritis – the carpus and tarsus are predilection sites; often bilateral (see 2.4.7 and Figure 2.4).
5. Cats – various feline polyarthritides; the carpus and tarsus are predilection sites.
6. Chinese Shar Pei fever syndrome/familial renal amyloidosis of Chinese Shar Pei dogs – usually young dogs; unknown aetiology; fever often accompanied by acute synovitis of tarsal (less commonly

carpal) joints; some dogs develop renal amyloidosis.
7. Tarsal fractures
   a. Distal tibia – Salter-Harris type I fractures of the distal tibial growth plate.
   b. Medial or lateral malleolar fractures of the distal tibia and fibula – often with subluxation of the tibiotarsal joint space; stressed views may be required to demonstrate subluxation.
   c. Central tarsal bone fractures – especially racing Greyhounds, right tarsus due to medial joint compression as running anticlockwise. May co-exist with other tarsal fractures. Five types are described (Figure 3.30):
      • Type 1 – non-displaced dorsal slab fracture; best seen on a ML view
      • Type 2 – displaced dorsal slab fracture
      • Type 3 – sagittal fracture; rare; best seen on a DPl view
      • Type 4 – combined dorsal plane and sagittal fractures; the most common type
      • Type 5 – severe comminution and displacement
   d. Fibular tarsal bone (calcaneal) fractures – especially racing Greyhounds, right tarsus; often seen with central tarsal bone fractures or with proximal intertarsal joint subluxation; various locations of fracture, both simple and comminuted. Fractures through the tuber calcis may be distracted by the Achilles tendon.
   d. Other tarsal bone fractures e.g. of tibial tarsal bone (talus) or T4.
8. Tarsal luxations and subluxations
   a. Tibiotarsal luxation – often with fracture of the medial or lateral malleolus of the tibia; stressed views may be needed (see 2.3.16 and Figure 2.2).
   b. Intertarsal and tarsometatarsal subluxation (Figure 3.31) – traumatic; also arise insidiously in the Rough Collie, Shetland Sheepdog and Border Collie and may be bilateral in these dogs; may also be associated with rheumatoid arthritis (see 2.4.7 and Figure 2.4) or systemic lupus erythematosus. Radiographic signs are best seen on a ML view and include soft tissue swelling, subluxation (stressed views may exacerbate), new bone (especially on the plantar aspect of the tarsus), enthesiophyte formation and dystrophic soft tissue mineralisation.
9. Lesions of the Achilles or common calcaneal tendon (common tendon of gastrocnemius and superficial digital flexor with minor contributions from semitendinosus, gracilis and biceps femoris; Figure 3.32) – strain, rupture or avulsion of one or more components at or near the insertion onto the tuber calcis; mature, large breed dogs, often overweight; may be bilateral. Radiographic signs include soft tissue swelling around the tendon and tuber calcis, a cap of proliferative new bone on the tuber calcis, avulsed fragments of bone and dystrophic mineralisation in the tendon. Ultrasonography of the tendon may be helpful in showing fibre disruption and areas of mineralisation.

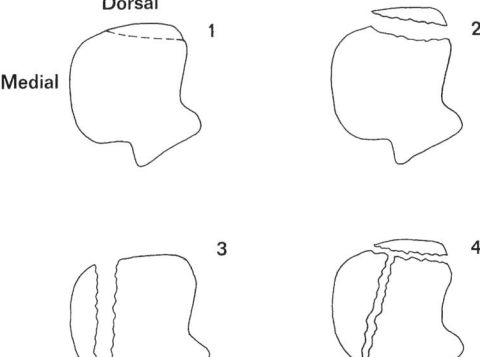

Figure 3.30 Classification of central tarsal bone fractures – cross-section of the right central tarsal bone.

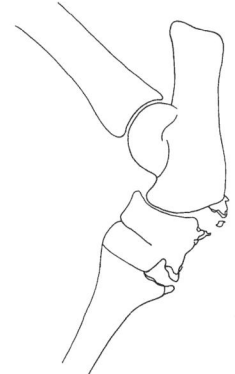

Figure 3.31 Chronic intertarsal subluxation with plantar new bone and soft tissue mineralisation.

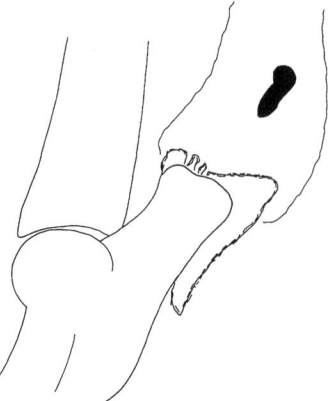

Figure 3.32 Chronic strain of the Achilles tendon – thickening of the tendon, dystrophic mineralisation (shown here black, but would be radio-opaque) and calcaneal new bone.

10. Lateral luxation of the superficial digital flexor tendon – lateral displacement of the tendon from the tip of the tuber calcis due to tearing of its medial attachment, predisposed to by flattening of the bone at this site as seen on the DPl view. Radiographs usually show soft tissue swelling only and no bony changes.
11. Tarsal osteoarthritis – usually secondary to osteochondrosis or other underlying disease; radiographic changes may be milder than the clinical signs suggest. Smooth spurs of new bone on the dorsal aspect of the central and third tarsal bones are often incidental findings in large breeds of dog.

FURTHER READING

Scapula

Jerram, R.M. and Herron, M.R. (1998) Scapular fractures in dogs. *Compendium of Continuing Education for the Practicing Veterinarian (Small Animal)* **20** 1254–1260.

Shoulder

Anderson, A., Stead, A.C. and Coughlan, A.R. (1993) Unusual muscle and tendon disorders of the forelimb in the dog. *Journal of Small Animal Practice* **34** 313–318.

Barthez, P.Y. and Morgan, J.P. (1993) Bicipital tenosynovitis in the dog – evaluation with positive contrast arthrography. *Veterinary Radiology and Ultrasound* **34** 325–330.

van Bree, H. (1992) Vacuum phenomenon associated with osteochondrosis of the scapulohumeral joint in dogs: 100 cases (1985–1991). *Journal of the American Veterinary Medical Association* **201** 1916–1917.

Flo, G.L. and Middleton, D. (1990) Mineralisation of the supraspinatus tendon in dogs. *Journal of the American Veterinary Medical Association* **197** 95–97.

Houlton, J.E.F. (1984) Osteochondrosis of the shoulder and elbow joints in dogs. *Journal of Small Animal Practice* **25** 399–413.

Krieglieder, H. (1995) Mineralisation of the supraspinatus tendon: clinical observations in 7 dogs. *Veterinary and Comparative Orthopaedics and Traumatology* **8** 91–97.

Long, C.D. and Nyland, T.G. (1999) Ultrasonographic evaluation of the canine shoulder. *Veterinary Radiology and Ultrasound* **40** 372–379.

Muir, P. and Johnson, K.A. (1994) Supraspinatus and biceps brachii tendinopathy in dogs. *Journal of Small Animal Practice* **35** 239–243.

Stobie, D., Wallace, L.J., Lipowitz, A.J., King, V. and Lund, E.M. (1995) Chronic bicipital tenosynovitis in dogs: 29 cases (1985–1992). *Journal of the American Veterinary Medical Association* **207** 201–207.

Elbow

Anderson, A., Stead, A.C. and Coughlan, A.R. (1993) Unusual muscle and tendon disorders of the forelimb in the dog. *Journal of Small Animal Practice* **34** 313–318.

Berry, C.R. (1992) Radiology corner: Evaluation of the canine elbow for fragmented medial coronoid process. *Veterinary Radiology and Ultrasound* **33** 273–276.

Houlton, J.E.F. (1984) Osteochondrosis of the shoulder and elbow joints in dogs. *Journal of Small Animal Practice* **25** 399–413.

Kirberger, R.M. and Fourie, S. (1998) Elbow dysplasia in the dog: pathophysiology, diagnosis and control. *Journal of the South African Veterinary Association* **69** 43–54.

Lowry, J.E., Carpenter, L.G., Park, R.D., Steyn, P.F. and Schwarz, P.D. (1993) Radiographic anatomy and technique for arthrography of the cubital joint in clinically normal dogs. *Journal of the American Veterinary Medical Association* **203** 72–77.

Mason, T.A., Lavelle, R.B., Skipper, S.C. and Wrigley, W.R. (1980) Osteochondrosis of the elbow joint in young dogs. *Journal of Small Animal Practice* **21** 641–656.

May, C. and Bennett, D. (1988) Medial epicondylar spur associated with lameness in dogs. *Journal of Small Animal Practice* **29** 797–803.

Miyabayashi, T., Takiguchi, M., Schrader, S.C. and Biller, D.S. (1995) Radiographic anatomy of the medial coronoid process of dogs. *Journal of the American Animal Hospital Association* **31** 125–132.

Murphy, S.T., Lewis, D.D., Shiroma, J.T., Neuwirth, L.A., Parker, R.B. and Kubilis, P.S. (1998) Effect of radiographic positioning on interpretation of cubital joint congruity in dogs. *American Journal of Veterinary Research* **59** 1351–1357.

Robins, G.M. (1980) Some aspects of the radiographical examination of the canine elbow joint. *Journal of Small Animal Practice* **21** 417–428.

Radius and ulna

Clayton-Jones, D.G. and Vaughan, L.C. (1970) Disturbance in the growth of the radius in dogs. *Journal of Small Animal Practice* **11** 453–468.

Ramadan, R.O. and Vaughan, L.C. (1978) Premature closure of the distal ulnar growth plate in dogs – a review of 58 cases. *Journal of Small Animal Practice* **19** 647–667.

Carpus

Anderson, A., Stead, A.C. and Coughlan, A.R. (1993) Unusual muscle and tendon disorders of the forelimb in the dog. *Journal of Small Animal Practice* **34** 313–318.

Guilliard, M.J. (1998) Enthesiopathy of the short radial collateral ligaments in racing greyhounds. *Journal of Small Animal Practice* **39** 227–230.

Johnson, K.A. (1987) Accessory carpal bone fractures in the racing greyhound: classification and pathology. *Veterinary Surgery* **16** 60–64.

Li, A., Bennett, D., Gibbs, C., Carmichael, S., Gibson, N., Owen, M. et al. (2000) Radial carpal bone fractures in 15 dogs. *Journal of Small Animal Practice* **41** 74–79.

Metacarpus, metatarsus and phalanges

Cake, M.A. and Read, R.A. (1995) Canine and human sesamoid disease: a review of conditions affecting the palmar metacarpal/metatarsal sesamoid bones. *Veterinary and Comparative Orthopaedics and Traumatology* **8** 70–75.

Homer, B.L., Ackerman, N., Woody, B.J. and Green, R.W. (1992) Intraosseous epidermoid cysts in the distal phalanx of two dogs. *Veterinary Radiology and Ultrasound* **33** 133–137.

Muir, P. and Norris, J.L. (1997) Metacarpal and metatarsal fractures in dogs. *Journal of Small Animal Practice* **38** 344–348.

Read, R.A., Black, A.P., Armstrong, S.J., MacPherson, G.C. and Peek, J. (1992) Incidence and clinical significance of sesamoid disease in Rottweilers. *Veterinary Record* **130** 533–535.

Voges, A.K., Neuwirth, L., Thompson, J.P. and Ackerman, N. (1996) Radiographic changes associated with digital, metacarpal and metatarsal tumors, and pododermatitis in the dog. *Veterinary Radiology and Ultrasound* **37** 327–335.

Hip

Adams, W.M., Dueland, R.T., Meinen, J., O'Brien, R.T., Guiliano, E. and Nordheim, E.K. (1998) Early detection of canine hip dysplasia: comparison of two palpation and five radiographic methods. *Journal of the American Animal Hospital Association* **34** 339–347.

Breur, G.J. and Blevins, W.E. (1997) Traumatic injury of the iliopsoas muscle in 3 dogs. *Journal of the American Veterinary Medical Association* **210** 1631–1634.

Gibbs, C. (1997) The BVA/KC scoring scheme for control of hip dysplasia: interpretation of criteria. *Veterinary Record* **141** 275–284.

Hauptman, J., Prieur, W.D., Butler, H.C. and Guffy, M.M. (1979) The angle of inclination of the canine femoral head and neck. *Veterinary Surgery* **8** 74–77.

Johnson, A.L. (1985) Osteochondrosis dissecans of the femoral head of a Pekingese. *Journal of the American Veterinary Medical Association* **187** 623–625.

Keller, G.G., Reed, A.L., Lattimer, J.C. and Corley, E.A. (1999) Hip dysplasia: a feline population study. *Veterinary Radiology and Ultrasound* **40** 460–464.

McDonald, M. (1988) Osteochondritis dissecans of the femoral head: a case report. *Journal of Small Animal Practice* **29** 49–53.

Nunamaker, D.M., Biery, D.N. and Newton, C.D. (1973) Femoral neck anteversion in the dog: its radiographic appearance. *Journal of the American Veterinary Radiological Society* **14** 45–48.

Perez-Aparicio, F.J. and Fjeld, T.O. (1993) Femoral neck fractures and capital epiphyseal separations in cats. *Journal of Small Animal Practice* **34** 445–449.

Queen J., Bennett D, Carmichael S., Gibson N., Li N., Payne-Johnson C.E. and Kelly D.F. (1998) Femoral neck metaphyseal osteopathy in the cat. *Veterinary Record* **142** 159–162.

Slocum B. and Devine T.M. (1990) Dorsal acetabular rim radiographic view for evaluation of the canine hip. *Journal of the American Animal Hospital Association* **26** 289–296.

Smith G.K., Biery D.N. and Gregor T.P (1990) New concepts of coxofemoral joint stability and the development of a clinical stress-radiographic method for quantitating hip joint laxity in the dog. *Journal of the American Veterinary Medical Association* **196** 59–70.

Stifle

Ferguson, J. (1997) Patellar luxation in the dog and cat. *In Practice* **19** 174–184.

Macpherson, G.C. and Allan, G.S. (1993) Osteochondral lesion and cranial cruciate ligament rupture in an immature dog stifle. *Journal of Small Animal Practice* **34** 350–353.

Montgomery, R.D., Fitch, R.B., Hathcock, J.T., LaPrade, R.F., Wilson, M.E. and Garrett, P.D. (1995) Radiographic imaging of the canine intercondylar fossa. *Veterinary Radiology and Ultrasound* **36** 276–282.

Muir, P. and Dueland, R.T. (1994) Avulsion of the origin of the medial head of the gastrocnemius muscle in a dog. *Veterinary Record* **135** 359–360.

Park, R.D. (1979) Radiographic evaluation of the canine stifle joint. *Compendium of Continuing Education for the Practicing Veterinarian (Small Animal)* **1** 833–841.

Prior, J.E. (1994) Avulsion of the lateral head of the gastrocnemius muscle in a working dog. *Veterinary Record* **134** 382–383.

Read, R.A. and Robins, G.M. (1982) Deformity of the proximal tibia in dogs. *Veterinary Record* **111** 295–298.

Reinke, J. and Mughannam, A. (1994) Meniscal calcification and ossification in six cats and two dogs. *Journal of the American Animal Hospital Association* **30** 145–152.

Robinson, A. (1999) Atraumatic bilateral avulsion of the origins of the gastrocnemius muscle. *Journal of Small Animal Practice* **40** 498–500.

de Rooster, H., Van Ryssen, B. and van Bree, H. (1998) Diagnosis of cranial cruciate ligament injury in dogs by tibial compression radiography. *Veterinary Record* **142** 366–368.

de Rooster, H. and van Bree, H. (1999) Popliteal sesamoid displacement associated with cruciate rupture in the dog. *Journal of Small Animal Practice* **40** 316–318.

de Rooster, H. and van Bree, H. (1999) Use of compression stress radiography for the detection of partial tears of the canine cranial cruciate ligament. *Journal of Small Animal Practice* **40** 573–576.

Skelly, C.M., McAllister, H. and Donnelly, W. (1997) Avulsion of the tibial tuberosity in a litter of greyhound puppies. *Journal of Small Animal Practice* **38** 445–449.

Soderstrom, M.J., Rochat, M.C. and Drost, W.T. (1998) Radiographic diagnosis: Avulsion fracture of the caudal cruciate ligament. *Veterinary Radiology and Ultrasound* **39** 536–538.

Tanno, F., Weber, U., Lang, J. and Simpson, D. (1996) Avulsion of the popliteus muscle in a Malinois dog. *Journal of Small Animal Practice* **37** 448–451.

Williams, J., Fitch, R.B. and Lemarie, R.J. (1997) Partial avulsion of the origin of the cranial cruciate ligament in a four year-old dog. *Veterinary Radiology and Ultrasound* **38** 380–383.

Tarsus

Carlisle, C.H. and Reynolds, K.M. (1990) radiographic anatomy of the tarsocrural joint of the dog. *Journal of Small Animal Practice* **31** 273–279.

Carlisle, C.H., Robins, G.M. and Reynolds, K.M. (1990) Radiographic signs of osteochondritis dissecans of the lateral ridge of the trochlea tali in the dog. *Journal of Small Animal Practice* **31** 280–286.

Dee, J.F., Dee, J. and Piernattei, D.L. (1976) Classification, management and repair of central tarsal fractures in the racing greyhound. *Journal of the American Animal Hospital Association* **12** 398–405.

Montgomery, R.D., Hathcock, J.T., Milton, J.L and Fitch, R.B. (1994) Osteochondritis dissecans of the canine tarsal joint. *Compendium of Continuing Education for the Practicing Veterinarian (Small Animal)* **16** 835–845.

Mughannam, A.J. and Reinke, J. (1994) Avulsion of the gastrocnemius tendon in three cats. *Journal of the American Animal Hospital Association* **30** 550–556.

Newell, S.M., Mahaffey, M.B. and Aron, D.N. (1994) Fragmentation of the medial malleolus of dogs with and without tarsal osteochondrosis. *Veterinary Radiology and Ultrasound* **35** 5–9.

Ost, P.C., Dee, J.F., Dee, L.G. and Hohn, R.B. (1987) Fractures of the calcaneus in racing greyhounds. *Veterinary Surgery* **16** 53–59.

Reinke, J.D. and Mughannam, A.J. (1993) Lateral luxation of the superficial digital flexor tendon in 12 dogs. *Journal of the American Animal Hospital Association* **29** 303–309.

Reinke, J.D., Mughannam, A.J. and Owens, J.M. (1993) Avulsion of the gastrocnemius tendon in 11 dogs. *Journal of the American Animal Hospital Association* **29** 410–418.

Rivers, B.J., Walter, P.A., Kramek, B. and Wallace, L. (1997) Sonographic findings in canine common calcaneal tendon injury. *Veterinary and Comparative Orthopaedics and Traumatology* **10** 45–53.

4

Head and neck

4.1 Radiographic technique for the skull
4.2 Breed and conformational variations of the skull and pharynx

CRANIAL CAVITY

4.3 Variations in shape of the cranial cavity
4.4 Variations in shape of the foramen magnum
4.5 Variations in radio-opacity of the cranium
4.6 Variations in thickness of the calvarial bones
4.7 Ultrasonography of the brain

MAXILLA AND PREMAXILLA

4.8 Maxillary and premaxillary bony proliferation or sclerosis
4.9 Maxillary and premaxillary bony destruction or rarefaction

MANDIBLE

4.10 Mandibular bony proliferation or sclerosis
4.11 Mandibular bony destruction or rarefaction
4.12 Mandibular fracture

TEMPOROMANDIBULAR JOINT

4.13 Temporomandibular joint not clearly seen
4.14 Malformation of the temporomandibular joint

THE EAR

4.15 Abnormalities of the external ear canal
4.16 Variations in the wall of the tympanic bulla
4.17 Increased radio-opacity of the tympanic bulla

NASAL CAVITY

4.18 Variations in shape of the nasal cavity

4.19 Increased radio-opacity of the nasal cavity
4.20 Decreased radio-opacity of the nasal cavity

FRONTAL SINUSES

4.21 Variations in shape of the frontal sinuses
4.22 Increased radio-opacity of the frontal sinuses
4.23 Variations in thickness of the frontal bone

TEETH

4.24 Variations in the number of teeth
4.25 Variations in the shape of teeth
4.26 Variations in structure or radio-opacity of the teeth
4.27 Periodontal radiolucency

PHARYNX AND LARYNX

4.28 Variations in the pharynx
4.29 Variations in the larynx
4.30 Changes in the hyoid apparatus

SOFT TISSUES OF THE HEAD AND NECK

4.31 Thickening of the soft tissues of the head and neck
4.32 Variations in radio-opacity of the soft tissues of the head and neck
4.33 Contrast studies of the nasolacrimal duct (dacryocystorhinography)
4.34 Ultrasonography of the eye and orbit
4.35 Contrast studies of the salivary ducts and glands (sialography)
4.36 Ultrasonography of the salivary glands
4.37 Ultrasonography of the thyroid and parathyroid glands
4.38 Ultrasonography of the carotid artery and jugular vein
4.39 Ultrasonography of lymph nodes of the head and neck

4 HEAD AND NECK

4.1 Radiographic technique for the skull

A basic radiographic examination of the head and neck should include lateral and ventrodorsal (VD) and/or dorsoventral (DV) projections. Great care should be taken to achieve accurate positioning, and to facilitate this general anaesthesia is usually required. Additional specialised projections are used to highlight specific areas of the head and neck and are described in the relevant section. A high definition film/screen system should be used and a grid is not necessary.

4.2 Breed and conformational variations of the skull and pharynx

Breeds of dog can be divided into three groups:

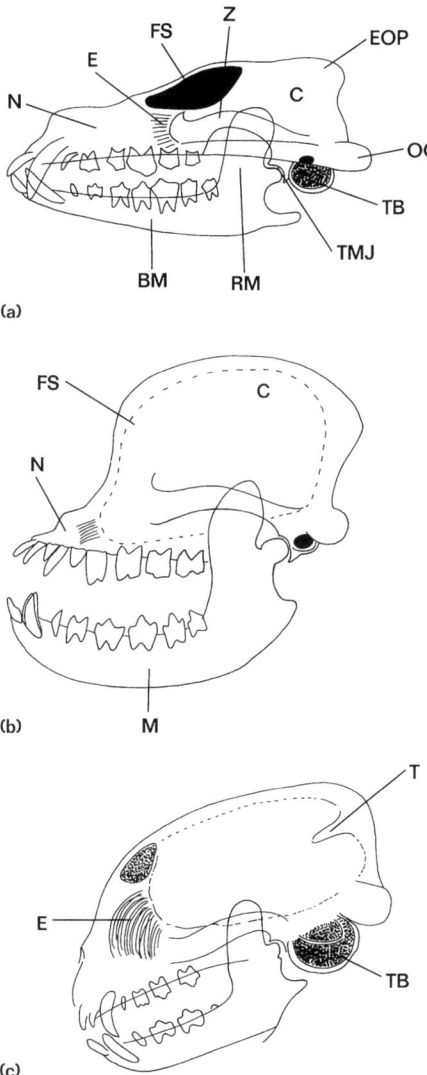

Figure 4.1 Normal lateral skulls. (a) Doliocephalic dog (BM = body of mandible; C = cranium/calvarium; E = ethmoturbinates; EOP = external occipital protuberance; FS = frontal sinus; N = nasal cavity; OC = occipital condyle; RM = ramus of mandible; TB = tympanic bulla; TMJ = temporomandibular joint; Z = zygomatic arch); (b) brachycephalic dog (C = domed cranium; FS = absent or reduced frontal sinus; M = curved body of mandible; N = reduced nasal cavity with crowding of teeth); (c) cat (E = ethmoturbinates; T = tentorium osseum; TB = large tympanic bulla with inner bony shell).

doliocephalic breeds, in which the nasal cavity is longer than the cranium (e.g. Irish Setter)

mesaticephalic breeds, in which the nasal cavity and cranium are of approximately equal length (e.g. Labrador)

brachycephalic breeds, in which the nasal cavity length is greatly reduced (e.g. Bulldog).

There are marked conformational variations in the skull, particularly between different breeds of dog, but also to a lesser extent between different breeds of cat (Figure 4.1). Brachycephalic breeds have a short maxilla, although the mandible may remain relatively long. The nasal cavity is correspondingly reduced in size and the teeth may be crowded and displaced. The cranium is more domed, and the occipital protuberance and frontal sinuses are less prominent than in the longer nosed breeds. Brachycephalic breeds of dog also show soft palate thickening, increased submandibular soft tissue mass and caudal displacement of the hyoid apparatus.

In cats, the cranium is relatively large and the *tentorium osseum* is prominent on the lateral view. The tympanic bullae are large and contain a characteristic inner bony shell which divides the bulla into two portions.

CRANIAL CAVITY

The cranial cavity is composed of the frontal, parietal, temporal and occipital bones, the cribriform plate of the ethmoid bone and those bones forming the base of the skull (the sphenoid and basioccipital bones). The roof of the cranial cavity, formed by the frontal and parietal bones and part of the occipital bone, is known as the calvarium.

Views: lateral, dorsoventral or ventrodorsal (DV/VD), lateral oblique, rostrocaudal (RCd), lesion-oriented oblique (LOO).

4.3 Variations in shape of the cranial cavity

1. Breed associated – brachycephalic breeds of dog and cat tend to have a domed calvarium.
2. Congenital hydrocephalus (Figure 4.2) – exaggeration of the domed shape, with thinning of the bones of the calvarium. The calvarial bones may have a more uniform radio-opacity than normal, lacking the usual "copper-beaten" appearance, and the fontanelle and suture lines are likely to remain open.
3. Trauma – usually flattening or concavity of the calvarium seen on a LOO view.

4.4 Variations in shape of the foramen magnum

1. Abnormal dorsal extension ("keyhole" shape) seen in occipital dysplasias; usually toy and miniature breeds of dog; may be associated with hydrocephalus, and/or atlantoaxial malformations. Seen on a well-penetrated RCd view.

4.5 Variations in radio-opacity of the cranium

1. Decreased radio-opacity of the cranium
   a. Generalised:
      * hyperparathyroidism – most commonly secondary to chronic renal disease, but also secondary to nutritional imbalance or primary parathyroid disease (see 1.16.4)
   b. Localised:
      * normal suture lines or vascular channels
      * fracture lines
      * neoplasia, e.g. plasma cell myeloma (multiple myeloma) – less common in the skull than in other flat bones.
2. Increased radio-opacity of the cranium
   a. Localised:
      * trauma leading to periosteal new bone formation
      * neoplasia – osteoma or multilobular tumour of bone (well defined, dense bony masses), osteochondroma/multiple cartilaginous exostoses (in

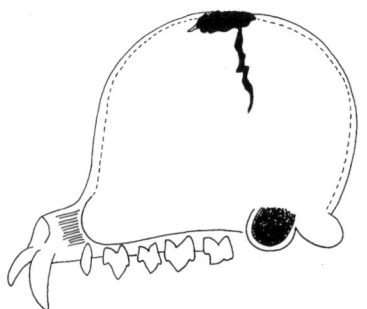

Figure 4.2 Congenital hydrocephalus – domed cranium with open fontanelle and suture lines.

cats often involve the skull; rounded, well mineralised juxta-cortical masses), osteosarcoma (often predominantly proliferative in the skull)
- overlapping fracture fragments
- foreign body reaction
- calcification of a meningioma or hyperostosis of overlying cranial bone (especially in cats)
- myelographic contrast in the ventricular system and subarachnoid space – characteristic pattern.

b. Generalised:
- increased radio-opacity due to cranial bone thickening (see 4.6.2).

3. Mixed or mottled radio-opacity of the cranial bones – usually due to a mixture of bone production or soft tissue mineralisation and osteolysis
   a. Neoplasia – primary bone and soft tissue tumours tend to have varying proportions of bone destruction and bone proliferation or soft tissue mineralisation. An example is osteosarcoma – tends to be predominantly proliferative at this site, but with some destruction; multilobular tumour of bone – soft tissue mass with speckled mineralisation and lysis of underlying bone, most often involving the temporo-occipital region
   b. Osteomyelitis:
   - bacterial
   - fungal (e.g. cryptococcosis*) – predominantly osteolytic.

4.6 Variations in thickness of the calvarial bones

1. Thinning of the bones of the calvarium
   a. Normal variant in small, brachycephalic breeds of dog, possibly due to subclinical hydrocephalus
   b. Hydrocephalus – usually with a domed calvarium, open suture lines and fontanelle and a homogeneous "ground-glass" radio-opacity. Most common in small breeds of dog. If there are open sutures, then it may be possible to examine the brain ultrasonographically (see 4.7)
   c. Erosion by an adjacent mass.
2. Increased thickness of the bones of the calvarium
   a. Normal variant in some breeds (e.g. Pit Bull Terrier)
   b. Healed fracture
   c. Craniomandibular osteopathy (may affect parietal, frontal, occipital and temporal bones as well as the mandible – see 4.10.1)
   d. Hyperostosis (thickening and sclerosis) of the calvarium in Bullmastiff puppies – mainly frontal and parietal bones, regresses at skeletal maturity; unknown aetiology
   e. Meningioma in cats – may cause localised hyperostosis adjacent to the tumour
   f. Acromegaly in cats.

4.7 Ultrasonography of the brain

Ultrasonographic examination of the brain is possible if there is an open fontanelle, and so is often possible in brachycephalic breeds of dog and in young dogs. The brain itself appears hypoechoic and loosely granular in texture, while the interior of the cranial cavity is outlined by a well-defined echogenic line. It may be possible to identify the lateral ventricles as small anechoic foci, usually bilaterally symmetrical in size, shape and position. MRI and CT are, however, superior techniques for imaging of intracranial structures.
1. Increased size of the lateral ventricles
   a. Breed associated, for example most brachycephalic breeds of dog have larger lateral ventricles than non-brachycephalic breeds
   b. Hydrocephalus
   - congenital
   - acquired, due to obstructive lesions or tumours causing increased production of cerebrospinal fluid.

MAXILLA AND PREMAXILLA

Views: lateral (right and left sides superimposed), lateral oblique, intra-oral DV, open mouth rostroventral–dorsocaudal oblique (RV – DcdO).

4.8 Maxillary and premaxillary bony proliferation or sclerosis

1. Osteomyelitis – usually a mixture of bone proliferation and destruction

a. Secondary to dental disease
b. Bacterial
c. Fungal.
2. Neoplasia – more often predominantly osteolytic (see below), but can be proliferative; some are exclusively proliferative, e.g. osteoma. Nasal cavity neoplasia may produce apparent increase in radio-opacity of the maxilla on the lateral radiograph.
3. Healing or healed maxillary or premaxillary fracture.

4.9 Maxillary and premaxillary bony destruction or rarefaction

1. Neoplasia – all types may show some degree of bone proliferation but are predominantly osteolytic
   a. Squamous cell carcinoma (Figure 4.5)
   b. Malignant melanoma
   c. Fibrosarcoma
   d. Primary bone tumours, primarily osteosarcoma
   e. Nasal cavity neoplasia eroding the surrounding bony case.
2. Odontogenic tumours or cysts – expansile, radiolucent lesions which may also contain tooth elements
   a. Ameloblastoma
   b. Adamantinoma
   c. Complex odontoma
   d. Dentigerous cyst.
3. Periodontal disease – radiolucent halo around the affected tooth (see 4.27.1 and Figure 4.14).

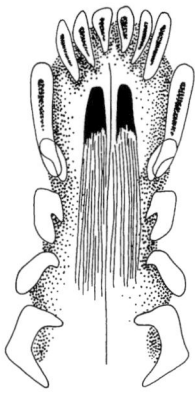

Figure 4.3 Renal secondary hyperparathryoidism. Rarefaction of bone produces ill-defined radiolucent haloes around the teeth, giving the impression of "floating teeth".

4. Renal secondary hyperparathyroidism ("rubber jaw") (Figure 4.3) – osteopenia secondary to chronic renal disease, especially renal dysplasia in young animals.
5. Nasolacrimal duct cysts – discrete radiolucency with a fine, sclerotic margin, communicating with the nasolacrimal duct on dacryocystorhinography (see 4.33).
6. Maxillary cholesterol granuloma – identical in appearance to nasolacrimal duct cyst but no communication with the nasolacrimal duct.
7. Maxillary giant cell granuloma – discrete osteolytic lesion, seen mainly in young dogs.

MANDIBLE

The mandibles of brachycephalic breeds are markedly curved when seen on the lateral view, suggesting an attempt at shortening in order for the incisor teeth to approach those of the premaxilla. In elderly cats, the mandibular symphysis appears irregular on the intraoral view.

Views: lateral (mandibles superimposed over each other), DV/VD (partly obscured by maxillae), lateral oblique, intraoral VD.

4.10 Mandibular bony proliferation or sclerosis

1. Craniomandibular osteopathy (CMO) (Figure 4.4) – florid periosteal new bone, which remodels with time; young dogs, primarily West Highland White Terrier, Cairn Terrier

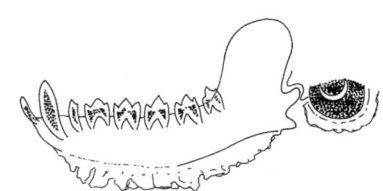

Figure 4.4 Craniomandibular osteopathy: florid periosteal new bone affecting the mandibles and tympanic bullae

and Scottish Terrier but occasionally large breeds; usually involves the mandible and/or the tympanic bullae, but also sometimes the calvarium and frontal bones.
2. Osteomyelitis – usually a mixture of bone proliferation and destruction

4 HEAD AND NECK

   a. Secondary to dental disease
   b. Bacterial
   c. Fungal.
3. Neoplasia – more often predominantly osteolytic (see below), but can be proliferative; some are exclusively proliferative, e.g. osteoma.
4. Healing or healed mandibular fracture.
5. Canine leucocyte adhesion deficiency (CLAD) – young Irish Red Setters – see 1.23.7.
6. Acromegaly (cats).

4.11 Mandibular bony destruction or rarefaction

1. Neoplasia – all types may show some degree of bone proliferation but are predominantly osteolytic
   a. Squamous cell carcinoma (Figure 4.5)
   b. Malignant melanoma
   c. Fibrosarcoma
   d. Also primary bone tumours, primarily osteosarcoma.
2. Odontogenic tumours or cysts – expansile, radiolucent lesions which may also contain tooth elements
   a. Ameloblastoma
   b. Adamantinoma
   c. Complex odontoma (Figure 4.6)
   d. Dentigerous cyst.

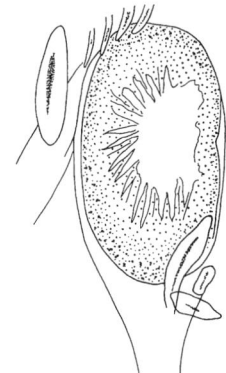

Figure 4.6 Tumour of dental origin: a complex odontoma in a young dog, seen as an expansile osteolytic bone lesion containing material of dental radio-opacity.

3. Periodontal disease – radiolucent halo around the affected tooth (see 4.27 and Figure 4.14).
4. Renal secondary hyperparathyroidism ("rubber jaw") – osteopenia secondary to chronic renal disease (see 4.9.4 and Figure 4.3).
5. Mandibular giant cell granuloma – discrete osteolytic lesion seen mainly in young dogs.

4.12 Mandibular fracture

1. Trauma
   a. Symphyseal injury – most common in the cat; "high rise syndrome" (falling from a height) typically results in symphyseal separation and splitting of the hard palate, in conjunction with limb and soft tissue injuries
   b. Fractures of the ramus
   c. Fractures involving the temporomandibular joint.
2. Pathological fracture
   a. Through an area of severe periodontal disease, especially in toy breeds of dog
   b. Osteolytic tumour
   c. Renal secondary hyperparathyroidism.

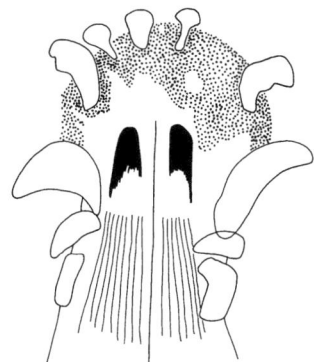

Figure 4.5 Squamous cell carcinoma of the premaxilla – mainly osteolytic with displacement, loss and erosion of teeth.

TEMPOROMANDIBULAR JOINT

Views: sagittal oblique (with mouth open and closed), VD or DV (Figure 4.7).

On the sagittal oblique views, the mandibular condyle should be smoothly rounded, fitting closely into the glenoid (the smooth concavity in the petrous temporal bone), just rostral to the tympanic bulla.

4.13 Temporomandibular joint not clearly seen

1. Incorrect positioning, especially if lateral oblique view is used (as for tympanic bullae) rather than sagittal oblique view.
2. Technical factors
   a. Underexposure
   b. Underdevelopment
3. Trauma
   a. Fracture
   b. Luxation/subluxation
4. Periarticular new bone
   a. Healing or healed fracture
   b. Osteoarthritis
   c. CMO (see 4.10.1 and Figure 4.4)
   d. CLAD; young Irish Red Setters (see 1.23.7).
5. Destruction of articular surfaces
   a. Infection – may extend from infection of the external or middle ear or a para-aural abscess
   b. Neoplasia.

4.14 Malformation of the temporomandibular joint

1. Irregular articular surfaces
   a. Trauma:
      - fracture
      - luxation/subluxation
   b. Osteoarthritis
   c. Infection
   d. Neoplasia.
2. Flattening +/– abnormal angulation of the articular surfaces – temporomandibular joint dysplasia; especially Basset Hound and Irish Red Setter. On an open mouth VD view may see the vertical ramus of the mandible impinging on the zygomatic arch, resulting in open mouth jaw locking.

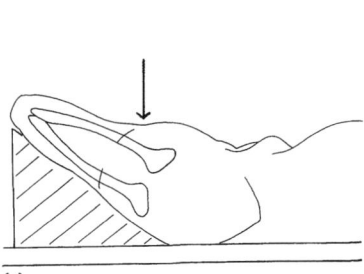
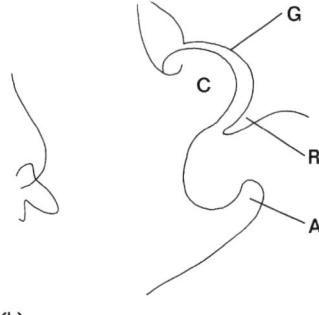

Figure 4.7 (a) Positioning for the sagittal oblique view of the temporomandibular joint. From a true lateral position the nose is tilted upwards 10–30°, depending on conformation (more tilt in brachycephalic breeds) (b) Normal appearance of the temporomandibular joint on a sagittal oblique view. (A = angular process of mandible; C = condyle; G = glenoid or mandibular fossa of temporal bone; R = retroarticular process).

4 HEAD AND NECK

THE EAR

Views: external ear canals – VD or DV; tympanic bullae – lateral oblique, open-mouth RCd, VD or DV (although in this view the petrous temporal bones and cranium are superimposed). In the cat, a special view – the rostro–10°–ventral–dorsocaudal oblique – has been described (Figure 4.8).

The normal external ear canals are seen as bands of gas lucency lateral to the tympanic bullae. The external ear canals and the pinnae may create confusing shadows on lateral radiographs. The walls of the tympanic bullae are seen as thin and regular bony structures, the cat also having an inner bony shell.

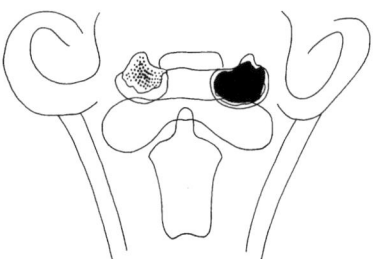

Figure 4.9 Otitis media – thickening of the bulla wall and increased radio-opacity of the bulla lumen, seen here on an open-mouth RCd radiograph.

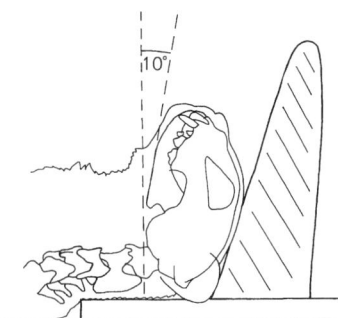

Figure 4.8 Positioning for the special view of the feline tympanic bullae.

4.15 Abnormalities of the external ear canal

1. External ear canal not visible
   a. Overexposure, overdevelopment or severe fogging of the film
   b. Congenital absence of the ear canal
   c. Previous surgical ablation of the canal
   d. Occlusion of the canal by wax, debris or purulent material
   e. Occlusion of the canal by a soft tissue mass:
      - neoplasm
      - polyp
2. Narrowing of the external ear canal
   a. Hypertrophy and/or inflammation of the lining of the canal – due to acute or chronic otitis externa
   b. Compression of the canal by a paraaural mass or swelling.
3. Calcification of the external ear canal
   a. Normal – a small amount of orderly calcification of the cartilages encircling the canal may be normal in older dogs
   b. Sequel to chronic otitis externa.

4.16 Variations in the wall of the tympanic bulla

1. Thickening of the wall of the tympanic bulla
   a. Otitis media (middle ear disease; see Figure 4.9)
   b. Polyp – check for nasopharyngeal polyp too, especially in cats
   c. CMO (see 4.10.1 and Fig. 4.4)
   d. Neoplasia (usually with osteolysis too)
      - squamous cell carcinoma
      - adenocarcinoma
   e. CLAD: young Irish Red Setters (see 1.23.7).
2. Destruction of the wall of the tympanic bulla
   a. Neoplasia
      - squamous cell carcinoma
      - adenocarcinoma
   b. Severe otitis media with osteomyelitis
   c. Previous bulla osteotomy.

4.17 Increased radio-opacity of the tympanic bulla

1. Artefactual due to poor positioning on the open mouth RCd view or superimposition of the tongue.
2. Increased radio-opacity of the bulla contents (Figure 4.9)
   a. Otitis media
   b. Polyp
   c. Neoplasia (see above)
   d. Cholesterol granuloma
   e. Cholesteatoma.
3. Increased radio-opacity due to thickening of the bony bulla wall (see 4.16.1).

SMALL ANIMAL RADIOLOGICAL DIFFERENTIAL DIAGNOSIS

NASAL CAVITY

Views: intraoral DV, open-mouth RV – DCd. VD or DV (mandibles are superimposed over the lateral parts of the nasal cavity), lateral (right and left sides superimposed over each other), lateral oblique.

The turbinate pattern should be clearly delineated, and broadly symmetrical when comparing the right and left nasal chambers. In the rostral third of the nasal chamber the turbinate pattern should consist of a fine linear pattern. In the middle third the pattern becomes woven into an irregular honeycomb. In the caudal third the pattern returns to a linear form. The bony part of the nasal septum (the vomer) divides the right and left nasal chambers. It is not unusual for the vomer to be curved or deviated in brachycephalic breeds and in cats. Rostrally, the paired palatine fissures are seen. On radiographs taken using a soft exposure, the soft tissues of the nostrils can also be assessed.

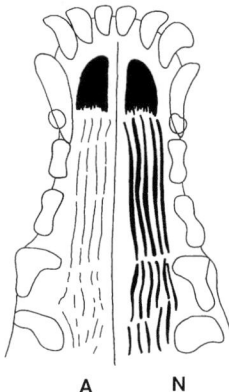

Figure 4.10 Unilateral rhinitis. The turbinate pattern is blurred compared with the normal side and there is an overall increase in radio-opacity. Confident diagnosis is more difficult if the changes are bilateral. (N = normal nasal cavity; A = affected side.)

4.18 Variations in shape of the nasal cavity

1. Breed variation.
2. Congenital deformity.
3. Trauma.
4. Mucopolysaccharidosis – inherited condition of the Domestic Shorthair cat, Siamese and Siamese crosses; broad, short maxilla, reduced or absent frontal sinuses, abnormal nasal conchae, hypoplasia of the hyoid apparatus (see also 1.12.7, 1.21.11 and 5.4.9).

4.19 Increased radio-opacity of the nasal cavity

1. Increased radio-opacity with retention of the underlying turbinate pattern – usually bilateral, occasionally unilateral (Fig. 4.10)
   a. Underexposure
   b. Underdevelopment
   c. Recent nasal flushing
   d. Non-specific rhinitis
   e. Hyperplastic rhinitis
   f. Rhinitis associated with dental disease
   g. Nasal haemorrhage
   h. Small or recent nasal foreign body (unilateral)
   i. Kartagener's syndrome (or immotile cilia syndrome; often associated with situs inversus and evidence of bronchitis/bronchiectasis – see 6.12.7)
   j. Primary ciliary dyskinesia (see 6.12.7)
   k. Cryptococcosis* (especially cats)
   l. Capillariasis* – may rarely cause rhinitis
   m. Fibrous osteodystrophy secondary to hyperparathyroidism (see 1.16.4).
2. Increased radio-opacity with destruction of the underlying turbinate pattern – usually begins unilaterally (there may also be destruction of the vomer and/or supporting bones)
   a. Neoplasia (Figure 4.11) – carcinoma most common; also sarcomas, including lymphosarcoma; usually starts in

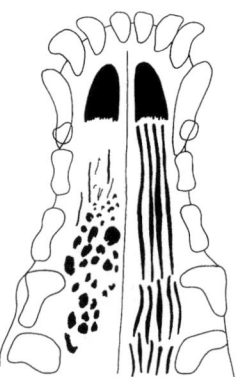

Figure 4.11 Nasal neoplasia: destruction of turbinate bones by a soft tissue radio-opacity. Osteolysis of the surrounding bones (maxilla, nasal bones and palate) may also occur.

4 HEAD AND NECK

the caudal or mid third of the nasal cavity, often near the carnassial tooth
b. Nasal polyp
c. Fungal rhinitis, especially aspergillosis* – with retention of necrotic material or fungal granuloma
d. Chronic nasal foreign body.

4.20 Decreased radio-opacity of the nasal cavity

1. Decreased radio-opacity with retention of the underlying turbinate pattern – bilateral
   a. Overexposure
   b. Overdevelopment
   c. Severe fogging of the film.
2. Decreased radio-opacity with destruction of the underlying turbinate pattern – unilateral or bilateral
   a. Fungal rhinitis (Figure 4.12) – especially *Aspergillus* spp., but also *Penicillium* and other species; usually starts in the rostral part of the nasal cavity; especially young dogs of dolicocephalic breed
   b. Viral rhinitis (cats)

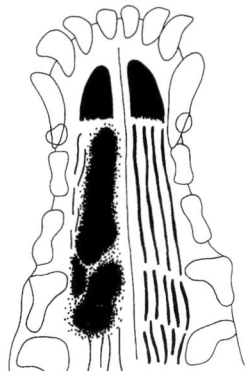

Figure 4.12 Destructive rhinitis (aspergillosis) – loss of the turbinate pattern with ill-defined and patchy increase in radio-opacity rather than diffuse nasal opacification.

   c. Nasal foreign body
   d. Destruction of the supporting palatine or maxillary bone
   e. Congenital defect of the hard palate
   f. Previous rhinotomy.

FRONTAL SINUSES

Views: RCd, lateral oblique, lateral (right and left frontal sinuses are superimposed), VD/DV (partially superimposed by the caudal nasal cavity and rostral calvarium).

Sinuses should be filled with air, which outlines the smooth bony folds of the walls. The frontal sinuses are more prominent in larger breeds of dog and in cats than in smaller breeds of dog; they may be absent in some brachycephalic breeds.

4.21 Variations in shape of the frontal sinuses

1. Breed and conformational variations – the frontal sinuses may be extremely large and prominent in some giant breeds of dog such as the St. Bernard.
2. Trauma
   a. Fracture of the walls of the sinus
   b. Occlusion of drainage due to a nasofrontal fracture, leading to accumulation of secretions and an expanded sinus (frontal sinus mucocoele)
3. Neoplasm involving the frontal bones.
4. Osteomyelitis involving the frontal bones.
5. Aplasia – mucopolysaccharidosis in cats.

4.22 Increased radio-opacity of the frontal sinuses

Increased radio-opacity of the frontal sinuses may be due to the presence of fluid or soft tissue within the sinus or to the superimposition of new bone or soft tissue swelling.

1. Sinusitis
   a. Bacterial
   b. Fungal – especially *Aspergillus* spp.
   c. Allergic
   d. Secondary to viral respiratory disease
   e. Kartagener's syndrome (see 6.12.7).
2. Occlusion of drainage of the frontal sinuses leading to mucus retention
   a. Trauma – occlusion of drainage due to a nasofrontal fracture, leading to accumulation of secretions and an expanded sinus (frontal sinus mucocoele)
   b. Mass in the caudal nasal cavity, usually neoplastic.
3. Neoplasia
   a. Extension of nasal neoplasia into the frontal sinuses
   b. Other soft tissue or bone neoplasia:
      • carcinoma – soft tissue radio-opacity; osteolytic

- osteosarcoma – mixed bone lesion
- osteoma or multilobular tumour of bone; mainly proliferative.
4. CMO – thickening of the frontal bones may occur, usually in conjunction with new bone in other typical locations (see 4.10.1) but occasionally in isolation.
5. CLAD – young Irish Red Setters (see 1.23.7).

4.23 Variations in thickness of the frontal bone

1. Increase in thickness of the frontal bone
   a. Healing or healed fracture
   b. Secondary to fungal sinusitis
   c. Neoplasm involving the frontal bones (see above)
   d. CMO (see 4.10.1 and Figure 4.4)
   e. CLAD; young Irish Red Setters (see 1.23.7)
   f. Acromegaly (cats).
2. Decrease in thickness or osteolysis of the frontal bone
   a. Neoplasm involving the frontal bones (see above)
   b. Osteomyelitis involving the frontal bones
   c. Erosion by an adjacent mass
   d. Secondary to a frontal sinus mucocoele – likely to be expansile.

TEETH

Views: lateral oblique, intraoral DV and VD projections of the maxilla and mandible, bisecting angle technique (incisors and canines), intraoral parallel technique (mandibular premolars and molars).

Each normal tooth has a well-defined crown and one or more clearly defined roots (Figure 4.13). The outer layer of the tooth, composed of enamel and dentine, is radio-opaque, while the inner pulp cavity is relatively radiolucent. In the immature animal, the pulp cavity is wider, with an open apical foramen; in the mature animal, the pulp cavity narrows and the apical foramina close. The tooth roots are embedded in the alveolar bone of the mandible or maxilla/incisive bone. They are surrounded by a radiolucent zone created by the periodontal membrane and outlined by a thin, radio-opaque line – the lamina dura.

The normal dental formulae for the dog and cat are given below:

	Immature (deciduous teeth)	Mature
Dog	$2 \times I\frac{3}{3} C\frac{1}{1} PM\frac{3}{3}$	$2 \times I\frac{3}{3} C\frac{1}{1} PM\frac{4}{4} M\frac{2}{3}$
Cat	$2 \times I\frac{3}{3} C\frac{1}{1} PM\frac{3}{2}$	$2 \times I\frac{3}{3} C\frac{1}{1} PM\frac{3}{2} M\frac{1}{1}$

4.24 Variations in the number of teeth

1. Decrease in the number of teeth
   a. Congenital anodontia (absence of teeth) or oligodontia (reduction in the number of teeth). Oligodontia is particularly common in brachycephalic breeds of dog and may be symmetrical or asymmetrical
   b. Previous tooth extraction or loss.
2. Increase in the number of teeth
   a. Retained temporary teeth
   b. Congenital polyodontia.

4.25 Variations in the shape of teeth

1. Change in shape of the crown
   a. Fracture of the crown
   b. Abnormal wear of the crown (e.g. stone chewing)
   c. Crown removed; one or more roots retained.
2. Change in shape of the root
   a. Periodontal disease leading to deformity or erosion of the root
   b. Deformation or displacement by an adjacent mass.

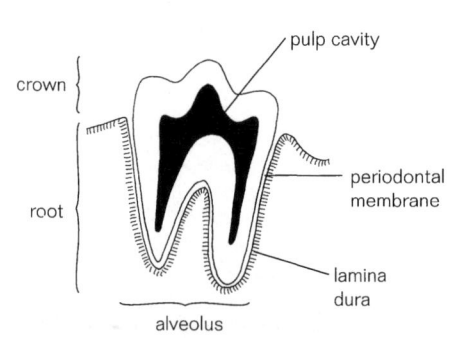

Figure 4.13 Anatomy of a normal tooth.

4.26 Variations in structure or radio-opacity of the teeth

1. Fracture of the tooth.
2. Caries – radiolucent defects in the crown.
3. Wide pulp cavity
   a. Immature tooth (all teeth appear similar)
   b. Dead tooth (other live teeth have a narrow pulp cavity)
   c. Inflammation of the pulp cavity
      • secondary to fracture of the tooth
      • secondary to periodontal disease.
4. Dentinogenesis imperfecta – thinning of dentine layer leading to multiple fractures; sometimes seen with osteogenesis imperfecta (see 1.16.13).

4.27 Periodontal radiolucency

1. Periodontal disease – destruction of alveolar bone and resorption of the alveolar crest between the tooth and its neighbours (Figure 4.14).

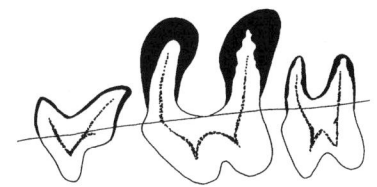

Figure 4.14 Peridontal disease – radiolucent halo around the affected tooth (the carnassial tooth, upper PM4), with irregularity of one of the tooth roots. Peridontal disease at this site is sometimes called "malar abscess".

2. Neoplasia
   a. Epulis (arises from periodontal membrane)
   b. Odontogenic tumours (arise from dental laminar epithelium, often contain dental structures – see 4.11.2 and Figure 4.6).
3. Primary or secondary hyperparathyroidism (generalised loss of bone radio-opacity although may be more severe around tooth roots – see 4.9.4 and Figure 4.3).

PHARYNX AND LARYNX

Views: lateral, VD/DV.

A true lateral projection, without an endotracheal tube in place, is essential for evaluation of the pharynx. The pharynx is divided into the oropharynx and nasopharynx by the soft palate, which should extend to the tip of the epiglottis (Figure 4.15). Mineralisation of the laryngeal cartilages in the dog is quite normal, and usually begins at 2–3 years of age (or earlier in large and chondrodystrophic breeds).

4.28 Variations in the pharynx

1. Reduction or obliteration of the air-filled nasopharynx
   a. Soft tissue mass in the nasopharynx

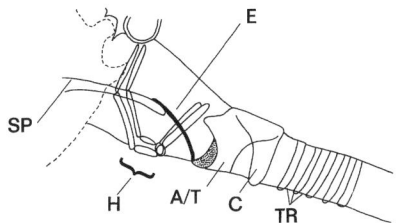

Figure 4.15 Normal lateral pharynx.
A/T = arytenoid and thyroid cartilages of larynx,
C = cricoid cartilage of larynx, E = epiglottis,
H = hyoid apparatus, SP = soft palate,
TR = tracheal rings.

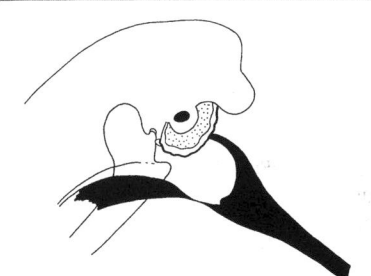

Figure 4.16 Nasopharyngeal polyp in a cat. A soft tissue mass is seen in the nasopharynx, depressing the soft palate. Bony changes are present in one of the tympanic bullae.

   • nasopharyngeal polyp (may be associated with radiological evidence of otitis media; increased radio-opacity of the bulla lumen and thickening of the bulla wall) (Figure 4.16)
   • neoplasia (most commonly carcinoma in dogs and lymphosarcoma in cats)
   • abscess or foreign body reaction
   • granuloma.
   b. Thickening of the soft palate
      • part of brachycephalic obstructive syndrome
      • palatine mass – tumour, cyst or granuloma
   c. Foreign body in the nasopharynx

SMALL ANIMAL RADIOLOGICAL DIFFERENTIAL DIAGNOSIS

   d. Excessive pharyngeal tissue – part of the brachycephalic obstructive syndrome
   e. Retropharyngeal mass
      - enlarged retropharyngeal lymph nodes (e.g. lymphosarcoma)
      - retropharyngeal abscess
      - retropharyngeal tumour
   f. Nasopharyngeal stenosis
      - congenital stenosis
      - acquired, secondary to trauma
   g. Obesity.
2. Ballooning of the pharynx
   a. Pharyngeal paralysis
   b. Respiratory obstruction.
3. Radio-opacities within the pharynx
   a. Radio-opaque foreign body
   b. Hyoid bones (see 4.30 and Figure 4.15)
   c. Mineralisation of laryngeal cartilages (see 4.29.3 and Figure 4.15)
   d. Dystrophic calcification within a mass
   e. Ossification within a mass
   f. Superimposed salivary calculi.

4.29 Variations in the larynx

1. Ventral displacement of the larynx and proximal trachea
   a. Enlargement of retropharyngeal lymph nodes
   b. Thyroid enlargement
   c. Cellulitis or abscessation of the retropharyngeal tissues
   d. Neoplasia involving the retropharyngeal tissues.
2. Caudal displacement of the larynx and proximal trachea
   a. Normal in brachycephalic dogs
   b. Extreme dyspnoea
   c. Disruption of the hyoid apparatus due to trauma or neoplasia.
3. Mineralisation of laryngeal cartilages
   a. Normal ageing changes
   b. Secondary to laryngeal neoplasia (mineralisation usually then more extensive and less ordered)
   c. Secondary to laryngeal chondritis.
4. Reduction or obliteration of the laryngeal airway
   a. Neoplasia
      - carcinoma most common in the dog
      - lymphosarcoma most common in the cat
   b. Laryngeal cyst
   c. Laryngeal granuloma.

4.30 Changes in the hyoid apparatus

1. Artefactual appearance of subluxation between hyoid bones due to positioning for radiography.
2. Fracture – choke chain injuries or other direct trauma.
3. Disruption of relationship between individual hyoid bones – 'hanging' injuries.
4. Bone proliferation and/or destruction
   a. Osteomyelitis
   b. Neoplasia, e.g. thyroid carcinoma.

SOFT TISSUES OF THE HEAD AND NECK

4.31 Thickening of the soft tissues of the head and neck

1. Focal thickening of the soft tissues of the head and neck
   a. Soft tissue tumour
   b. Abscess
   c. Haematoma
   d. Granuloma
   e. Cyst
   f. Recent administration of subcutaneous fluids into the neck area.
2. Diffuse thickening of the soft tissue of the head and neck
   a. Obesity (fat is more radiolucent than other soft tissues)
   b. Cellulitis
   c. Oedema
   d. Diffuse neoplasia.

4.32 Variations in radio-opacity of the soft tissues of the head and neck

1. Decreased radio-opacity of soft tissues
   a. Gas within soft tissues
      - secondary to pharyngeal or oesophageal perforation
      - secondary to tracheal perforation
      - discharging sinus or fistulous tract
      - secondary to pneumomediastinum (gas tracks cranially along cervical fascial planes)
      - abscess cavity
      - puncture or laceration of skin leading to subcutaneous emphysema
   b. Fat within soft tissues
      - normal subcutaneous and fascial plane fat

- obesity
- lipoma or liposarcoma.
2. Increased radio-opacity of soft tissues
   a. Artefactual (e.g. wet hair, dirty coat)
   b. Calcification
      - calcinosis circumscripta (rounded deposits of amorphous mineralisation) (see 12.2.2 and Figure 12.1). Mainly large breeds of dog, especially German Shepherd dog
      - calcinosis cutis (secondary to hyperadrenocorticism; linear streaks in fascial planes or granular deposits near skin surface)
      - dystrophic calcification in a tumour, haematoma, abscess or granuloma
   c. Radio-opaque foreign body
   d. Microchip
   e. Leakage of barium sulphate into soft tissues through a pharyngeal or oesophageal tear.

4.33 Contrast studies of the nasolacrimal duct (dacryocystorhinography)

Dacryocystorhinography is not often performed, but may be used to demonstrate occlusion or leakage of the nasolacrimal duct. A fine catheter is placed within either the upper or lower punctum of the eyelids and, while digital pressure is used to occlude the other punctum, 1–1.5 ml of a water-soluble, iodinated contrast medium are slowly injected into the duct. A radiograph is then taken immediately, usually with the patient in lateral recumbency.
1. Contrast column does not fill the duct
   a. Poor technique
      - leakage of contrast from one or both puncta
      - inadequate volume of contrast medium used
   b. Nasolacrimal duct not patent

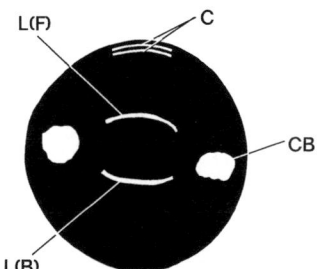

Figure 4.17 Normal ocular ultrasonogram (C = front and back of cornea; CB = ciliary body; L(B) = back of lens; L(F) = front of lens).

- aplasia of a segment of the nasolacrimal duct
- occlusion of the nasolacrimal duct by foreign material, mucus, purulent material, stricture formation or neoplasia.
2. Irregular contrast column in the nasolacrimal duct
   a. Contrast mixing with mucus or purulent material
   b. Contrast outlining foreign material in the nasolacrimal duct
   c. Inflammation of the nasolacrimal duct
   d. Neoplasia involving the nasolacrimal duct.
3. Leakage of contrast medium from the nasolacrimal duct
   a. Rupture of the nasolacrimal duct
   b. Entry into a nasolacrimal duct cyst.

4.34 Ultrasonography of the eye and orbit

Radiography of the eye is of limited value, so ultrasound is increasingly used to image this region. A high-frequency (7.5–10 MHz) sector or curvilinear transducer is placed directly on the cornea or nictitating membrane following topical anaesthesia. A stand-off is useful when examining the anterior chamber. The eye should be examined in both horizontal and vertical planes, taking care to sweep through the whole volume of the globe and the retrobulbar structures.

The globe of the eye is approximately spherical, with a smooth, thin, well-defined wall (Figure 4.17). Separate layers of the sclera, retina and choroid are not normally recognised. A small depression or elevation may be seen posteriorly, representing the optic disc. The aqueous and vitreous humours in the chambers of the eye are normally anechoic. The surface of the lens is identified by echoes only at those points where the incident sound beam is perpendicular to the lens surface; at other points the smooth curve of the lens surface scatters echoes away from the transducer. The substance of the lens is anechoic. The hypoechoic ciliary body and iris may be visible on either side of the lens.

The retrobulbar tissues usually form an orderly cone behind the eye. The retrobulbar muscles are hypoechoic, while the retrobulbar fat is hyperechoic. A dark tract running through the retrobulbar tissues was at one time thought to represent the optic nerve but is now thought more likely to be acoustic shadowing deep to the optic disc.

SMALL ANIMAL RADIOLOGICAL DIAGNOSIS

1. Increased size of the globe
   a. Breed associated (bilaterally symmetrical)
   b. Glaucoma – hydrophthalmos.
2. Decreased size of the globe
   a. Breed associated (bilaterally symmetrical) e.g. Rough Collie
   b. Congenital microphthalmos
   c. Phthisis bulbi
      - following trauma
      - after inflammatory disease
      - end-stage glaucoma.
3. Thickening of the wall of the globe
   a. Generalised thickening
      - scleritis
      - chorioretinitis
   b. Localised thickening
      - tumour
      - subretinal haemorrhage
      - granuloma (see below).
4. Echogenicities within the chambers of the eye
   a. Generalised increase in echogenicity
      - haemorrhage (secondary to trauma, neoplasia, coagulopathy, hypertension, chronic glaucoma)
      - inflammatory exudate (endophthalmitis)
      - vitreal degeneration
      - vitreous 'floaters'
      - asteroid hyalosis (middle aged and older dogs)
      - gain settings inappropriately high
   b. Localised 'mass' effect
      - blood clot
      - sediment of inflammatory cells
      - intraocular tumour – melanoma (usually arise from ciliary body); ciliary body adenoma or adenocarcinoma; lymphosarcoma (often bilateral, may be associated with intraocular haemorrhage); metastatic tumour
      - intraocular granuloma – blastomycosis* (usually choroidal in origin); coccidioidomycosis*; cryptococcosis*; histoplasmosis*; feline infectious peritonitis (FIP); toxoplasmosis*
      - subretinal haemorrhage
      - retinal detachment – occasionally gives rise to a mass effect, but more often produces (curvi)linear echogenicities (see below)
      - intraocular foreign body – there may be acoustic shadowing, or if metallic may see reverberation

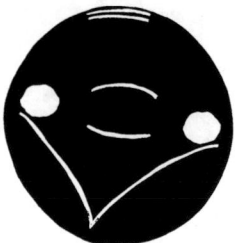

Figure 4.18 Total retinal detachment on ultrasonography.

   c. Linear or curvilinear echogenicities
      - retinal detachment (Figure 4.18) – when complete, appears as 'sea gull's wings', with attachments at optic disc and ciliary body. Partial detachments may also be visible as linear or curvilinear echoes within the vitreous
      - posterior vitreous detachment – similar in appearance to detached retina but not attached at the optic disc
      - vitreous membranes – fibrous strands which sometimes develop secondary to clot formation; can lead to tractional retinal detachment.
5. Change in position of the lens – luxation or subluxation. The lens may move anteriorly or posteriorly
   a. Trauma
   b. Hereditary predisposition
   c. Displacement by an adjacent mass
   d. Glaucoma.
6. Increased echogenicity of the lens – cataract formation. Increased echogenicity may be generalised or focal, and may be capsular and/or within the body of the lens
   a. Trauma
   b. Hereditary predisposition
   c. Diabetes mellitus
   d. Inflammation
   e. Radiation exposure
   f. Intraocular tumours
   g. Posterior polar cataract associated with persistent hyperplastic primary vitreous (PHPV).
7. Enlargement of the ciliary body
   a. Inflammation
   b. Neoplasia
      - melanoma
      - adenoma
      - adenocarcinoma.

8. Changes in the retrobulbar tissues
    a. Diffuse disturbance – heterogeneous in echogenicity and echotexture
        • cellulitis
        • neoplasia
    b. Mass – varying echogenicity, often deforming the back of the globe
        • retrobulbar abscess (bacterial, fungal, parasitic, secondary to foreign body)
        • neoplasia (lymphosarcoma – often bilateral; other primary and metastatic neoplasms)
    c. Focal echogenicity(ies) +/– acoustic shadowing
        • retrobulbar foreign body (NB: a metallic foreign body may give rise to reverberation rather than shadowing)
        • dystrophic calcification
        • bone proliferation arising from the bones of the orbit
    d. Enlargement of the optic nerve +/– protruding optic disc
        • optic neuritis (numerous causes including toxoplasmosis*, cryptococcosis*, canine distemper, blastomycosis*, FIP, trauma).

4.35 Contrast studies of the salivary ducts and glands (sialography)

Sialography is occasionally undertaken to characterise further the nature of swellings around the head and neck. A fine cannula is introduced into the appropriate duct opening:
parotid (on the mucosal ridge opposite the caudal margin of the upper fourth premolar tooth)
zygomatic (about 1 cm caudal to the parotid opening)
mandibular (lateral surface of the lingual caruncle at the frenum linguae)
sublingual (may be common with the mandibular opening, or 1–2 mm caudal to it).

Water-soluble iodinated contrast medium (1–2 ml) is carefully injected, taking care to avoid leakage back around the cannula, and radiographs of the appropriate region of the head and neck are taken immediately.
1. Salivary duct not filled
    a. Inadequate technique
        • too little contrast medium used
        • leakage of contrast back around cannula
    b. Occlusion of the salivary duct
        • sialolith
        • stricture
        • foreign body
        • compression of the salivary duct by an adjacent mass.
2. Spillage of contrast medium into surrounding soft tissues
    a. Rupture of the salivary duct
    b. Salivary mucocoele.
3. Irregular filling of the salivary duct
    a. Inflammation
    b. Neoplasia
    c. Sialolith
    d. Foreign material.
4. Uneven filling of the salivary gland
    a. Insufficient contrast medium used
    b. Abscessation of the salivary gland
    c. Neoplasia of the salivary gland e.g. adenocarcinoma
    d. Salivary gland cyst
    e. Infarction of the salivary gland
    f. Compression of the salivary gland by an adjacent mass.

4.36 Ultrasonography of the salivary glands

The mandibular salivary gland is the only salivary gland that can be consistently imaged. It is located superficially, caudal to the angle of the mandible. Ultrasonographically it appears well defined, oval and hypoechoic with a more echogenic capsule. There may be thin echogenic streaks within the substance of the gland.
1. Hypoechoic or anechoic foci in the salivary gland
    a. Salivary gland cyst
    b. Salivary gland abscess
    c. Neoplasm.
2. Echogenic foci in the salivary gland – sialolith (often with acoustic shadowing).
3. Heterogeneous foci in the salivary gland
    a. Neoplasm
        • benign papillomatous tumour
        • carcinoma
    b. Salivary gland abscess.

4.37 Ultrasonography of the thyroid and parathyroid glands

A high-frequency transducer is required. The two lobes of the thyroid gland may be identified lying on each side of the trachea, caudal to the larynx, and medial to the ipsilateral common carotid artery. The lobes should

be smooth, well defined, hypoechoic, and finely granular in texture. Each lobe of the normal thyroid gland in a medium-sized dog is around 2.5–3 cm long, and 0.4–0.6 cm wide. In the cat, the normal dimensions are about 2 cm long and 0.2–0.3 cm wide.
1. Nodules within the thyroid gland – may be of variable echogenicity
   a. Thyroid tumour
      - adenoma
      - carcinoma
   b. Parathyroid tumour
      - adenoma
      - carcinoma
   c. Parathyroid hyperplasia
   d. Thyroid cyst (irregularly marginated cysts with hyperechoic septations may be seen in hyperthyroid cats).
2. Enlargement of the thyroid gland
   a. Well marginated, low echogenicity – thyroid adenoma
   b. Poorly marginated, heterogeneous mass – thyroid carcinoma; may see invasion of common carotid artery and/or jugular vein, and involvement of regional lymph nodes.

4.38 Ultrasonography of the carotid artery and jugular vein

The external jugular veins lie in a groove on the ventrolateral aspect of the neck. The common carotid arteries lie deep to the jugular veins, bifurcating near the head into external and internal carotid arteries. The vein is thin walled and compressible, with anechoic contents, while the arteries have thicker walls and are less compressible. Doppler ultrasound may be used to confirm the arterial or venous nature of the blood flow.
1. Intraluminal mass in the carotid artery or jugular vein
   a. Thrombus
   b. Invasion by adjacent tumour.
2. Multiple abnormal vessels associated with the carotid artery or jugular vein
   a. Collateral vessels
      - secondary to obstruction of normal vessels
      - supplying an abnormal mass
   b. Arteriovenous malformation
      - secondary to trauma
      - secondary to neoplasia
      - congenital malformation.

4.39 Ultrasonography of lymph nodes of the head and neck

Most lymph nodes in the head and neck of the dog and cat are small (<5 mm diameter) and are not consistently seen ultrasonographically. Based on work in humans, lymph nodes in the head and neck are considered enlarged if they are over 1 cm in diameter. Enlarged lymph nodes usually remain hypoechoic, but may become heterogeneous, especially if cavitation occurs. In humans, reactive lymph nodes tend to retain their oval or flat shape, whilst neoplastic lymph nodes are more likely to become round. It is not clear if this applies to small animals.
1. Enlarged lymph nodes
   a. Reactive
   b. Neoplasia
      - lymphosarcoma
      - metastases.

FURTHER READING

General

Gibbs, C. (1976) Radiological refresher: The head part I – Traumatic lesions of the skull. *Journal of Small Animal Practice* **17** 551–554.

Johnston, G.R. and Feeney, D.A. (1980) Radiology in ophthalmic diagnosis. *Veterinary Clinics of North America; Small Animal Practice* **10** 317–337.

Konde, L.J., Thrall, M.A., Gasper, P., Dial, S.M., McBiles, K., Colgan, S. and Haskins, M. (1987) Radiographically visualized skeletal changes associated with mucopolysaccharidosis VI in cats. *Veterinary Radiology* **28** 223–228.

Cranial cavity

Hudson, J.A., Cartee, R.E., Simpson, S.T. and Buxton, D.F. (1989) Ultrasonographic anatomy of the canine brain. *Veterinary Radiology* **30** 13–21.

Hudson, J.A., Simpson S.T., Buxton D.F., Cartee, R.F. and Steiss, J.E. (1990) Ultrasonographic diagnosis of canine hydrocephalus. *Veterinary Radiology* **31** 50–58.

Muir, P. Dubielzig, R.R., Johnson, K.A. and Shelton, D.G. (1996) Hypertrophic osteodystrophy and calvarial hyperostosis. *Compendium of Continuing Education for the Practicing Veterinarian (Small Animal)* **18** 143–151.

4 HEAD AND NECK

Spaulding, K.A. and Sharp, N.J.H. (1990) Ultrasonographic imaging of the lateral cerebral ventricles in the dog. *Veterinary Radiology* **31** 59–64.

Maxilla and premaxilla

Frew, D.G. and Dobson, J.M. (1992) Radiological assessment of 50 cases of incisive or maxillary neoplasia in the dog. *Journal of Small Animal Practice* **33** 11–18.

Mandible

Gibbs, C. (1977) Radiological refresher: The head part II – Traumatic lesions of the mandible. *Journal of Small Animal Practice* **18** 51–54.

Watson, A.D.J., Adams, W.M. and Thomas, C.B. (1995) Craniomandibular osteopathy in dogs. *Compendium of Continuing Education for the Practicing Veterinarian (Small Animal)* **17** 911–921.

Temporomandibular joint

Lane, J.G. (1982) Disorders of the canine temporomandibular joint. *Veterinary Annual* **22** 175–187.

Sullivan, M. (1989) Temporomandibular ankylosis in the cat. *Journal of Small Animal Practice* **30** 401–405.

The ear

Eom, K-D., Lee, H-C., Yoon, J-H. (2000) Canalographic evaluation of the external ear canal in dogs. *Veterinary Radiology and Ultrasound* **41** 231–234.

Gibbs, C. (1978) Radiological refresher: The head part III – Ear disease. *Journal of Small Animal Practice* **19** 539–545.

Hofer, P., Meisen, N., Bartholdi, S. and Kaser-Hotz, B. (1995). Radiology Corner – A new radiographic view of the feline tympanic bulla. *Veterinary Radiology and Ultrasound* **36** 14–15.

Hoskinson, J.J. (1993) Imaging techniques in the diagnosis of middle ear disease. *Seminars in Veterinary Medicine & Surgery* **8** 10–16.

Trower, N.D., Gregory, S.P., Renfrew, H. and Lamb, C.R. (1998) Evaluation of the canine tympanic membrane by positive contrast ear canalography. *Veterinary Record* **142** 78–81.

Nasal cavity and frontal sinuses

Coulson, A. (1988) Radiology as an aid to diagnosis of nasal disorders in the cat. *Veterinary Annual* **28** 150–158.

Gibbs, C., Lane, J.G. and Denny, H.R. (1979) Radiological features of intra-nasal lesions in the dog: a review of 100 cases. *Journal of Small Animal Practice* **20** 515–535.

O'Brien, R.T., Evans, S.M., Wortman, J.A. and Hendrick, M.J. (1996) Radiographic findings in cats with intranasal neoplasia or chronic rhinitis: 29 cases (1982–1988). *Journal of the American Veterinary Medical Association* **208** 385–389.

Sullivan, M., Lee, R., Jakovljevic, S. and Sharp, N.J.H. (1986) The radiological features of aspergillosis of the nasal cavity and frontal sinuses of the dog. *Journal of Small Animal Practice* **27** 167–180.

Sullivan, M., Lee, R. and Skae, C.A. (1987) The radiological features of sixty cases of intra-nasal neoplasia in the dog. *Journal of Small Animal Practice* **28** 575–586.

Teeth

Eisner, E.R. (1998) Oral-dental radiographic examination technique. *Veterinary Clinics of North America; Small Animal Practice* **28** 1063–1087.

Gibbs, C. (1978) Radiological refresher: The head part IV – Dental disease. *Journal of Small Animal Practice* **19** 701–707.

Gorrel, C. (1998) Radiographic evaluation. *Veterinary Clinics of North America; Small Animal Practice* **28** 1089–1110.

Harvey, C.E. and Flax, B.M. (1992) Feline oral-dental radiographic examination and interpretation. *Veterinary Clinics of North America; Small Animal Practice* **22** 1279–1295.

Hooft, J., Mattheeuws, D. and van Bree, P. (1979) Radiology of deciduous teeth resorption and definitive teeth eruption in the dog. *Journal of Small Animal Practice* **20** 175–180.

Lommer, M.L., Verstraete, F.J.M. and Terpak, C.H. (2000) Dental radiographic technique in cats. *Compendium of Continuing Education for the Practicing Veterinarian (Small Animal)* **22** 107–117.

Zontine, W.J. (1975) Canine dental radiology: radiographic technique, development and anatomy. *Veterinary Radiology* **16** 75–83.

Pharynx, larynx and other soft tissues of the neck

Bray, J.P., Lipscombe, V.J., White, R.A.S. and Rudorf, H. (1998) Ultrasonographic examination of the pharynx and larynx of the normal dog. *Veterinary Radiology and Ultrasound* **39** 566–571.

Gallagher, J.G., Boudrieau, R.J., Schelling, S.H. and Berg, J. (1995) Ultrasonography of the brain and vertebral canal in dogs and cats: 15 cases (1988–1993). *Journal of the American Veterinary Medical Association* **207** 1320–1324.

Gelatt, K.N., Cure, T.H., Guffy, M.M. and Jessen, C. (1972) Dacryocystorhinography in the dog and cat. *Journal of Small Animal Practice* **13** 381–397.

Gibbs, C. (1986) Radiographic examination of the pharynx, larynx and soft tissue structures of the neck in dogs and cats. *Veterinary Annual* **26** 227–241.

Glen, J.B. (1972) Canine salivary mucocoeles: Results of sialographic examination and surgical treatment of fifty cases. *Journal of Small Animal Practice* **13** 515–526.

Harvey, C.E. (1969) Sialography in the dog. *Journal of the American Veterinary Radiological Society* **10** 18–27.

Hudson, J.A., Finn-Bodner, S.T. and Steiss, J.E. (1998) Neurosonography. *Veterinary Clinics of North America; Small Animal Practice* **28** 943–972.

Rudorf, H. (1997) Ultrasound imaging of the tongue and larynx in normal dogs. *Journal of Small Animal Practice* **38** 349–444.

Rudorf, H., Herrtage, M.E. and White, R.A.S. (1997) Use of ultrasonography in the diagnosis of tracheal collapse. *Journal of Small Animal Practice* **38** 513–518.

Rudorf, H. (1998) Ultrasonography of laryngeal masses in six cats and one dog. *Veterinary Radiology and Ultrasound* **39** 430–434.

Solano, M. and Penninck, D.G. (1996) Ultrasonography of the canine, feline and equine tongue: normal finding and case history reports. *Veterinary Radiology and Ultrasound* **37** 206–213.

Williams, J. and Wilkie, D.A. (1996) Ultrasonography of the eye. *Compendium of Continuing Education for the Practicing Veterinarian (Small Animal)* **18** 667–676.

Wisner, E.R., Mattoon, J.S., Nyland, T.G. and Baker, T.W. (1991) Normal ultrasonographic anatomy of the canine neck. *Veterinary Radiology* **32** 185–190.

Wisner, E.R., Nyland T.G. and Mattoon J.S. (1994) Ultrasonographic examination of cervical masses in the dog and cat. *Veterinary Radiology and Ultrasound* **35** 310–315.

Wisner, E.R., Penninck, D., Biller, D.S., Feldman, E.C., Drake, C. and Nyland, T.G. (1997) High resolution parathyroid sonography. *Veterinary Radiology and Ultrasound* **38** 462–466.

Wisner, E.K. and Nyland, T.G. (1998) Ultrasonography of the thyroid and parathyroid glands. *Veterinary Clinics of North America; Small Animal Practice* **28** 973–992.

Yakely, W.L. and Alexander, J.E. (1971) Dacryocystorhinography in the dog. *Journal of the American Veterinary Medical Association* **159** 1417–1421.

5

Spine

5.1 Radiographic technique for the spine
5.2 Variations in vertebral number
5.3 Variations in vertebral size and shape – congenital or developmental
5.4 Variations in vertebral size and shape – acquired
5.5 Variations in vertebral alignment
5.6 Diffuse changes in vertebral opacity
5.7 Localised changes in vertebral opacity
5.8 Abnormalities of the intervertebral disc space
5.9 Abnormalities of the intervertebral foramen
5.10 Abnormalities of the articular facets
5.11 Lesions in the paravertebral soft tissues
5.12 Spinal contrast studies – technique and normal appearance
5.13 Technical errors during myelography
5.14 Extradural spinal cord compression on myelography
5.15 Intradural extramedullary spinal cord compression on myelography
5.16 Intramedullary spinal cord enlargement on myelography
5.17 Miscellaneous myelographic findings
5.18 Neurological deficits involving the spinal cord or proximal nerve roots with normal survey radiographs and myelogram radiographs.

5.1 Radiographic technique for the spine

Optimal radiographs are obtained with the patient under sedation or general anaesthesia to minimise motion blur and allow accurate positioning.

True lateral and ventrodorsal (VD) positioning should be ensured by the use of positioning aids (Figure 5.1). Horizontal VD views are desirable when severe instability or spinal fractures are suspected, to avoid additional injury on manipulation of the patient. Detail-intensifying screens are preferred, and a grid should be used if the tissue thickness is greater than 10 cm. Close collimation will also improve image definition by reducing the production of scattered radiation. If neurological deficits are present or if disc disease is suspected, the primary beam must be centred at the level of the suspected lesion.

Myelography is the most commonly used contrast medium technique for the evaluation of the spinal cord or cauda equina. Epidurography, discography and lumbar sinus venography are additional techniques which are sometimes used to evaluate the cauda equina. More advanced diagnostic modalities are usually only available at academic institutions or human facilities. Linear tomography is useful in

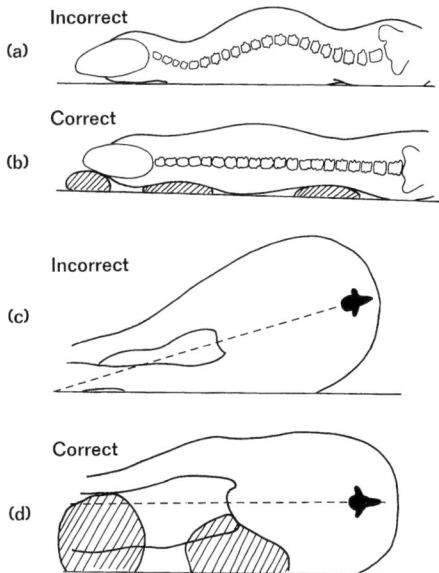

Figure 5.1 Achieving accurate positioning with the use of foam wedges.

the thoracic and lumbosacral regions to eliminate superimposition of the ribs and ilial wings, respectively. Cross-sectional images can be obtained by means of computed tomography

83

(CT) and magnetic resonance imaging (MRI); CT provides better definition of bone and joint abnormalities whereas MRI provides high soft tissue contrast and is ideal for cases with no survey film abnormalities such as spinal tumours, early infectious processes or ligamentous pathology. Scintigraphy is occasionally used to identify the location of inflammatory or neoplastic processes.

Optimal interpretation of spinal radiographs requires a systematic evaluation, which involves assessing radiographic quality and technique, extravertebral soft tissue structures, osseous vertebral structures, disc spaces and intervertebral foramina. Each vertebra, disc space and intervertebral foramen should be compared with those adjacent to them. Disc spaces normally appear narrower towards the periphery of the film due to divergence of the primary X-ray beam.

5.2 Variations in vertebral number

The normal vertebral formula in the dog and cat is seven cervical, thirteen thoracic, seven lumbar, three sacral and a variable number of caudal vertebrae. Numerical alterations may be genuine or may be accompanied by other congenital vertebral abnormalities which may result in apparent vertebral number alterations ("transitional" vertebrae – see 5.3.2).
1. Six or eight lumbar vertebrae (especially Dachshund).
2. Four sacral vertebrae – vestigial disc spaces may be visible.
3. Twelve thoracic vertebrae.
    a. twelve genuine thoracic vertebrae and seven lumbar vertebrae
    b. T13 lacks ribs, giving the appearance of twelve thoracic and eight lumbar vertebrae
4. Fourteen thoracic vertebrae – usually due to the presence of rib-like structures on L1 rather than a genuine increase in number.

5.3 Variations in vertebral size and shape – congenital or developmental

More than one abnormality may be present.
1. Normal variants
    a. C7 and L7 may be shorter than the adjacent vertebrae
    b. the ventral margins of L3 and L4 vertebral bodies are often poorly defined due to bony roughening at the origins of the diaphragmatic crura.

2. Transitional vertebrae – these are vertebrae that have anatomical features of two adjacent regions. They are commonly seen and may accompany numerical abnormalities, but other than those at the lumbosacral junction they are not usually clinically significant. The transitional segment may show unilateral or bilateral changes
    a. Sacralisation of the last lumbar vertebra (Figure 5.2a) – the transverse process fuses to the wing of the sacrum and may also articulate with the ilium. This may predispose to lumbosacral instability and disc degeneration with secondary cauda equina syndrome. If rotational malalignment is present it may predispose to unilateral hip dysplasia and result in an inability to obtain pelvic symmetry during positioning for hip dysplasia radiographs. Common in the German Shepherd dog but also seen in the Dobermann, Rhodesian Ridgeback and Brittany Spaniel
    b. Lumbarisation of S1 vertebra, which fails to fuse to the rest of the sacrum
    c. Partial or complete fusion of S3 to Cd1. Pseudoarticulation of the transverse processes may be present. Often seen with (b) in an attempt to restore three sacral segments
    d. Transitional T13 vertebra (Figure 5.2b) – a rib develops into a transverse process; a vestigial rib may be seen as a mineralised line in the soft tissues
    e. Transitional L1 vertebra – a transverse process develops into a rib
    f. Transitional C7 vertebra – a transverse process develops into a rib
    g. Occipitalisation of the atlas.
3. Hemivertebrae (Figure 5.3) – malformation of the vertebral body; a common abnormality in the thoracic and tail regions, particularly in screw-tailed breeds and the German Short-haired Pointer. Rare in cats. Multiple vertebrae are often affected. Clinical signs (neurological deficits due to spinal cord compression) are uncommon and usually occur in the first year of life during the growth phase
    a. Dorsal hemivertebra – ventral half did not develop, producing kyphosis
    b. Lateral hemivertebra – left or right half did not develop, producing scoliosis
    c. Ventral hemivertebra – dorsal half did not develop, producing lordosis.

5 SPINE

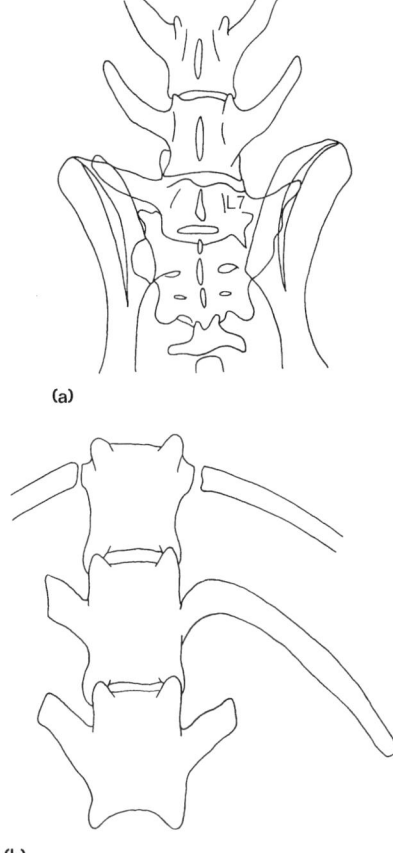

(a)

(b)

Figure 5.2 (a) Unilateral sacralisation of L7; a transverse process at one side and articulation with the ilium on the other. (b) Transitional vertebra at the thoracolumbar junction, with one rib and one transverse process.

4. Block or fused vertebrae – usually only two, and rarely three, segments are fused; reduced or absent disc space with vertebrae of normal length. The degree of fusion varies. The increased

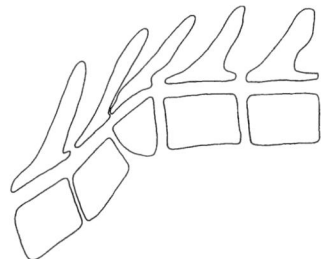

Figure 5.3 Typical mid-thoracic hemivertebra – a wedge-shaped vertebral body resulting in kyphosis and narrowing of the vertebral canal.

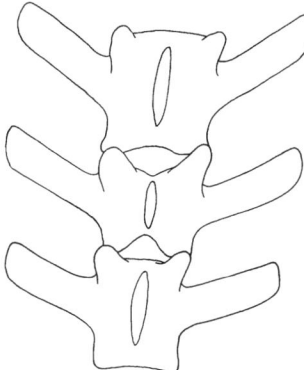

Figure 5.4 Butterfly vertebra, seen on the VD view.

stress on adjacent disc spaces predisposes to subsequent disc herniation. DDx old trauma and bony remodelling
   a. Lumbar region
   b. Cervical region.
5. Butterfly vertebrae (Figure 5.4) – particularly brachycephalic breeds of dog, rare in cats. Unlikely to cause clinical signs. Seen on the VD view, particularly in the caudal thoracic and caudal lumbar regions as a cleft of the cranial and caudal vertebral end-plates due to partial sagittal cleavage of the vertebral body.
6. Incomplete fusion of sacral segments.
7. C2 – dens (odontoid peg) abnormalities
   a. Agenesis, hypoplasia or non-fusion leading to atlantoaxial instability (see 5.5.5)
   b. Dorsal angulation of the dens.
8. Cervical vertebral malformation malarticulation syndrome (CVMM or "Wobbler" syndrome; Figure 5.5) – malformed cer-

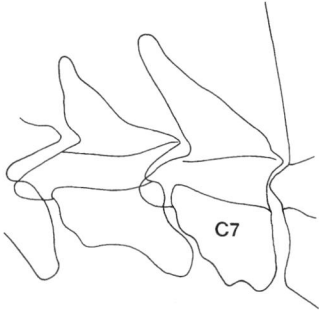

Figure 5.5 Typical vertebral malformation seen with the cervical vertebral malformation malarticulation syndrome ("Wobbler" syndrome) – deformity and upward tilting of the vertebral body with vertebral canal stenosis.

85

vical vertebrae, often with a "ploughshare" appearance of lower cervical vertebrae and wedge-shaped disc spaces; may be accompanied in middle age by changes such as spondylosis deformans and secondary disc prolapse. Especially Dobermann. Most cases present in middle age due to secondary disc protrusion but in cases of severe deformity neurological signs are evident at a younger age.
9. Narrowed vertebral canal (spinal stenosis) – needs myelography to demonstrate the degree of stenosis
    a. Secondary to hemivertebrae or block vertebrae
    b. CVMM ("Wobbler") syndrome
    c. Thoracic stenosis
        - T3–6 usually with no cord compression – Dobermann
        - individual thoracic vertebrae – Bulldog
    d. Congenital lumbosacral stenosis in small and medium-sized dogs.
10. Congenital metabolic disease affecting vertebrae at a young age
    a. Pituitary dwarfism – especially German Shepherd dog; proportionate dwarfism +/– epiphyseal dysgenesis
    b. Congenital hypothyroidism – especially Boxer; disproportionate dwarfism with epiphyseal dysgenesis leading in the spine to delayed vertebral end-plate ossification and growth plate closure; end plates show characteristic ventral spikes. Pathological fracture through unfused growth plate has been reported. Long bone changes also occur (see 1.21.9).
11. Fused dorsal spinal processes.
12. Spina bifida – results in a split or absent dorsal spinous process or absent lamina, most common in the lumbar region, especially the Bulldog. A widened vertebral canal may be seen on the lateral view. May be accompanied by spinal dysraphism, a defective closure of the neural tube
    a. Spina bifida occulta – normal spinal cord and intact skin. Common in short-tailed breeds
    b. Meningocoele – herniated meninges, skin intact
    c. Myelomeningocoele – herniated spinal cord and meninges, skin intact
    d. Spina bifida manifesta – herniated spinal cord and meninges exposed to the exterior
    e. Spina bifida cystica – herniated spinal cord and meninges elevated above the skin.
13. Occipitoatlantoaxial malformation.
14. Other occasional complex vertebral anomalies.
15. Cervical articular facet aplasia.
16. Perocormus – severe shortening of the vertebral column.
17. Cats – sacrococcygeal (sacrocaudal) dysgenesis; varies from spina bifida to complete sacrococcygeal agenesis. Especially in Manx cats, in which it may be accompanied by other anomalies such as shortened cervical vertebrae, butterfly vertebrae and fusion of lumbar vertebrae.
18. Cats – mucopolysaccharidosis: congenital lysosomal storage diseases but lesions do not manifest until later in life (see 5.4.9).

5.4 Variations in vertebral size and shape – acquired

For articular facet variations see 5.10.

Increased vertebral size

1. Spondylosis deformans – varying sizes of ventral and lateral bony spurs that may bridge the disc space (Figure 5.6). Usually clinically insignificant unless so extensive as to result in nerve root involvement
    a. Initiated by degeneration of annulus fibrosis – an incidental finding which may start as young as 2 years, is very common and increases in incidence with age
    b. Secondary to
        - chronic disc prolapse
        - CVMM ("Wobbler") syndrome
        - disc fenestration
        - discospondylitis
        - hemivertebrae
        - fracture/luxation injuries
    c. Syndesmitis ossificans – extensive ossification of the ventral longitudinal ligament – young Boxers.

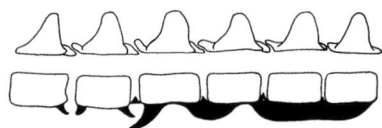

Figure 5.6 Varying degrees of spondylosis; small spurs of new bone progressing to ankylosis.

2. Fracture and enlarged vertebra due to callus formation
   a. Trauma
   b. Pathological fracture (extensive callus unlikely)
      • nutritional secondary hyperparathyroidism (juvenile osteoporosis – see 1.16.4 and Figure 1.21)
      • osteolytic tumour e.g. plasma cell myeloma
      • aneurysmal bone cyst (see 1.18.9).
3. Neoplasia
   a. Benign neoplasia
      • single or multiple cartilaginous exostoses, often involving the dorsal spinous processes. Growth ceases after the active growth phase in dogs but lesions may arise after the active growth phase in cats (see 1.15.2 and Figure 1.19)
   b. Malignant neoplasia
      • osteosarcoma
      • other primary or metastatic tumours
   c. Metastatic or infiltrative tumours resulting in ventral periosteal reaction on caudal lumbar and sacral vertebrae; DDx spondylitis (see below)
      • prostatic tumour – the most common cause of such new bone
      • bladder/urethral tumour
      • peri-anal tumour
      • mammary tumour.
4. Spondylitis (Figure 5.7) – usually characterised by vertebral body periosteal reactions, particularly ventrally, and which may progress to osteomyelitis of the vertebral body. Conversely osteomyelitis may also originate haematogenously within the vertebra and extend peripherally

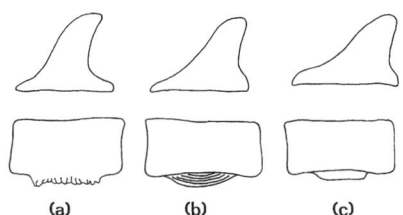

Figure 5.7 New bone on the ventral margins of vertebral bodies due to metastatic neoplasia (usually L5–7) or spondylitis (usually L1–3). The new bone may be brushlike (a), lamellar (b) or solid (c). See 1.6 for further description of periosteal reactions.

   a. Bacterial
      • migrating grass awns – especially ventral to L3 and L4. Medium and large-sized dogs aspirate grass awns which migrate through the lung and diaphragm to the origin of the crura at L3 and L4
      • other foreign bodies
      • haematogenous infection
      • bite wounds
      • iatrogenic due to surgical complications
   b. Parasitic
      • *Spirocerca lupi** – spondylitis of caudal thoracic vertebrae
   c. Fungal
      • actinomycosis*
      • coccidiodomycosis*
      • aspergillosis*
   d. Protozoal
      • hepatozoonosis* – there may be extensive new bone formation, including other bones of the body.
5. Baastrup's disease – bony proliferation between dorsal spinous processes. Larger dog breeds, especially Boxer.
6. Disseminated idiopathic skeletal hyperostosis (DISH) – the main changes are in the spine with extensive new bone formation along the ventral and lateral margins of the vertebral bodies and at sites of ligamentous attachments; also extremital periarticular new bone and enthesiophyte formation.
7. Aneurysmal bone cyst (see 1.18.9).
8. Cats – hypervitaminosis A; extensive new bone formation on cervical and cranial thoracic vertebrae and rarely further caudally. Mainly ventrally, mimicking severe spondylosis, but may also involve the sides and dorsum of the vertebrae. Long bone joints may also be affected, especially the elbow and stifle. Usually young cats on raw liver diets; DDx mucopolysaccharidosis.
9. Mucopolysaccharidosis; lysosomal storage diseases causing new bone on the vertebrae which may lead to spinal fusion; also dwarfism, facial deformity, pectus excavatum and hip dysplasia. More common in the cat, especially those with Siamese ancestry; rare in the dog; DDx hypervitaminosis A.

Decreased vertebral size

10. Fractures – may result in shortened vertebra due to compression
    a. Trauma

SMALL ANIMAL RADIOLOGICAL DIFFERENTIAL DIAGNOSIS

    b. Pathological fracture
- nutritional secondary hyperparathyroidism (juvenile osteoporosis) (see 1.16.4 and Figure 1.21)
- osteolytic tumour (e.g. plasma cell myeloma).

11. Discospondylitis – osteolysis of vertebral end plates eventually results in a shortened vertebral body, with secondary spondylosis deformans and even fusion in the later stages (see 5.8.3 and Figure 5.9).
12. Sacral osteochondrosis – defect of the craniodorsal aspect of S1 +/– an osteochondral fragment; young German Shepherd dogs.
13. Indented vertebral end-plates
    a. Intravertebral disc herniation (Schmorl's node) – particularly L7 and/or S1; medium and large breeds, especially German Shepherd dog
    b. Nutritional secondary hyperparathyroidism (juvenile osteoporosis) – bony deformity from pathological fractures may remain for life.
14. Mucopolysaccharidosis; the vertebrae may be shortened or misshapen because dwarfism may be a feature; also vertebral body new bone and fusion, facial deformity, pectus excavatum and hip dysplasia; more common in the cat, especially those with Siamese ancestry; rare in the dog. DDx hypervitaminosis A.

Altered vertebral shape

15. CVMM ("Wobbler") syndrome – congenitally malformed cervical vertebrae; may be accompanied by acquired changes such as remodelling of the centrum, spondylosis deformans and secondary disc prolapse. Especially Dobermann (see 5.3.8 and Figure 5.5).
16. Fractures – the vertebrae may be misshapen due to malunion or asymmetric compression
    a. Trauma
    b. Pathological fracture
       - nutritional secondary hyperparathyroidism (juvenile osteoporosis)
       - osteolytic tumour e.g. plasma cell myeloma
       - aneurysmal bone cyst (see 1.18.9).
17. Neoplasia (see 5.4.3).
18. Mucopolysaccharidosis (see 5.4.9 and 5.4.14).

Vertebral canal changes

19. Widened vertebral canal
    a. Normal at the level of the cervical (C5–T2) and lumbar (L2–5) intumescentia
    b. Enlarged spinal cord due to chronic pathology
       - tumour e.g. astrocytoma, ependymoma
       - hydromyelia, especially at the level of C2
       - syringomyelia
    c. Spinal arachnoid cyst.
20. Narrowed vertebral canal
    a. CVMM ("Wobbler") syndrome
       - lateral view: dorsoventral narrowing at the cranial end of the affected vertebra
       - VD/DV view: medially deviating pedicles of the caudal vertebral canal
    b. Expansile or healing lesions of adjacent bone
    c. Lumbosacral stenosis
    d. Calcium phosphate deposition disease in Great Dane pups – dorsal displacement of C7 accompanied by deformation of the articular facets.

5.5 Variations in vertebral alignment

The floor of the vertebral canal of adjacent vertebrae should form a continuous straight to gently curved line. Malalignment may be constant and visible on survey radiographs or intermittent and require radiographs to be taken whilst the region is flexed or extended (stress radiography) to demonstrate instability.

1. Scoliosis (lateral curvature)
    a. Muscular spasm
    b. Congenital spinal abnormalities e.g. hemivertebrae, butterfly vertebrae (see 5.3.3, 5.3.5 and Figures 5.3 and 5.4)
    c. Spinal cord abnormalities leading to functional scoliosis
       - Dandy–Walker syndrome
       - spinal dysraphism – Weimaraner
       - hydromyelia/syringomyelia.
2. Lordosis (ventral curvature)
    a. Normal conformational variant
    b. Muscular spasm
    c. Congenital spinal abnormalities, e.g. hemivertebrae (see 5.3.3 and Figure 5.3)
    d. Loss of fibrotic vertebral support – old and heavy dogs
    e. Nutritional secondary hyperparathyroidism (juvenile osteoporosis) (see 1.16.4).

5 SPINE

3. Kyphosis (dorsal curvature)
   a. Normal conformational variant
   b. Muscular spasm
   c. Congenital spinal abnormalities – (see 5.3)
   d. Thoracolumbar disc disease
   e. Discospondylitis
   f. Nutritional secondary hyperparathyroidism (juvenile osteoporosis) (see 1.16.4).
4. Trauma
   a. Fracture
   b. Subluxation
   c. Luxation.
5. Atlantoaxial instability (Figure 5.8) – widening of the space between the roof of C1 and the cranioventral aspect of the spine of C2 which is exacerbated by mild neck flexion. Usually due to defects of the dens (odontoid peg); evaluation of which is best achieved on oblique or VD views of the neck or a RCd open mouth view (taken with care to avoid spinal cord damage).
   a. Congenital atlantoaxial instability – younger miniature and toy breeds, rarely large breed dogs (especially Yorkshire Terrier, Miniature Poodle, Chihuahua, Pomeranian and Maltese). May present clinically at a later age due to superimposed trauma
      • dens agenesis
      • dens hypoplasia
      • non-fusion of the dens to C2 (fusion normally completed at 7–9 months)
      • absence of the dens ligaments
      • cats – dens agenesis resulting from mucopolysaccharidosis
   b. Acquired atlantoaxial instability
      • fracture of the dens or cranial part of C2
      • rupture of the transverse ligament of the atlas.
6. CVMM ("Wobbler") syndrome
   a. Static – malformed caudal cervical vertebrae with craniodorsal subluxation (tipping) of one or more vertebrae and a dorsoventrally narrowed cranial vertebral canal opening. Often accompanied by wedge-shaped or narrowed disc spaces and spondylosis. Very common in the middle aged Dobermann
   b. Dynamic – malalignment only evident with ventroflexion of the neck.
7. Lumbosacral instability – step formation between the last lumbar and first sacral vertebrae. May be seen only on stress radiography of the region. Common in the German Shepherd dog in which transitional lumbosacral vertebrae may predispose to instability.
8. Calcium phosphate deposition disease in Great Dane pups – dorsal displacement of C7 accompanied by deformation of the articular facets.

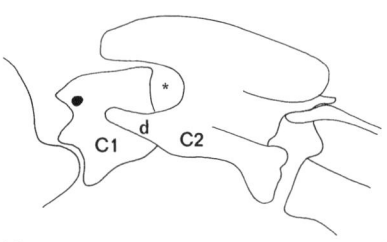

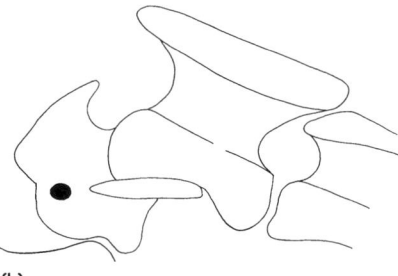

Figure 5.8 Atlantoaxial instability. (a) In the lateral view of a normal spine the spinous process of C2 overhangs the arch of C1, producing a comma-shaped intervertebral foramen *; no alteration is seen on flexion. (b) In atlantoaxial instability flexion occurs at this joint and the intervertebral foramen widens. In this case, C2 lacks a dens (d).

5.6 Diffuse changes in vertebral opacity

Generalised decrease in radio-opacity of the vertebrae [see also 1.16]

1. Artefactual generalised decrease in vertebral radio-opacity
   a. Overexposure
   b. Long scale exposure techniques (high kV, low mAs)
   c. Obese or large patients allowing large amounts of scattered radiation to reach the film, especially if a grid was not used or with inadequate collimation
   d. Overdevelopment
   e. Fogging of the film (numerous causes).

SMALL ANIMAL RADIOLOGICAL DIFFERENTIAL DIAGNOSIS

2. Metabolic bone disease
   a. Secondary hyperparathyroidism
   b. Primary hyperparathyroidism
   c. Corticosteroid excess
      - hyperadrenocorticism – Cushing's disease
      - iatrogenic – long-term corticosteroid administration
   d. Hyperthyroidism
   e. Diabetes mellitus
   f. Congenital hypothyroidism – especially Boxer; delayed closure of vertebral physes and dysgenesis of end plates
   g. Pseudohyperparathyroidism; hypercalcaemia of malignancy
   h. Osteogenesis imperfecta – long bone changes usually predominate.
3. Senile osteoporosis – especially aged cats.
4. Neoplastic
   a. Plasma cell myeloma (multiple myeloma) – genuine osteopenia as well as multiple osteolytic lesions (see 1.18.1 and Figure 1.24).
5. Cats – hypervitaminosis A (raw liver diets); although proliferative bony changes predominate and mask the osteopenia.
6. Cats – mucopolysaccharidosis; likewise.

Generalised increase in radio-opacity of the vertebrae
[see also 1.13]

7. Artefactual generalised increase in vertebral radio-opacity
   a. Underexposure
   b. Underdevelopment.
8. Osteopetrosis – hereditary in the Basenji.
9. Fluorosis.
10. Cats – FeLV-associated medullary sclerosis.

5.7 Localised changes in vertebral opacity

Localised decrease in radio-opacity of one or more vertebrae
[see also 1.18]

1. Artefactual localised decrease in vertebral radio-opacity
   a. Superimposed bowel or lung air on VD or rotated lateral views
   b. Superimposed subcutaneous gas.
2. Decreased radio-opacity of the vertebral endplate
   a. Discospondylitis – end plate also irregular, and sclerotic in chronic cases (see 5.8.3 and Figure 5.9)
   b. Neoplasia – see below
   c. Intravertebral disc herniation (Schmorl's node) – particularly at L7 and/or S1; medium and large breeds, especially German Shepherd dog.
3. Irregular or discrete radiolucencies – single or multiple radiolucent areas involving single or multiple vertebrae and which may be accompanied by bone production
   a. Primary tumour – usually only one vertebra involved
      - osteosarcoma
      - solitary plasma cell myeloma
      - chondrosarcoma
      - fibrosarcoma
   b. Metastatic or infiltrative tumours – may involve multiple vertebrae and may be accompanied by an adjacent soft tissue mass
      - multiple myeloma (plasma cell myeloma)
      - osteosarcoma
      - lymphosarcoma
      - haemangiosarcoma
   c. Aneurysmal bone cyst
4. Linear radiolucencies
   a. Fractures
   b. Widened vertebral physis
      - Salter-Harris fractures in skeletally immature animals
      - vertebral physitis – younger dogs, caudal lumbar physes; may also be associated with portosystemic shunts
      - congenital hypothyroidism – delayed closure of vertebral physes with dysgenesis of end plates; especially Boxer
   c. Dermoid sinus extending to cranial cervical vertebrae – Rhodesian Ridgeback.

Localised increase in radio-opacity of one or more vertebrae

5. Artefactual localised increase in vertebral radio-opacity
   a. Superimposed structures
   b. Underexposure of thicker areas of tissue.
6. Superimposed periosteal or bony reactions
   a. Spondylosis
   b. Discospondylitis
   c. Spondylitis
   d. Neoplasia
      - osteogenic osteosarcoma
      - chondrosarcoma.

7. Fractures
    a. Compression fracture
    b. Healed fracture.
8. Vertebral end-plate sclerosis
    a. With collapsed disc space
        - old disc prolapse, especially at the lumbosacral junction
        - old surgically fenestrated disc
    b. Relative sclerosis compared with osteopenic vertebra (see 1.16 for causes)
    c. Hemivertebra
    d. Adjacent to sacral osteochondrosis – especially German Shepherd dog.
9. Metallic radio-opacity in vertebrae
    a. Bullets and air gun pellets.
10. Lead poisoning – metaphyseal sclerosis.
11. Ossifying pachymeningitis (dural osseous metaplasia) – fine, horizontal lines dorsally and ventrally in the vertebral canal, seen in old age.

Mixed radio-opacity of one or more vertebrae

12. Neoplasia
    a. Primary
    b. Metastatic
    c. Infiltration from adjacent soft tissue tumour.
13. Osteomyelitis/spondylitis
    a. Bacterial
    b. Fungal.

5.8 Abnormalities of the intervertebral disc space

1. Disc space widened
    a. Normal variants
        - lumbar disc spaces are wider than thoracic disc spaces
        - the lumbosacral disc space may be wider than adjacent lumbar disc spaces
    b. Artefactual widening – traction during stress radiography
    c. Apparent widening due to vertebral end-plate erosion
        - discospondylitis
        - osteolytic tumour of adjacent vertebral body
        - intravertebral disc herniation (Schmorl's node) – particularly at L7 and/or S1; medium and large breeds, especially German Shepherd dog
    d. Trauma
        - subluxation
        - luxation
    e. Adjacent to hemivertebra
    f. Cats – mucopolysaccharidosis, due to shortened vertebral bodies.
2. Disc space narrowed or of irregular width
    a. Normal at T10–11 (anticlinal junction)
    b. Artefactual narrowing
        - disc spaces narrow towards the periphery of a radiograph due to divergence of the primary X-ray beam
        - spine not positioned parallel to cassette as result of muscular spasm or incorrect positioning
        - on VD views where the disc space is not parallel to the primary beam (e.g. cervical disc spaces and at the lumbosacral junction)
    c. Prolapsed disc – rare in the cat
        - disc degeneration in middle-aged chondrodystrophic breeds, especially Dachshund – spinal pain or neurological signs tend to have an acute onset due to rupture of the annulus fibrosus and extrusion of calcified disc material into the vertebral canal (Hansen Type I disc disease)
        - disc degeneration in older dogs of other breeds – clinical signs often gradual in onset due to dorsal bulging of disc material and hypertrophy of the overlying annulus fibrosus (Hansen Type II disc disease)
        - trauma – acute onset
    d. CVMM ("Wobbler") syndrome, with malformed lower cervical vertebrae; disc space cranial to the malformed vertebra usually wedge-shaped
    e. After surgical fenestration
    f. Associated with advanced spondylosis
    g. Subluxation due to trauma (orthogonal view may show greater displacement)
    h. Discospondylitis – (see below)
        - early phase before vertebral end-plate osteolysis
        - healing phase
    i. Collapse of disc space due to adjacent vertebral neoplasm
    j. Very narrow disc space within block vertebra – (see 5.3.4)
    k. Adjacent to hemivertebra
    l. Intravertebral disc herniation (Schmorl's node) – particularly L7 and/or S1; medium and large breeds, especially German Shepherd dog.
3. Disc space irregularly marginated
    a. Discospondylitis (Figure 5.9) – end-plate osteolysis creates irregular margins to

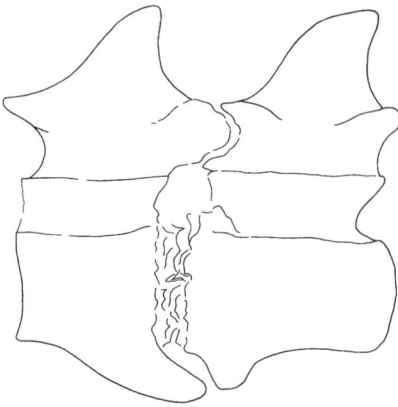

Figure 5.9 Discospondylitis – irregularity of the disc space due to erosion of adjacent vertebral end plates; secondary spondylotic new bone and facet arthropathy.

the disc space, which may be either narrowed or widened. In the early stages the end plates may show decreased radio-opacity but later become sclerotic with surrounding spondylosis. A source of infection should be sought (e.g. cystitis, prostatitis or vegetative endocarditis). At the lumbosacral junction early discospondylitis must be distinguished from intravertebral disc herniation (Schmorl's nodes). Survey lateral radiographs of the rest of the spine should be obtained as multiple disc spaces may be involved
- bacterial – *Staphylococcus aureus* and *S. intermedius*, *Escherichia coli*, *Corynebacterium diphtheria*, *Brucella canis* (mainly USA), *Streptococcus* spp.
- fungal – especially *Aspergillus** spp. in immunocompromised German Shepherd dogs
- viral – bacterial infection secondary to transient immunosuppression with canine parvovirus infection
- iatrogenic – complication of intervertebral disc surgery or discogram
b. Advanced spondylosis
c. Remodelled vertebrae following nutritional secondary hyperparathyroidism
d. Old cats – indentations of multiple end plates are commonly seen
e. Mucopolysaccharidosis.
4. Increased radio-opacity of the disc space
a. Artefactual increased radio-opacity
- superimposed rib or transverse process on lateral radiographs
- vertebral end plate seen obliquely

b. Mineralisation of the nucleus pulposus in chondrodystrophic breeds and older dogs of other breeds (often an incidental finding)
c. Contrast medium deposition during a discogram.
5. Increased radiolucency of the disc space
a. Gas due to vacuum phenomenon – indicative of disc degeneration
- may be consistently present
- may be present only during traction.

5.9 Abnormalities of the intervertebral foramen

The lumbar intervertebral foramina are readily seen on the lateral views, although the thoracic ones are mostly obscured by the ribs. The cervical intervertebral foramina open ventrolaterally and are not seen on the routine lateral view except to a limited extent for that at C2–3. They are best evaluated by making a VD radiograph and tilting the spine 45° to the left and right sides.
1. Opacified intervertebral foramen
a. Normal – superimposition of accessory processes in the thoracolumbar region
b. Artefactual
- superimposed bony rib nodules
- superimposed skin opacities
c. Dorsally prolapsed calcified nucleus pulposus from the disc space
d. Dorsally bulging calcified annulus fibrosus
e. Ossifying pachymeningitis (dural osseous metaplasia) – fine, horizontal linear opacity ventrally or dorsally; more often in larger breeds
f. Expansile or proliferative bony lesions of adjacent vertebrae
g. Bullets, air gun pellets or other missiles.
2. Enlarged intervertebral foramen
a. Neoplasia of nerve root
- neurofibroma
- meningioma
b. After surgery
- foraminotomy or pediculectomy
c. Trauma
- fracture of adjacent vertebra
- vertebral subluxation.
3. Reduced intervertebral foramen size
a. Artefactual due to opacification (see 5.9.1)
b. Disc prolapse with associated narrowing of the disc space
c. Bony proliferative tumour of adjacent vertebra

d. Trauma
   - fracture of adjacent vertebra
   - subluxation
   - callus of a healing/healed vertebral fracture
   e. Block vertebra (see 5.3.4).

5.10 Abnormalities of the articular facets

1. Widened joint space
   a. Normal with ventroflexion of spine
   b. Subluxation
   c. Joint effusion
   d. Severe kyphosis.
2. Narrowed joint space
   a. Associated with narrowed disc space and intervertebral foramen
      - disc disease
      - trauma with (sub)luxation
   b. Spondylarthrosis – see below.
3. Irregular joint space
   a. Spondylarthrosis – degenerative changes of the facetal synovial joint with osteophyte formation. Most commonly seen in the lumbar region, occasionally cervically
      - idiopathic – single or multiple joints in older dogs
      - secondary to trauma – usually a single joint
      - CVMM ("Wobbler") syndrome – in the Great Dane due to malformed and malpositioned articular facets which often show secondary arthrosis
   b. Infection – irregularity of facets is seen in some cases of discospondylitis.

5.11 Lesions in the paravertebral soft tissues

Soft tissue changes in the tissues surrounding the spine may be indicative of trauma, neoplastic or infectious changes which could involve the spine.
1. Gas accumulation in paravertebral soft tissues
   a. Trauma with an open wound
   b. Gas-producing bacterial infection.
2. Metallic foreign bodies
   a. Bullets, air-gun pellets and other missiles
   b. Needles etc. that may have been ingested and exited the gut.
3. Swelling of paravertebral soft tissues – more likely in the sublumbar and lumbosacral region, often displacing the descending colon ventrally
   a. Reactive lymph nodes
   b. Neoplasia
      - osseous
      - soft tissue
   c. Abscess
   d. Granuloma
   e. Haematoma.
4. Mineralisation in the paravertebral soft tissues
   a. Dystrophic mineralisation in a tumour
   b. Calcinosis circumscripta – in soft tissues at the level of C1–2 and C5–6 and occasionally elsewhere near the spine. Especially affects young German Shepherd dogs (see 12.2.2 and Figure 12.1).

5.12 Spinal contrast studies – technique and normal appearance

Myelography

Myelography involves opacification of the subarachnoid space which may be performed via either the cervical or the lumbar route. The latter is regarded as safer for the patient but is more difficult to perform. Reliability of results can be improved by injecting the contrast medium at the site closest to the suspected lesion.

The patient is anaesthetised and the site prepared for aseptic injection. The normal dosage rate is 0.3 ml/kg of iopamidol or iohexol at a concentration of 250–300 mg iodine/ml, with a minimum of 2 ml for cats and small dogs. Cerebrospinal fluid may be collected before injecting the contrast medium. The contrast medium should be warmed to reduce its viscosity.

CERVICAL (CISTERNA MAGNA) MYELOGRAPHY

An assistant holds the animal's head at right angles to the neck with the median plane of the nose and skull parallel to the table. The spinal needle must penetrate the skin at a point in the midline midway between the levels of the external occipital protuberance of the skull and the cranial edges of the wings of the atlas, these landmarks being palpated.

In small dogs and cats a 4–5 cm 22-gauge spinal needle is used; once the skin has been penetrated the stilette should be removed and the needle advanced slowly. In larger dogs a 6–9-cm needle is required and the stilette is left in the needle until the resistance offered by the strong dorsal atlanto-occipital ligament is felt or until the ligament has been perforated. When the needle enters the subarachnoid space cerebrospinal fluid will begin to flow from the needle and may be collected for analysis. The needle should be held firmly at its point of entrance through the skin to prevent movement of the tip when the syringe is attached. The contrast medium is injected slowly over about 1 minute.

LUMBAR MYELOGRAPHY

Injection may be made with the patient in lateral or sternal recumbency; many operators prefer the spine to be flexed. The site of injection should be L5–6 in dogs, L6–7 in cats (Figure 5.10). The dorsal spinous process of L6 is located just cranial to a line through the wings of the ilium and the spinal needle is introduced flush against its cranial edge in a direction perpendicular to the long axis of the spine and parallel or vertical to the table top (depending on the patient's position) until solid resistance by the bony vertebral canal floor is felt. The spinal cord is deliberately penetrated to reach the more voluminous ventral subarachnoid space. Penetration of the cauda equina often results in a hindquarter jerk or anal twitch indicating correct needle placement. If the needle will not enter the vertebral canal it must be redirected slightly. The stilette is removed when the needle tip is in the vertebral canal. Free flow of cerebrospinal fluid confirms correct needle position, although the amount of fluid obtained is usually much less than with cervical puncture and lack of cerebrospinal fluid flow does not necessarily indicate incorrect placement of the needle.

If severe spinal cord compression or swelling is suspected the contrast medium must be injected rapidly over 10 seconds and exposures made immediately and again after 30 seconds. The first exposure will show the caudal edge of the lesion to best advantage and the slightly delayed one the cranial end.

NORMAL MYELOGRAPHIC APPEARANCE

On the lateral radiograph dorsal and ventral contrast columns are visible; on the VD view the lateral columns are seen. The columns are of even width along the vertebral canal except cranially, within C1 and C2, where they are dilated due to the cisterna magna. The spinal cord creates a non-opacified band between the columns, with mild diffuse enlargement at the brachial and lumbar intumescentia. The spinal cord is relatively large compared with the size of the vertebral canal in small dogs and cats, and appears relatively smaller in large breeds of dog. The ventral contrast column is often slightly indented over the disc spaces without effect on the diameter of the spinal cord. From the midlumbar area, the spinal cord tapers and is surrounded by the nerves forming the cauda equina, creating a converging, striated appearance. Extension of the dural sac across the lumbosacral disc space is variable among dogs. In cats, the spinal cord extends more caudally.

COMPLICATIONS OF MYELOGRAPHY

1. Seizures.
2. Aggravation of clinical signs may occur within the first day – these are related to manipulation during positioning.
3. Injection into the central canal of the spinal cord may cause severe paresis or paralysis depending on the quantity of contrast medium injected. Such injections usually occur with lumbar puncture performed cranial to L5–6 (Figure 5.10).
4. Apnoea can occur if the injection is given too rapidly via the cisternal route.
5. Death – penetrating the spinal cord with the needle during cisternal myelography.

Epidurography

Epidurography is used mainly to investigate cauda equina syndrome. The patient may be positioned in sternal or lateral recumbency. A spinal needle is introduced into the epidural space via the sacrocaudal junction or between caudal vertebrae 1 and 2 or 2 and 3. The lumbosacral junction should usually be avoided as pathology is often located at this site. In large breed dogs about 4–8 ml of contrast medium is injected and immediate lateral and DV or VD radiographs taken.

The normal epidurogram creates an undulating or scalloped appearance, with the ventral contrast column elevated over each disc space and draped more ventrally in between. It is much harder to interpret than a myelogram.

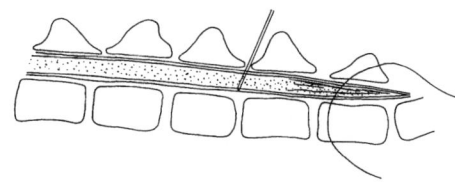

Figure 5.10 Normal lumbar myelogram with correct needle placement at L5–6.

Discography

Discography is most often performed at the lumbosacral junction in order to detect disc degeneration. The normal nucleus pulposus is difficult to inject whilst degenerate discs accommodate more contrast medium and may show dorsal leakage. Needle placement is facilitated by the use of fluoroscopy with image intensification. However, discography is being superseded by the use of CT and MRI.

5.13 Technical errors during myelography

General myelography: technical errors (Figure 5.11)

1. Single or multiple 1–3-mm diameter radiolucent filling defects – air bubbles due to air in syringe during injection.
2. Contrast medium in soft tissues dorsal to injection site – leakage of contrast medium up the needle tract.

Cervical myelogram: technical errors

1. Poor distribution of contrast medium in the subarachnoid space resulting in an uneven or bizarre myelographic appearance; DDx – severe meningitis, diffuse neoplasia (e.g. lymphosarcoma)
   a. Inadequate subarachnoid volume of contrast medium
      - initial volume too small
      - marked extradural injection or leakage (see below)
   b. Contrast medium not warmed to body temperature; poor mixing with cerebrospinal fluid may contribute
   c. Injecting too slowly may contribute
2. Subdural contrast medium injection or leakage – contrast medium lies mainly dorsally, is very dense and has an undulating, scalloped inner margin and a knife-shaped distal termination.
3. Contrast medium in the central canal
   a. Central canal >2 mm wide
      - inadvertent injection into hydromyelic cord. Unlikely to result in additional neurological effects
   b. Central canal 0.5–2 mm wide
      - reflux into the canal if the spinal needle accidentally penetrated the spinal cord and passed through or close to the canal.
4. Contrast medium accidentally injected into the spinal cord parenchyma – the prognosis for patient survival is volume dependent.
5. Contrast medium does not pass an obstructive lesion – try elevating head and neck further to gravitate the contrast medium past the obstructive site
   a. Lack of pressure of cisterna magna injection does not allow contrast medium to force its way past lesions totally obstructing the subarachnoid space. An additional lumbar puncture myelogram should be performed
   b. Inadequate volume of contrast medium
   c. If contrast medium does not outline the caudal cervical region on a VD radiograph, obtain a DV radiograph to encourage pooling of contrast medium in this area.

Lumbar myelogram: technical errors

1. Scalloped appearance of contrast medium
   a. Epidural injection
      - needle tip too deep when in the ventral part of the vertebral canal
      - multiple dural punctures with contrast leaking out of the subarachnoid space
      - needle tip in an extradural mass lesion.
2. Subdural contrast medium injection or leakage – contrast medium lies mainly dorsally, is very dense and has an undulating, scalloped inner margin and a knife-shaped termination.
3. Contrast medium pooling in the intervertebral foramina and around nerve roots – epidural injection.
4. Contrast medium in sublumbar vasculature, lymphatics and lymph nodes – epidural injection.
5. Contrast medium in the central canal – more likely to occur with needle place-

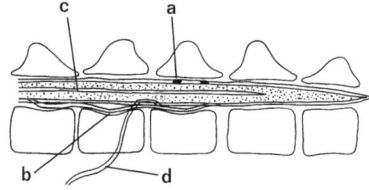

Figure 5.11 Lumbar myelogram showing technical errors. (a) Air bubbles in the contrast medium; (b) epidural leakage of contrast medium; (c) contrast medium in the central canal of the spinal cord; and (d) leakage of contrast medium into vessels.

SMALL ANIMAL RADIOLOGICAL DIFFERENTIAL DIAGNOSIS

ment cranial to the recommended L5–6 interarcuate space
  a. Central canal 0.5–2 mm wide
     - reflux into the canal if the spinal needle passed through or close to the canal
     - aberrant communication between the subarachnoid space and the central canal due to tumour, prolapsed disc or malacic cord
  b. Central canal >2 mm wide
     - iatrogenic distension of the central canal due to direct injection. Depending on the extent, the dog may go into respiratory or cardiac arrest and will develop neurological deficits, which are likely to improve over time
     - hydromyelia.
6. Contrast medium injected into the spinal cord parenchyma.

5.14 Extradural spinal cord compression on myelography

The spinal cord is narrowed on one view and widened on the orthogonal projection (Figure 5.12). Occasionally an hour-glass compression is seen with neoplasia or haematoma which may encircle the cord.

1. Normal variants – slight compression of the ventral subarachnoid space with no attenuation of the opposite contrast medium column or spinal cord
   a. Ventrally over C2–3 disc space
   b. Dorsally at the C3–4–5–6–7 articulations
   c. Ventrally over other disc spaces, especially in large breeds of dog.
2. Disc extrusion (Hansen Type I disc disease). Spinal cord compression may be from any direction.
   a. Thoracolumbar region (T11–L2), especially in chondrodystrophic breeds; more caudal lumbar disc spaces are less often affected. Extrusion of disc material, and thus spinal compression, may be ventral, ventrolateral, lateral, dorsolateral and occasionally dorsal, or in combinations of these locations. Oblique views are helpful to localise disc material, which is usually at or cranial to the affected disc space.
      Disc lesions T1–T10 are unusual due to the presence of the intercapital ligament between the heads of the ribs.

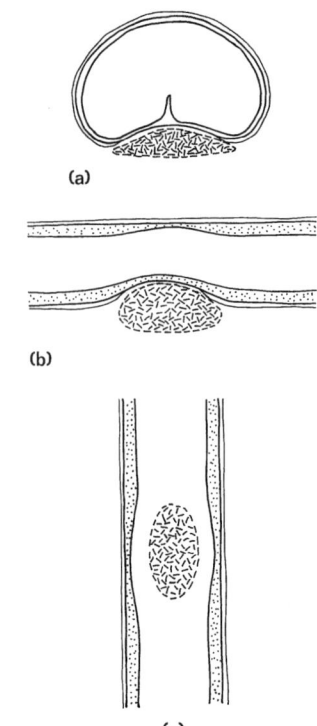

Figure 5.12 Schematic representation of an extradural lesion. (a) mass position, lying outside the meninges; (b) myelogram view tangential to the lesion shows spinal cord compression; (c) the orthogonal view shows apparent spinal cord widening.

   b. Cervical region (C2–C7) in any breed of dog, mainly smaller breeds. The major clinical sign is often neck pain rather than a neurological deficit. The disc material usually lies ventrally or ventrolaterally.
   c. CVMM ("Wobbler") syndrome – lower cervical region in large breed dogs, especially Dobermann and Rottweiler. Mainly ventrally. Traction or ventroflexion of the neck has minimal effect on the compression. However, disc lesions secondary to

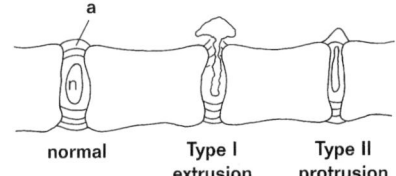

Figure 5.13 Normal disc (n = nucleus pulposus; a = annulus fibrosus); Type I disc disease (extrusion); Type II disc disease (protrusion).

CCVM are more often protrusions than extrusions – see below
   d. Lumbosacral disc, particularly larger breeds, especially German Shepherd dog. Disc material lies ventrally. Again, disc protrusions are more common than extrusions
   e. Adjacent to deformed vertebrae or rigid sections of the spine (e.g. hemivertebrae, block vertebra and areas of ankylosed spondylosis).
3. Hypertrophied annulus fibrosis/disc protrusion (Hansen Type II disc disease) – ventral compression of spinal cord
   a. CVMM ("Wobbler") syndrome – lower cervical region; large breed dogs, especially Dobermann and Rottweiler. Traction or ventroflexion of the neck decreases the compression by "flattening" the bulging soft tissue
   b. Lumbosacral region, especially larger breeds such as the German Shepherd dog.
4. Hypertrophied ligamentum flavum (interarcuate ligament) – dorsal compression of spinal cord
   a. CVMM ("Wobbler") syndrome – large-breed dogs. Ventroflexion of the neck decreases the compression, dorsiflexion of the neck aggravates the compression. C5–C7 especially Great Dane, C2–C3 Rottweiler
   b. Lumbosacral instability.
5. Extradural neoplasia with or without bony changes
   a. Primary or metastatic tumour in surrounding bone – often osteolytic lesions and may be accompanied by pathological fractures
      • various histological types in adults
      • in young animals, consider osteochondroma (may be multiple)
   b. Originating from soft tissues within the vertebral canal
      • neurofibroma
      • myxoma/myxosarcoma
      • meningioma
      • lymphosarcoma
      • lipoma/angiolipoma
      • haemangiosarcoma
   c. Paraspinal tumour from the soft tissues surrounding the vertebral column
      • phaeochromocytoma, usually cranial lumbar region
   d. Cats – lymphosarcoma from as young as 6 months, often thoracolumbar region.
6. Extradural bony lesions
   a. Neoplasia – see above
   b. Congenital vertebral malformations (see 5.3)
   c. Trauma
      • fracture; acute fracture or fracture healing with callus formation
      • spinal luxation or subluxation
   d. CVMM ("Wobbler") syndrome
      • ventral or dorsal compression – especially lower cervical region, seen on lateral view (see 5.3.8 and Figure 5.5)
      • dorsolateral compression – malformation of articular facets; especially lower cervical region; Great Danes
      • medially converging caudal cervical pedicles – only visible on VD view
   e. Cats – hypervitaminosis A – occasionally causes spinal cord compression (see 5.4.8).
7. Extradural haematoma/haemorrhage
   a. Trauma
      • external trauma e.g. road traffic accident
      • internal trauma due to acute disc prolapse or dural tearing
      • post-surgical haemorrhage
      • iatrogenic haemorrhage caused by spinal needle
   b. Coagulopathy
      • haemophilia A, especially young male German Shepherd dogs
      • anticoagulant poisoning
      • thrombocytopenia
   c. Haemorrhage secondary to
      • tumour
      • vascular malformation
      • parasitic migration
      • meningitis
      • necrotising vasculitis – Bernese Mountain dog, German Shorthaired Pointer and Beagle
   d. Subperiosteal vertebral haematoma.
8. Extradural infectious process, focal abscess or more diffuse empyema
   a. Extension from discospondylitis (see 5.8.3)
      • bacterial
      • fungal
   b. Haematogenous infection
      • bacterial
      • fungal
   c. Extension from spondylitis (see 5.4.4)
      • bacterial
      • fungal
      • parasitic e.g. *Spirocerca lupi**.

SMALL ANIMAL RADIOLOGICAL DIFFERENTIAL DIAGNOSIS

9. Membrane disease (epidural scarring) – weeks to months after laminectomy or hemilaminectomy.
10. Synovial joint lesions – dorsolateral compression
    a. CVMM ("Wobbler") syndrome – synovitis of joints between articular facets especially in the lower cervical region
    b. Synovial cysts.
11. Parasites
    a. Granuloma from aberrant migration of *Spirocerca lupi** in the caudal thoracic region
    b. Aberrant migration of heartworm (*Dirofilaria immitis**).
12. Aneurysm of venous sinus.
13. Calcinosis circumscripta – extradural location reported; especially young German Shepherd dogs.
14. Extradural foreign body e.g. pieces of wood from pharyngeal stick injuries.

5.15 Intradural extramedullary spinal cord compression on myelography

The column of contrast medium splits ("golf tee sign") or widens ("tear drop" shape) and often shows abrupt termination (Figure 5.14). A split contrast column must be differentiated from focal extradural compression by utilising oblique views.
1. Neoplasia – nerve root tumours may also cause enlargement of the intervertebral foramen
    a. Neurofibroma (Schwannoma) – mainly lower cervical region and often near an intervertebral foramen
    b. Meningioma – mainly lower cervical region and often near an intervertebral foramen
    c. Neurofibrosarcoma
    d. Nephroblastoma – caudal thoracic to cranial lumbar region in young dogs
    e. Myxoma/myxosarcoma
    f. Ependymoma
    g. Lymphosarcoma – especially cats (although more often extradural).
2. Prolapsed disc material that ruptures dural membranes.
3. Subdural haematoma/haemorrhage (see 5.14.7 for causes of spinal haemorrhage).
4. Spinal arachnoid cyst – bulbous or tear drop shaped contrast medium filled cavity compressing the adjacent spinal cord. Usually dorsally in C2–C3 or T8–T10 region.

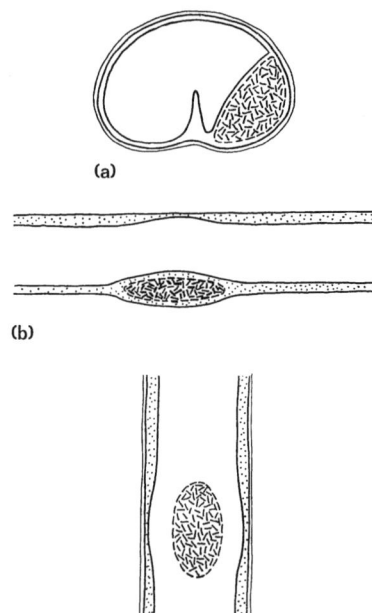

Figure 5.14 Schematic representation of an extramedullary, intradural lesion. (a) Mass position, lying within the meninges but outside the spinal cord; (b) myelogram view tangential to the lesion shows spinal cord compression but splitting of the contrast column, which often terminates; (c) the orthogonal view shows apparent spinal cord widening due to spinal cord compression in the other plane.

5.16 Intramedullary spinal cord enlargement on myelography

The spinal cord is widened on all views with internal attenuation of contrast columns and general reduction of contrast opacity in the area (Figure 5.15).
1. Normal spinal cord enlargement
    a. Brachial intumescence – lower neck
    b. Lumbar intumescence – mid lumbar area
    c. The spinal cord-to-canal ratio is larger in cats and small-breed dogs than in large-breed dogs.
2. Neoplasia – most commonly seen at the cervicothoracic and thoracolumbar junctions
    a. Primary spinal cord tumours
        • astrocytoma
        • oligodendroglioma
        • ependymoma

5 SPINE

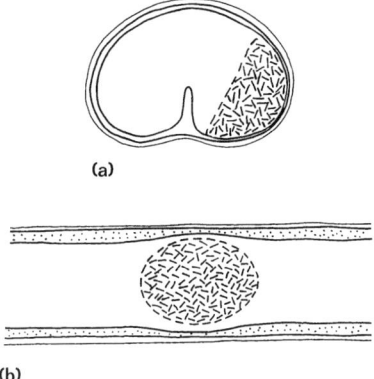

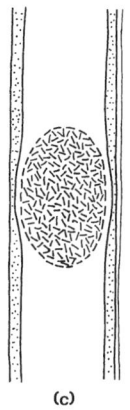

Figure 5.15 Schematic representation of an intramedullary lesion. (a) Mass position, lying within the spinal cord; (b) and (c) myelogram views from any angle show spinal cord widening.

- neurofibroma
- lymphosarcoma
  b. Metastatic spinal cord tumours
  c. Intradural extramedullary tumour infiltrating the spinal cord.
3. Haemorrhage and/or oedema of the spinal cord
  a. Acute spinal cord injury
     - external trauma (e.g. road traffic accident)
     - internal trauma due to acute disc prolapse
     - post-surgical effects on the spinal cord
  b. Coagulopathy
     - haemophilia A, especially in young male German Shepherd dogs
     - anti-coagulant poisoning
     - thrombocytopenia
  c. Haemorrhage secondary to
     - tumour

- vascular malformation
- parasitic migration.
4. Fibrocartilagenous infarct – rarely causes spinal cord swelling; diagnosis often made based on typical history and lack of myelographic findings.
5. Granulomatous meningoencephalomyelitis (GME) – rarely causes spinal cord swelling; diagnosis often made based on clinical signs and cerebrospinal analysis.
6. Hydromyelia – especially cervical area associated with Chiari malformation in Cavalier King Charles Spaniel.
7. Syringomyelia.
8. Dermoid or epidermoid cysts.

5.17 Miscellaneous myelographic findings

1. Narrowed spinal cord with no external compression
   a. Spinal cord atrophy due to chronic compression, e.g. at site of Type II disc protrusion
   b. Progressive haemorrhagic myelomalacia – often in non-responding acute disc prolapse. Contrast medium is retained within damaged cord tissue
   c. Spinal dysraphism – Weimaraner.
2. Myelomalacia – contrast medium migrates into damaged cord tissue.
3. Spina bifida – contrast medium extends dorsally beyond the normal dural confines into a meningocoele or myelomeningocoele (see 5.3.12).

5.18 Neurological deficits involving the spinal cord or proximal nerve roots with normal survey radiographs and myelogram radiographs

Ensure that the clinical signs are not due to an orthopaedic problem, myopathy, muscular dystrophy, neuromuscular transmission disorder, peripheral neuropathy or infectious agent.

Congenital/hereditary diseases

DOGS

1. Neuroaxonal dystrophy – starts 1+ year in Rottweiler and 6+ weeks in Papillon.
2. Canine giant axonal neuropathy – starts 14+ months. Megaoesophagus may develop. German Shepherd dog.
3. Central peripheral neuropathy – starts 2+ months. Boxer.

4. Spinal muscular atrophy – starts 6+ weeks. Swedish Lapland dog, Brittany Spaniel, German Shepherd dog, Rottweiler, English Pointer.
5. Globoid cell leucodystrophy – starts 4+ months. West Highland White terrier, Cairn terrier, Poodle, Pomeranian, Beagle and Basset hound.
6. Spinal dysraphism – Weimaraner.
7. Hereditary myelopathy – 6–13 months. Afghan hound.
8. Hereditary ataxia – 2–6 months. Fox Terrier and Jack Russell Terrier.
9. Progressive neuronopathy – 5+ months. Cairn Terrier.
10. Sensory neuropathy – 3–8 months. English Pointer.
11. Inherited hypertrophic neuropathy – 7–12 weeks. Tibetan Mastiff.
12. Hydromyelia.
13. Syringomyelia.

CATS

14. Distal polyneuropathy – 6+ weeks. Birman.
15. Globoid cell leucodystrophy – Domestic Shorthaired cat.
16. Neuroaxonal dystrophy – 6 weeks.

Acquired diseases

DOGS

1. Degenerative myelopathy – 6+ years. German Shepherd dogs and cross-breeds and occasionally other large-breed dogs.
2. Fibrocartilagenous embolism with secondary necrotising myelopathy. Usually middle-aged large and giant breeds.
3. Acute idiopathic polyradiculoneuritis – adults of any breed.
4. Coonhound paralysis – acute polyradiculoneuritis after a racoon bite – adults of any breed.
5. GME – 1+ years. Smaller breeds, especially Poodle types.
6. Corticosteroid responsive meningitis (aseptic meningitis) – young medium to large-breed dogs.
7. Secondary to modified live rabies vaccine – 7–10 days post-vaccination.
8. Ischaemic neuromyopathy due to caudal aorta thromboembolism.
9. Leucoencephalomyelopathy – 1.5–4 years +. Rottweiler.
10. Hound ataxia – 2–7 years. Fox Hound, Harrier Hound and Beagle.
11. Meningeal fibrosis with axonal degeneration secondary to necrotising vasculitis – 5–13 months. Bernese Mountain dog, German Short-haired Pointer and Beagle.
12. Chronic relapsing idiopathic polyradiculoneuritis.
13. Demyelinating myelopathy – 2–4 months. Miniature Poodles.
14. Hydromyelia.
15. Syringomyelia.

CATS

16. Ischaemic neuromyopathy due to caudal aorta thromboembolism – secondary to cardiac disease.
17. Fibrocartilagenous embolism with secondary necrotising myelopathy.
18. Secondary to modified live rabies vaccine – 7–10 days post-vaccination.
19. Feline polioencephalomyelitis – 6+ months.
20. Degenerative myelopathy.
21. Chronic relapsing idiopathic polyradiculoneuritis.
22. Hydromyelia.
23. Syringomyelia.

FURTHER READING

General

Dennis, R. (1987) Radiographic examination of the canine spine. *Veterinary Record* **121** 31–35.

McKee, M. (1993) Differential diagnosis of cauda equina syndrome. *In Practice* **15** 243–250.

McKee, M. (1996) Cervical pain in small animals. *In Practice* **18** 169–184.

Morgan, J.P. and Bailey, C.S. (1990) Cauda equina syndrome in the dog: Radiographic evaluation. *Journal of Small Animal Practice* **31** 69–77.

Congenital and developmental diseases; diseases of young animals

Bailey, C.S. and Morgan, J.P. (1992) Congenital spinal malformations. *Veterinary Clinics of North America; Small Animal Practice* **22** 985–1015.

Braund, K.G. (1994) Pediatric neuropathies. *Seminars in Veterinary Medicine and Surgery (Small Animals)* **9** 86–98.

Lang, J., Haeni, H., and Schawalder, P. (1992) A sacral lesion resembling osteochondrosis in the

German Shepherd dog. *Veterinary Radiology and Ultrasound* **33** 69–76.

Morgan, J.P. (1999) Transitional lumbosacral vertebral anomaly in the dog: a radiographic study. *Journal of Small Animal Practice* **40** 167–172.

Sharp, N.J.H., Wheeler, S.J., Cofone, M. (1992) Radiological evaluation of 'wobbler' syndrome – caudal cervical spondylomyelopathy. *Journal of Small Animal Practice* **33** 491–499.

Metabolic diseases (some overlap with above)

Konde, L.J., Thrall, M.A., Gasper, P., Dial, S.M., McBiles, K., Colgan, S. and Haskins, M. (1987) Radiographically visualized skeletal changes associated with mucopolysaccharidosis VI in cats. *Veterinary Radiology* **28** 223–228.

Infective and inflammatory conditions

Dvir, E., Kirberger, R.M. and Mallaczek, D. (2001) Radiographic and computed tomographic changes and clinical presentation of spirocercosis in the dog. *Veterinary Radiology and Ultrasound* In press.

Jimenez, M.M. and O'Callaghan, M.W. (1995) Vertebral physitis: a radiographic diagnosis to be separated from discospondylitis. *Veterinary Radiology and Ultrasound* **36** 188–195.

Kornegay, J.N., Barber, D.L. (1980) Discospondylitis in dogs. *Journal of the American Veterinary Medical Association* **177** 337–341.

Neoplasia

Gilmore, D.R. (1983) Intraspinal tumours in the dog. *Compendium of Continuing Education for the Practicing Veterinarian* **5** 55–64.

Levy, M.S., Kapatkin, A.S., Patnaik, A.K., Mauldin, G.E. (1997) Spinal tumours in 37 dogs: Clinical outcome and long-term survival (1987–1994). *Journal of the American Animal Hospital Association* **33** 307–312.

Morgan, J.P., Ackerman, N., Bailey, C.S., Pool, R.R. (1980) Vertebral tumors in the dog: A clinical, radiologic, and pathologic study of 61 primary and secondary lesions. *Veterinary Radiology* **21** 197–212.

Trauma

Anderson, A. and Coughlan, A.R. (1997) Sacral fractures in dogs and cats: a classification scheme and review of 51 cases. *Journal of Small Animal Practice* **38** 404–409.

Hay, C.W. and Muir, P. (2000) Tearing of the dura mater in three dogs. *Veterinary Record* **146** 279–282.

Roush, J.K., Douglass, J.P., Hertzke, D. and Kennedy, G.A. (1992) Traumatic dural laceration in a racing greyhound. *Veterinary Radiology and Ultrasound* **33** 22–24.

Yarrow, T.G. and Jeffery, N.D. (2000) Dura mater laceration associated with acute paraplegia in three dogs. *Veterinary Record* **146** 138–139.

Miscellaneous conditions

Cauzinille, L. and Kornegay, J.N. (1996) Fibrocartilagenous embolism of the spinal cord in dogs: Review of 36 histologically confirmed cases and retrospective study of 26 suspected cases. *Journal of Veterinary Internal Medicine* **10** 241–245.

Chrisman, C.L. (1992) Neurological diseases of Rottweilers: Neuroaxonal dystrophy and leucoencephalomalacia. *Journal of Small Animal Practice* **33** 500–504.

Dyce, J., Herrtage, M.E., Houlton, J.E.F. and Palmer, A.C. (1991) Canine spinal "arachnoid cysts". *Journal of Small Animal Practice* **32** 433–437.

Dyce, J. and Houlton, J.E.F. (1993) Fibrocartilaginous embolism in the dog (review). *Journal of Small Animal Practice* **34** 332–336.

Gaschen, L., Lang, J. and Haeni, H. (1995) Intravertebral disc herniation (Schmorl's node) in five dogs. *Veterinary Radiology and Ultrasound* **36** 509–516.

Kirberger, R.M., Jacobson, L.S., Davies, J.V. and Engela, J. (1997) Hydromyelia in the dog. *Veterinary Radiology and Ultrasound* **38** 30–38.

Morgan, J.P. and Stavenborn, M. (1991) Disseminated idiopathic skeletal hyperostosis (DISH) in a dog. *Veterinary Radiology* **32** 65–70.

Contrast radiography of the spine

Barthez, P.Y., Morgan, J.P. and Lipsitz, D. (1994) Discography and epidurography for evaluation of the lumbosacral junction in dogs with cauda equina syndrome. *Veterinary Radiology and Ultrasound* **35** 152–157.

Kirberger, R.M., Roos, C.J. and Lubbe, A.M. (1992) The radiological diagnosis of thoracolumbar disc disease in the dachshund. *Veterinary Radiology and Ultrasound* **33** 255–261.

Kirberger, R.M. and Wrigley, R.H. (1993) Myelography in the dog: Review of patients with contrast medium in the central canal. *Veterinary Radiology and Ultrasound* **34** 253–258.

Kirberger, R.M. (1994) Recent developments in canine lumbar myelography. *Compendium of Continuing Education for the Practicing Veterinarian (Small Animal)* **16** 847–854.

Lamb, C.R. (1994) Common difficulties with myelographic diagnosis of acute intervertebral disc prolapse in the dog. *Journal of Small Animal Practice* **35** 549–558

Lang, J. (1988) Flexion-extension myelography of the canine cauda equina. *Veterinary Radiology* **29** 242–257.

Matteucci, M.L., Ramirez III, O. and Thrall, D.E. (1999) Radiographic diagnosis: effect of right versus left lateral recumbency on myelographic appearance of a lateralized extradural mass. *Veterinary Radiology and Ultrasound* **40** 351–352.

Penderis, J., Sullivan, M., Schwarz, T. and Griffiths, I.R. (1999) Subdural injection of contrast medium as a complication of myelography. *Journal of Small Animal Practice* **40** 173–176.

Ramerez III, O. and Thrall, D.E. (1998) A review of imaging techniques for cauda equina syndrome. *Veterinary Radiology and Ultrasound* **39** 283–296.

Roberts, R.E. and Selcer, B.A. (1993) Myelography and epidurography. *Veterinary Clinics of North America; Small Animal Practice* **23** 307–328.

Scrivani, P.V., Barthez, P.Y. and Leveille, R. (1996) Radiology corner: The fallibility of the myelographic "double line" sign. *Veterinary Radiology and Ultrasound* **37** 264–265.

Scrivani, P.V., (2000) Myelographic artefacts. *Veterinary Clinics of North America; Small Animal Practice* **30** 303–314.

Stickle, R., Lowrie, C. and Oakley, R. (1998) Radiology corner: Another example of the myelographic "double line" sign. *Veterinary Radiology and Ultrasound* **39** 543.

Weber, W.J. and Berry, C.R. (1994) Radiology corner: Determining the location of contrast medium on the canine lumbar myelogram. *Veterinary Radiology and Ultrasound* **35** 430–432.

6

Lower respiratory tract

6.1 Radiographic technique for the thorax
6.2 Ultrasonographic technique for the thorax
6.3 Poor intrathoracic ultrasonographic visualisation
6.4 Thoracic radiographic changes associated with ageing
6.5 Border effacement in the thorax
6.6 Tracheal displacement
6.7 Variations in tracheal diameter
6.8 Tracheal lumen opacification
6.9 Variations in tracheal wall visibility
6.10 Ultrasonography of the trachea
6.11 Changes of the main-stem bronchi
6.12 Bronchial lung pattern
6.13 Artefactual increase in lung opacity
6.14 Alveolar lung pattern
6.15 Poorly marginated pulmonary opacities or areas of consolidation
6.16 Ultrasonography of areas of alveolar filling
6.17 Single consolidated lung lobe
6.18 Ultrasonography of consolidated lung lobes
6.19 Solitary pulmonary nodules or masses
6.20 Nodular lung pattern
6.21 Ultrasonography of pulmonary nodules or masses
6.22 Diffuse, unstructured, interstitial lung pattern
6.23 Linear or reticular interstitial lung pattern
6.24 Vascular lung pattern
6.25 Mixed lung pattern
6.26 Generalised pulmonary hyperlucency
6.27 Focal areas of pulmonary hyperlucency (including cavitary lesions)
6.28 Intrathoracic mineralised opacities
6.29 Hilar masses
6.30 Increased visibility of lung or lobar edges

6.1 Radiographic technique for the thorax

Precise positioning using artificial aids is required, with the front limbs pulled forwards to avoid overlay of the cranial thorax. True lateral and DV/VD positioning should be ensured. In lateral recumbency the upper lung lobes are seen better, due to relatively increased aeration. The dependent lobes are poorly aerated, meaning that smaller lesions may be overlooked. In dorsal recumbency for the VD view the cardiac silhouette tends to displace cranially, allowing greater visualisation of the accessory lung lobe region; the divergence of the X-ray beam plus the shape of the diaphragm also means that more of the caudal lung field will be visible. However, the VD view may be less accurate than the DV for assessment of cardiac size and shape.

A minimum of two views are required to build up a three-dimensional image (i.e. a right or left lateral recumbent and a DV or VD radiograph). Some radiologists prefer left lateral recumbency (LLR) and VD for general thoracic evaluation and right lateral recumbency (RLR) and DV for assessment of the heart, but consistency of technique is probably more important. A combination of RLR and LLR +/− VD views is recommended for suspected metastases or small, poorly-defined pulmonary lesions. Dorsal recumbency for a VD view is contraindicated in patients with severe dyspnoea. Additional radiographs taken using a horizontal X-ray beam utilising the effect of gravity may be required to highlight certain types of pathology such as mediastinal masses, small amounts of free fluid or air and emphysema.

A fast film/screen combination should be used to minimise motion blur and a grid should be employed if the chest is greater than 12 cm thick or in smaller, obese dogs. A long scale contrast technique (high kV, low mAs) will reduce the naturally high contrast in the thorax and increase the lung detail visible, as well as reducing the exposure time.

Exposure should be made at the end of inspiration to maximise lung aeration and optimise contrast, using manual inflation if necessary in anaesthetised patients (allowing for radiation safety).

Optimal evaluation of thoracic radiographs requires a systematic approach which involves assessing radiographic technique, extrathoracic structures (soft tissues, osseous structures, thoracic inlet and diaphragm) and intrathoracic structures, and then re-evaluating abnormalities and areas indicated by clinical history. Intrathoracic evaluation is done on a system basis: respiratory, cardiovascular, pleural space and mediastinum (including the oesophagus). On placing radiographs on the viewing box, the standard convention is that lateral views are positioned with the thoracic inlet facing to the left; DV/VD views are placed with the thoracic inlet uppermost and the left side of the patient on the right side of the viewing box.

6.2 Ultrasonographic technique for the thorax

Sector or curvilinear transducers allow optimal access to intrathoracic structures. As high a frequency as possible should be selected whilst still achieving adequate tissue penetration (e.g. 7.5 MHz for cats/small dogs and 5 MHz for medium/large dogs). An acoustic window that overlies the area of interest is chosen, avoiding intervening skeletal structures and minimising the amount of interposed air-filled lung. In general this means placing the transducer in an appropriate intercostal space, but parts of the thorax may also be imaged from a cranial abdominal approach through the liver, or from the thoracic inlet. When the patient is in lateral recumbency, the dependent lung lobes become compressed, and less interference from air-filled lung then occurs if the thorax is imaged from beneath. The position of the animal can be altered if necessary to make use of the effects of gravity on the distribution of free fluid or free air in the thoracic cavity. Free fluid acts as an excellent acoustic window and thoracic ultrasound should be performed before any thoracocentesis.

The chosen acoustic window should be carefully prepared by clipping hair from the area, cleaning the skin with surgical spirit to remove dirt and grease, and applying liberal quantities of acoustic gel.

6.3 Poor intrathoracic ultrasonographic visualisation

May be due to any combination of the following factors.
1. Poor preparation of the scanning site.
2. Poor skin–transducer contact.
3. Rib interposed between the transducer and the region of interest.
4. Too much aerated lung interposed between the transducer and the region of interest.
5. Free air in the thoracic cavity.
6. Subcutaneous emphysema.
7. Obesity.
8. Calcification of intrathoracic structures sufficient to result in acoustic shadowing.

6.4 Thoracic radiographic changes associated with ageing

1. Calcification of costochondral junctions and chondral cartilages
   a. "Rosette" appearance around costochondral junctions in old dogs
   b. Appearance of fragmentation of calcified costal cartilages in old cats.
2. Tracheal ring calcification – especially chondrodystrophic breeds.
3. Bronchial wall calcification – especially chondrodystrophic breeds.
4. Spondylosis and sternal new bone.
5. Pleural thickening.
6. Pulmonary osteomata (heterotopic bone formation) and calcified pleural plaques in older, large-breed dogs – 2–4-mm diameter nodules of varying number and slightly irregular outline, very radio-opaque and distributed randomly throughout the lungs although often in greatest numbers ventrally; DDx miliary neoplasia when present in large numbers.
7. Fine, diffuse reticular to reticulonodular interstitial lung pattern.
8. More horizontal orientation of the heart in aged cats, with exaggerated cranial curvature of the aortic arch.

6.5 Border effacement in the thorax

Border effacement, previously referred to as the "silhouette sign", occurs when a pathological soft tissue/fluid opacity comes into direct contact with normal thoracic soft tissue structures (Figure 6.1a). This eliminates the air usually present between the two structures, resulting in the creation of a single

6 LOWER RESPIRATORY TRACT

shadow with loss of visibility of the adjacent margins of the individual structures. This can affect the cardiac silhouette, vascular markings and diaphragmatic line and may be generalised or localised. Conversely if the individual borders of two superimposing soft tissue structures are visible it implies that these two structures are not touching each other and that air-filled lung is interposed (Figure 6.1b). Border effacement must not be confused with fat deposits (pleural, pericardial and epicardial) lying adjacent to soft tissues. Accumulations of fat are less radio-opaque than soft tissue and can be differentiated on good-quality radiographs.

1. Artefactual border effacement due to technical factors
   a. Underexposure due to inadequate penetration of tissues (kV too low)
   b. Underdevelopment of the film
   c. Poor aeration of the lungs.
2. Pleural effusion.
3. Pleural masses.
4. Alveolar lung pattern.
5. Severe interstitial lung pattern.
5. Pulmonary masses.
6. Diaphragmatic rupture or hernia.
7. Large mediastinal masses.

6.6 Tracheal displacement

1. Dorsal displacement of the trachea (the normal position of the trachea is shown in Figures 6.2a and 6.2e)
   a. Artefactual
      - ventral flexion of the head or neck (elevation of cranial thoracic trachea, dipping ventrally towards the carina)
      - expiration; cranial movement of intrathoracic structures
      - rotated lateral positioning
   b. Conformation (e.g. Bulldog and Yorkshire Terrier)
   c. Whole trachea elevated (Figure 6.2b)
      - generalised cardiomegaly (see 7.5)
      - right heart enlargement (see 7.11 and 7.12)
      - left heart enlargement (see 7.8 and 9)
      - extensive cranial mediastinal mass (see 8.11.1 and Figure 8.9)
   d. Cranial thoracic trachea elevated, dipping ventrally towards the carina (Figure 6.2c)
      - cranial mediastinal mass (see 8.11.1 and Figure 8.9)
      - tracheobronchial lymphadenopathy (see 8.11.3 and Figure 8.9)
      - right atrial enlargement (see 7.11 and Figure 7.7)
      - heart-base tumour (see 7.16.2).
2. Ventral displacement of the trachea (Figure 6.2d)
   a. Oesophageal dilation (see 8.16)
   b. Oesophageal foreign body (see 8.19)
   c. Tracheobronchial lymphadenopathy (see 8.11.3 and Figure 8.9)
   d. Craniodorsal mediastinal mass or loculated fluid (see 8.11.2 and Figure 8.9)
   e. Massive cervicothoracic spondylosis or other bony mass
   f. Post-stenotic aortic dilation distal to coarctation of the aorta (see 7.10.1).
3. Lateral displacement of the trachea – displacement is usually to the right as the aorta prevents displacement to the left (Figure 6.2f)

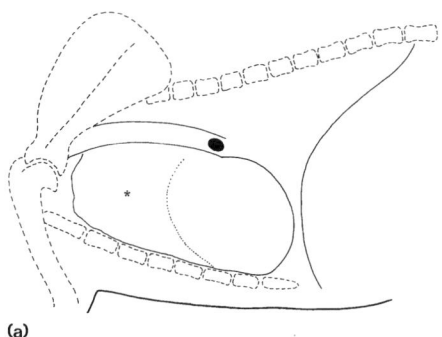
(a)

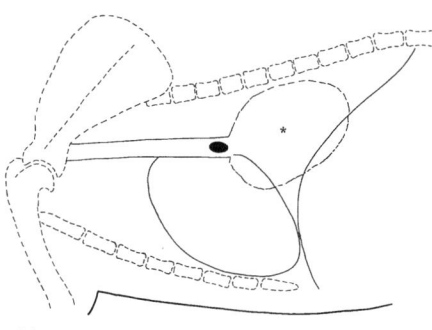
(b)

Figure 6.1 (a) Effacement of the cranial heart border due to a mediastinal mass (*); the mass is touching the heart and no air-filled lung lies between the two structures. The dotted line shows the location of the cranial heart border. (b) A large caudal lobe mass (*) with no border effacement of the heart, indicating that air-filled lung is interposed.

SMALL ANIMAL RADIOLOGICAL DIFFERENTIAL DIAGNOSIS

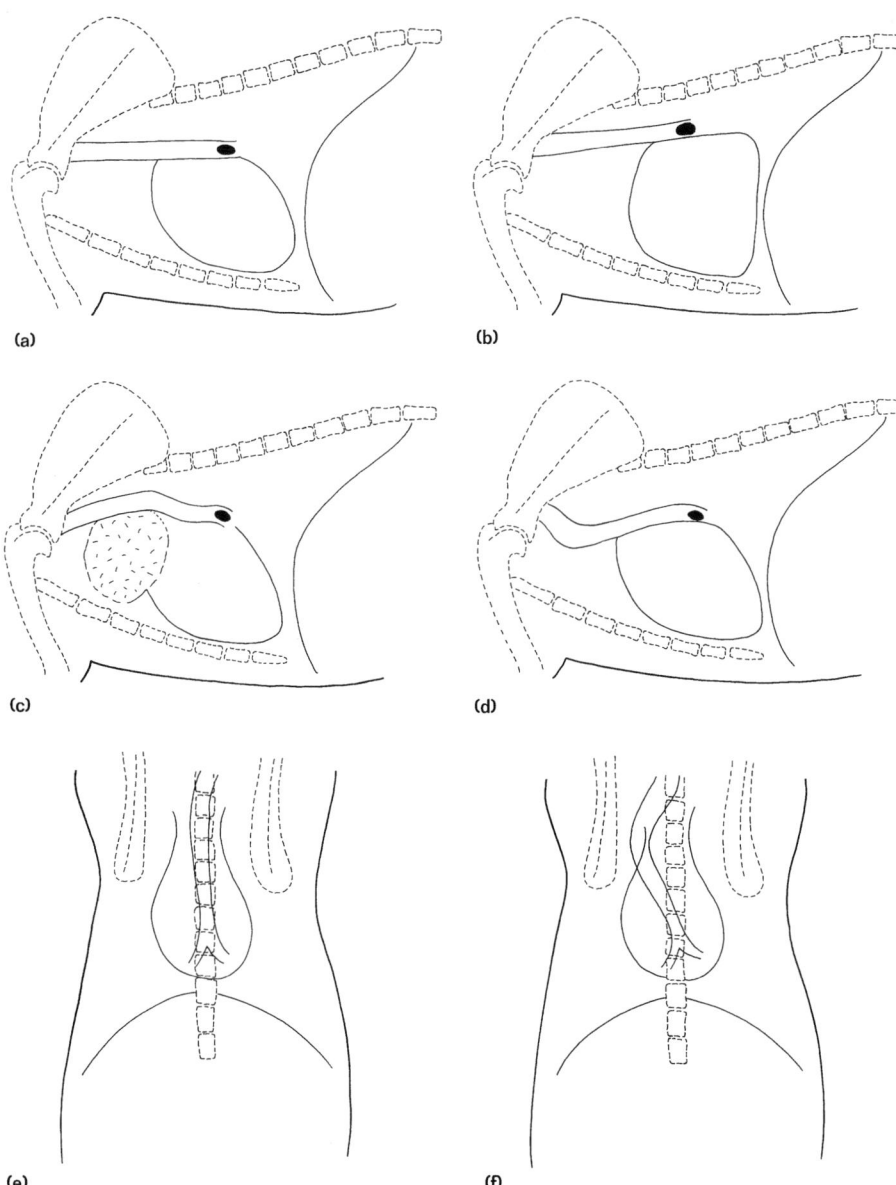

Figure 6.2 (a) Normal tracheal position (lateral view). In most breeds of dogs and in cats the trachea diverges slightly from the spine. (b) The trachea is elevated throughout its length, in this case due to generalised cardiomegaly. (c) The trachea is elevated cranial to the heart but the carina is in a normal position, in this case due to a cranial mediastinal mass. (d) Ventral tracheal displacement. (e) Normal tracheal position (DV view); slight curvature to the right through the thoracic inlet, especially in chondrodystrophic dogs. (f) Lateral displacement of the trachea, usually to the right.

a. Artefactual
   - ventral flexion of the head or neck
   - expiration; cranial movement of intrathoracic structures
   - rotated DV/VD positioning
b. Normal in chondrodystrophic dogs, especially if obese
c. Cranial mediastinal mass (see 8.11.1 and 2 and Figure 8.9)
d. Oesophageal dilation (see 8.16)
e. Cranial mediastinal shift (see 8.8)
f. Heart base tumour (see 7.16.2).

6 LOWER RESPIRATORY TRACT

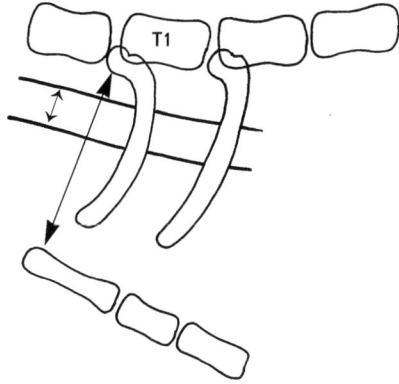

Figure 6.3 Measurement of the trachea at the thoracic inlet: the tracheal diameter is usually at least 20% of the thoracic inlet depth.

6.7 Variations in tracheal diameter

The tracheal diameter as a ratio to the thoracic inlet, measured at the thoracic inlet on the lateral view, should not be less than 0.20 in normal dogs (Figure 6.3). In the Bulldog the normal ratio can be as low as 0.14.
1. Narrowing of the trachea
   a. Artefactual
      - superimposition of the longus colli muscle or oesophagus at the level of and cranial to the thoracic inlet
      - hyperextension of the neck
   b. Congenital hypoplasia – Bulldog and other brachycephalic breeds, Bull Mastiff and occasionally the Labrador Retriever, German Shepherd dog, Weimaraner, Basset Hound and in cats. May be accompanied by other congenital abnormalities, megaoesophagus and secondary aspiration bronchopneumonia
   c. Tracheal collapse syndrome – due to deformed tracheal cartilage rings and invagination of the dorsal tracheal membrane. Often there is dynamic narrowing of the cervical trachea during inspiration and of the intrathoracic trachea during expiration. The tangential view of the thoracic inlet is more reliable for detection of collapse than lateral radiographs. Fluoroscopy and endoscopy are useful ancillary imaging techniques
      - congenital – Yorkshire Terrier and Chihuahua; may not manifest until older age
      - acquired – obese, older, small and miniature breeds (Pomeranian and Toy Poodle) often secondary to chronic bronchitis; rare in large dog breeds and cats
   d. Mucosal thickening
      - tracheitis due to respiratory viral infections, inhalation of gases, smoke and dust, allergies, bacterial and parasitic infections
      - submucosal haemorrhage – anticoagulant poisoning
      - cats – feline infectious peritonitis (FIP)
   e. Extrinsic pressure – the tracheal rings are fairly rigid and tracheal displacement is more likely than narrowing
      - oesophageal foreign body (see 8.19)
      - oesophageal dilation (see 8.16)
      - cranial mediastinal mass (see 8.11.1 and Figure 8.9)
      - hilar mass (see 8.11.3 and Figure 8.9)
      - vascular ring anomaly with oesophageal dilation cranial to the anomaly
   f. Tracheal stricture or segmental stenosis
      - old traumatic injury
      - prolonged intubation with excessive cuff pressure
      - congenital
   g. Focal mass lesions of the tracheal wall (see 6.8.2–5).
2. Widening of the trachea
   a. Respiratory difficulty
   b. Adjacent to tracheal collapse or during the opposite phase of respiration
   c. Scarring adjacent to the trachea.

6.8 Tracheal lumen opacification

1. Aspirated foreign body.
2. *Oslerus osleri** (previously *Filaroides osleri*) – soft tissue nodules on the floor of the terminal trachea and main stem bronchi. More common in young dogs; does not occur in cats.
3. Abscess or granuloma involving the tracheal mucosa
   a. Infectious
   b. Eosinophilic.
4. Neoplasia
   a. Osteochondroma – young large breeds, may mineralise (see 1.15.2 and Figure 1.19)
   b. Mast cell tumour

SMALL ANIMAL RADIOLOGICAL DIFFERENTIAL DIAGNOSIS

  c. Leiomyoma
  d. Chondrosarcoma
  e. Osteosarcoma
  f. Infiltrative tumour (e.g. thyroid carcinoma)
  g. Lymphosarcoma – especially cats
  h. Adenocarcinoma – especially cats.
5. Tracheal polyp.
6. Positive contrast agents – mineral opacity
   a. Inadvertent aspiration during gastrointestinal contrast studies
   b. Oral contrast studies in dysphagic animals
   c. Gastrointestinal contrast studies with an oesophagotracheal fistula present.

6.9 Variations in tracheal wall visibility

The tracheal wall is a soft tissue opacity that blends in with the surrounding cranial mediastinal structures and is not usually visible.
1. Mineralisation of cartilage rings – a normal ageing change, especially in chondrodystrophic dogs.

2. Tracheo-oesophageal stripe sign – the dorsal wall of the trachea and adjacent ventral oesophageal wall summate and become visible due to the presence of air in the oesophagus – usually due to oesophageal dilation (see 8.16).
3. Pneumomediastinum (see 8.9.1–6).

6.10 Ultrasonography of the trachea

Because the trachea is air filled, ultrasonographic imaging is limited. However, the shape of the air column in the cervical trachea may be evaluated.
1. Flattening of the air column in the cervical trachea
   a. Dynamic, on hyperextension of the neck
      • tracheal collapse syndrome
   b. Static
      • traumatic stricture
      • congenital stenosis
      • mass lesions of the bracheal wall (see 6.8.2–5)

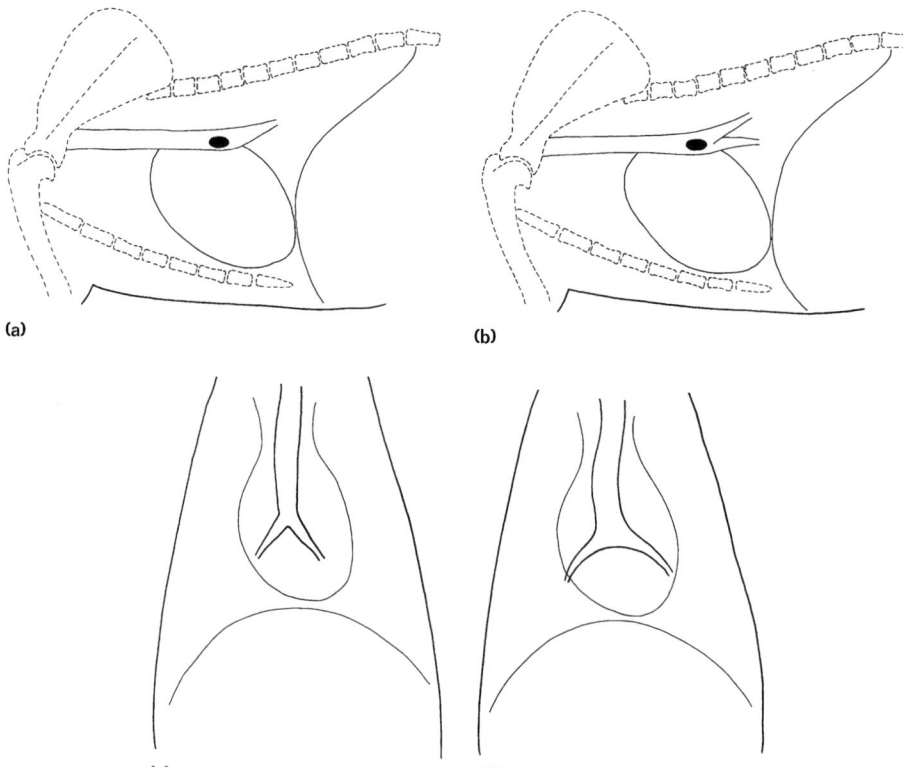

Figure 6.4 (a) Normal superimposed main-stem bronchi on the lateral view. (b) Displacement or "splitting" of the main stem bronchi on the lateral view. (c) Normal main stem bronchi on the DV view, diverging at 50–60°. (d) Widened angle of the main stem bronchi on the DV view.

6.11 Changes of the main-stem bronchi

The main-stem bronchi are visible for a short distance caudal to the carina, as superimposed air-filled structures on the lateral view and diverging at an angle of about 60–90° on the DV view (Figures 6.4a and c).
1. Displacement of the main-stem bronchi
   a. Artefactual – rotated lateral view (Figure 6.4b)
   b. Enlarged left atrium (see 7.8) (Figures 6.4b and 6.4d)
   c. Hilar lymphadenopathy (see 8.12.1–6) (Figures 6.4b and 6.4d).
2. Narrowing of the main-stem bronchi
   a. May accompany displacement due to external compression
   b. Loss of bronchial wall rigidity resulting in dynamic airway collapse and secondary chronic obstructive pulmonary disease (COPD) is frequently observed in association with tracheal collapse syndrome (see 6.7.1)
3. Opacification of the main-stem bronchi – similar to the trachea and the rest of the bronchial tree (see 6.8 and 6.12).

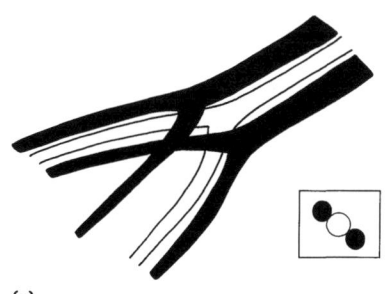

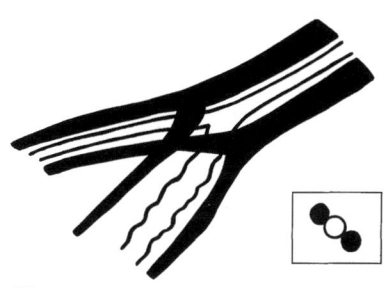

Figure 6.5 (a) Normal lung pattern – the bronchus runs between the artery and vein and is barely visible (inset shows a cross-section). (b) Bronchial lung pattern, producing "tramline" and "doughnut" markings. Bronchiectasis results in widened or irregular bronchi as shown.

6.12 Bronchial lung pattern

A bronchial pattern implies increased visibility of the bronchial walls and may be accompanied by changes in size and shape of the lumen and diminished visualisation of adjacent vascular structures (Figure 6.5). It is often accompanied by an interstitial lung pattern. In young animals only the mineralised wall of the main stem bronchi may be visible. As the animal ages, this mineralisation may extend more peripherally along the bronchial tree and may be accompanied by pulmonary fibrosis.

Increased bronchial wall visibility

1. Normal in aged and chondrodystrophic dogs – thin, mineralised wall.
2. Chronic bronchitis – mucosal inflammation and peribronchial cuffing produce thickened, soft tissue opacity walls (acute bronchitis usually lacks radiographic changes). Often a component of bronchopneumonia (see 6.14.2)
   a. Bacterial
   b. Viral
   c. Allergic
      - pulmonary infiltrate with eosinophilia (PIE)
      - cats – feline bronchial asthma
   d. Fungal (see 6.15.5)
   e. Parasitic; usually a component of a pneumonic pattern (see 6.15.5), also *Crensoma vulpis* infection*
   f. Protozoal
      - toxoplasmosis*
   g. Secondary to primary ciliary dyskinesia. May be accompanied by situs inversus (mirror-image inversion of thoracic and abdominal structures).
3. Neoplasia
   a. Lymphosarcoma, accompanied by a diffuse or reticulonodular interstitial lung pattern and lymphadenopathy
   b. Bronchogenic carcinoma, possibly accompanied by pulmonary nodules or masses.
4. Bronchial wall oedema – may be part of alveolar or interstitial oedema (see 6.14.1 and 6.14.7).
5. Bronchiectasis – see below.
6. Hyperadrenocorticism (Cushing's disease) or long-term corticosteroid administration – thin, mineralised bronchial walls.

Bronchial dilation

7. Bronchiectasis – usually cranioventrally; uncommon in dogs and rare in cats. Saccular or cylindrical

SMALL ANIMAL RADIOLOGICAL DIFFERENTIAL DIAGNOSIS

a. Congenital predisposition
- primary ciliary dyskinesia – inherited abnormality of ciliary function leading to chronic rhinitis and severe pneumonia +/– bronchiectasis; especially young Rottweilers and Newfoundlands
- Kartagener's syndrome – inherited condition as above but also associated with total situs inversus (mirror-image transposition of heart and abdominal viscera)

b. Acquired bronchiectasis – usually middle-aged patients.

Bronchial lumen opacification

8. Ill-defined opacities: mucus or exudate due to pneumonia (see 6.14.2) or bronchiectasis.
9. Single foreign body, especially grass awns in working dogs – caudal lobes, often right bronchus. Chronic cases show secondary lobar bronchopneumonia.
10. *Oslerus osleri** (previously *Filaroides osleri*) nodules in main-stem bronchi – usually also tracheal nodules. More common in young dogs; does not occur in cats.

6.13 Artefactual increase in lung opacity

The following factors all contribute to an artefactual increase in lung opacity, which may result in false-negative or false-positive diagnoses.

1. Poorly inflated lungs
   a. Exposure made on expiration
   b. Abdominal distension
   c. Laryngeal paralysis or other upper respiratory tract obstruction.
2. Obesity.
3. Motion blur.
4. Underexposure.
5. Underdevelopment.
6. Cranial thorax – overlying musculature if the front limbs are not pulled cranially.
7. Bandages.
8. Wet or dirty hair coat.
9. Thymus in young animals (especially cats) – an ill-defined radio-opacity blurring the cranial heart margin in the lateral view.

6.14 Alveolar lung pattern

The acini become airless, either by being filled with fluid and/or cells (alveolar consolidation) or by collapsing (atelectasis). The pattern is characterised by ill-defined, poorly demarcated amorphous infiltrates in the early stages progressing to more extensive lung opacification with air bronchograms and border effacement (see 6.5) in more advanced cases (Figure 6.6). It may be widespread, lobar or as single or multiple poorly marginated regions. A severe alveolar pattern may give rise to poorly marginated apparent pulmonary masses or areas of consolidation, which are described in Section 6.15. The changes are fairly labile and frequent repeat radiography may be necessary to monitor the course of a disease. Alveolar lung patterns may arise from, or give rise to, interstitial lung patterns (see 6.22, 6.23 and 6.25).

1. Cardiogenic pulmonary oedema – associated with cardiomegaly and possibly a hypervascular pattern (see 6.24.1–4).
   a. Perihilar and symmetrical distribution in dogs
   b. Perihilar to peripheral distribution in cats; the consolidations are often patchy and asymmetrical; may affect the right caudal lobe only.
2. Pneumonia
   a. Bronchopneumonia – asymmetrical, mainly cranioventral lung lobes; starts

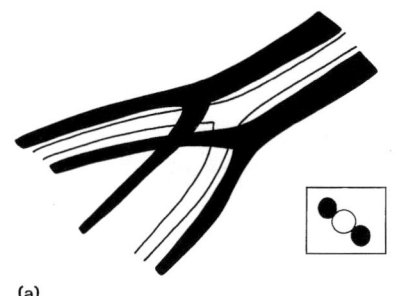

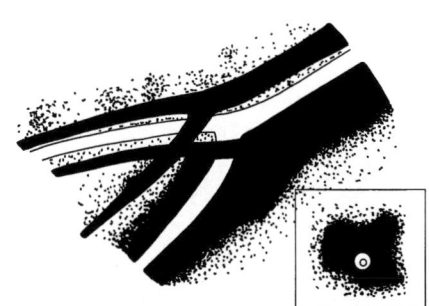

Figure 6.6 (a) Normal lung pattern – the bronchus runs between the artery and vein and is barely visible (inset shows cross-section).
(b) Alveolar lung pattern with blurring or loss of normal lung detail, patchy or diffuse increase in radio-opacity and air bronchogram formation.

peripherally and then spreads inwards. Often involves the right middle lobe. Usually initiated by viral infections (e.g. tracheobronchitis and distemper) or mycoplasma and then complicated by a bacterial infection. Usually also a pronounced bronchial lung pattern. Uncommon in cats
b. Aspiration pneumonia – observed along the bronchial tree, more commonly in the ventral parts of the middle and caudal lobes. Secondary to:
- regurgitation and vomiting especially if oesophageal dilation is present
- iatrogenic aspiration – force feeding, medication, anaesthesia and the administration of contrast media
- swallowing disorders
- weakness and debilitation
- cleft palate
- oesophagotracheal/bronchial fistula
- gastrobronchial fistula
c. Aspirated foreign body pneumonia – caudodorsal segments of caudal lobes, usually affecting a single lobe and with bronchial pattern too
d. Fungal pneumonia (see 6.15.5); often with mediastinal lymphadenopathy too
- also diffuse fungal pneumonia due to *Pneumocystis carinii** in immunocompromised dogs; especially in younger Miniature Dachshunds and Cavalier King Charles Spaniels
e. Parasitic pneumonia
- dirofilariasis* (heartworm); with right heart enlargement, prominence of the main pulmonary artery and a hypervascular lung pattern
- angiostrongylosis* ("French" heartworm); as above, but may be less severe
- *Filaroides hirthi** and *F. milksi**
- aelurostrongylosis* (feline lungworm) – usually younger cats but mostly asymptomatic; initial alveolar or bronchoalveolar pattern progresses to a miliary nodular pattern
f. Secondary to primary ciliary dyskinesia or as part of Kartagener's syndrome – especially Newfoundland and Rottweiler (see 6.12.7)
g. Radiation pneumonitis – in, and adjacent to, irradiated areas
h. Tuberculosis – often also with cavitary lung lesions, mediastinal lymphadenopathy and/or pleural effusion
i. *Francisella* (*Pasteurella*) *tularensis** (tularaemia) – very rare, potential contact with rodents.

3. Pulmonary haemorrhage – usually asymmetrical and less homogeneous than cardiogenic oedema
a. Trauma – look for fractured ribs and subcutaneous emphysema also
b. Coagulopathy
- disseminated intravascular coagulation (DIC)
- anti-coagulant poisoning
- haemophilia, von Willebrand's disease (especially Dobermann) and other inherited coagulopathies
- immune-mediated diseases
- bone marrow depression.
4. Atelectasis (reduced aeration of a lung lobe), recognised by mediastinal shift on DV/VD views (see 8.8). Air bronchograms are only observed with moderate to severe lung collapse
a. Peracute collapse of dependent lobes under gaseous anaesthesia
b. External compression of a lobe
- extended periods in lateral recumbency
- severe pneumothorax
- severe pleural effusion
- large pleural, rib or soft tissue mass
c. Minor airway obstruction due to chronic bronchitis – especially middle and cranial lobes
d. Major airway obstruction – any single lobe; usually no air bronchograms visible
- intrinsic obstruction due to a foreign body or tumour blocking the bronchus
- extrinsic obstruction due to compression
e. Cicatrisation due to chronic pleural and pulmonary disease
f. Adhesive atelectasis – lack of surfactant; airways are patent
- new-born animal
- acute respiratory distress syndrome (ARDS – see 6.14.7)
g. Lung lobe torsion (see 6.17.4)
h. Cats – right middle lobe atelectasis often occurs in feline bronchial asthma; usually with a bronchointerstitial pattern and pulmonary overinflation too.
5. Allergic pulmonary disease – pulmonary infiltrate with eosinophilia (PIE); rarely see an alveolar pattern, more often interstitial or nodular.
6. Neoplasia
a. Primary lung tumour – an alveolar-type pattern is occasionally seen in cases of diffuse bronchogenic carcinoma; air bronchograms are rare

b. Malignant histiocytosis (see 6.15.3)
   c. Pulmonary lymphomatoid granulomatosis – rare neoplastic disorder; often with pulmonary nodules or masses and hilar lymphadenopathy too.
7. Non-cardiogenic pulmonary oedema
   a. Perihilar to peripheral – more likely in the caudodorsal area, often asymmetrical and more on the right side
      • airway obstruction (e.g. many Bulldogs, strangulation, laryngeal paralysis)
      • head trauma and other central nervous system disease
      • near drowning – more severe with salt water than fresh water
      • electric shock
      • post-ictal
      • allergic
      • uraemic
      • reactions to intravenous contrast media
      • aspirated hyperosmolar contrast medium
      • acute pancreatitis
      • toxins, e.g. alphanapthylthiourea (ANTU), snake venom and endotoxin
      • inhaled irritants (e.g. smoke and phosphorus)
      • re-expansion pulmonary oedema after treatment of, for example, pneumothorax
   b. Symmetrical – entire lung
      • acute respiratory distress syndrome (ARDS or "shock lung"). Causes include trauma, infection, severe babesiosis*, pancreatitis, inhalation, disseminated intravascular coagulation (DIC), ingested toxins and iatrogenic causes such as oxygen therapy, overhydration, cardioversion and drug reactions. Initial interstitial pattern progresses to a patchy alveolar pattern with reduced lung volume
   c. One hemithorax
      • hypostasis from extended lateral recumbency or anaesthesia
      • hilar mass blocking pulmonary drainage mechanisms
   d. Perihilar
      • hilar mass blocking pulmonary drainage mechanisms
      • iatrogenic overhydration with intravenous fluids.
8. Pulmonary thromboembolism – localised hypovascular pattern too
9. Lung lobe torsion (see 6.17.4).

6.15 Poorly marginated pulmonary opacities or areas of consolidation

Lesions may be single or multiple, and are generally greater than 4 cm in diameter (Figure 6.7). For smaller lesions see 6.14; for well-defined lesions see 6.19 and 6.20.

1. Artefactual – food material in a distended oesophagus
2. Pneumonia – a mixed bronchial/alveolar lung pattern +/– larger areas of consolidation or poorly marginated opacities (see 6.14.2).
3. Neoplasia – may cavitate or calcify
   a. Primary lung tumours
      • bronchogenic carcinoma most common – may be a solitary nodule or may be multicentric. More often well defined or lobar in shape than poorly marginated
      • adenocarcinoma and squamous cell carcinoma – especially cats (may be associated with multiple digital metastases – see 3.7.11 and Figure 3.16)
   b. Metastatic lung tumours – a single metastatic nodule tends to be smaller than a single primary tumour; again, more likely to be well defined, or ill defined but small; usually multiple when diagnosed
   c. Malignant histiocytosis – middle-aged, large breed dogs with male preponderance – mainly Bernese Mountain dog but also Rottweiler and Golden and Flatcoated retrievers.
4. Pulmonary oedema – usually produces an alveolar or interstitial lung pattern if cardiogenic in dogs, but in cats cardiogenic pulmonary oedema can lead to patchy and asymmetric consolidations, especially in the

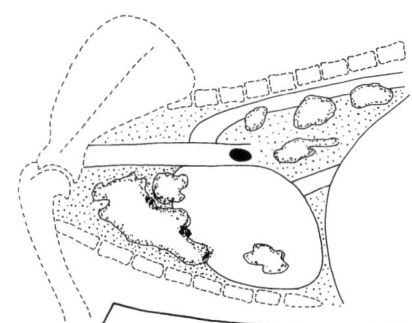

Figure 6.7 Poorly marginated pulmonary opacities or areas of consolidation.

right caudal lobe; oedema due to other causes may also produce poorly marginated areas of consolidation (see 6.14.7).
5. Pulmonary granulomatous diseases – cellular rather than exudative inflammatory reaction, often accompanied by thoracic lymphadenopathy. Granulomata may cavitate
   a. Aspirated foreign body, especially grass awns in working dogs; usually solitary and in the caudal or intermediate lobes
   b. Fungal and fungal-like diseases – in endemic areas and more likely in working and hunting dogs. No typical radiographic appearance; may also be a nodular to interstitial lung pattern. Additional foci of infection may be present elsewhere in the body (e.g. osteomyelitis, chorioretinitis, dermatitis and central nervous system involvement). There may also be a pleural effusion.

Specific obligate pathogens:
   - histoplasmosis* – with moderate to marked lymphadenopathy which tends to calcify during healing; rare in cats
   - blastomycosis* – moderate lymphadenopathy occurs occasionally; rare in cats in which a nodular pattern is more likely
   - coccidioidomycosis* – moderate to marked lymphadenopathy; rare in cats
   - cryptococcosis* – uncommon in dogs but the most common fungal infection in cats. Often associated with sternal lymphadenopathy

Opportunistic infections:
   - actinomycosis* – severe or mild pleural effusions. Pleural, mediastinal and pulmonary abscesses are more common; rare in cats
   - nocardiosis* – uncommon. Often younger dogs, also in cats; may be associated with migrating plant material. Severe or mild pleural effusions and moderate lymphadenopathy
   - aspergillosis* – most likely in immune incompetent animals and a predisposition to the German Shepherd dog
   - sporotrichosis* – rare
   c. Exogenous lipid pneumonia – aspirated mineral or vegetable oil
   d. Parasites
   - dirofilariasis* (heartworm); with right heart enlargement, prominence of the main pulmonary artery and a hypervascular pattern too
   - angiostrongylosis* ("French" heartworm); as above but may be less severe
   - *Paragonimus kellicotti* (lung fluke); amorphous consolidations in the caudal lobes that progress to thin-walled cysts, which may be septated
   - toxoplasmosis*
   - larval migrans, changes very subtle
   - capillariasis* – rare
   - *Filaroides hirthi* and *F. milksi*; Beagles in breeding colonies
   - cats – aelurostrongylosis* (feline lungworm): an initial bronchoalveolar pattern tends to become nodular with time
   e. Eosinophilic pulmonary granulomatosis – often marked hilar lymphadenopathy
   f. Lymphomatoid granulomatosis – rare neoplastic disease; often with an interstitial/alveolar lung pattern and hilar lymphadenopathy
   g. Bacterial granulomatous diseases
   - tuberculosis, rare due to the reduction in incidence of bovine tuberculosis. The source of infection may include humans and birds. Pleural effusion and lymphadenopathy occur in dogs; pleural effusion is less common and milder in cats, in which a nodular pattern is more likely
   - *Corynebacterium.*
6. Allergic lung disease – especially cats; although more usually a bronchointerstitial pattern with pulmonary overinflation.
7. Thromboembolic pneumonia – most likely peripherally in the caudal lobes
   a. From a non-respiratory abscess or infection
   b. In immunocompromised animals
   - animals with lymphosarcoma
   - animals on immunosuppressive therapy
   - associated with autoimmune haemolytic anaemia
   c. From bacterial endocarditis
   d. In animals with fever of unknown origin
   e. From inflammatory joint disease.

6.16 Ultrasonography of areas of alveolar filling

Regions of alveolar filling may be imaged ultrasonographically if they lie adjacent to the

SMALL ANIMAL RADIOLOGICAL DIFFERENTIAL DIAGNOSIS

thoracic wall, the heart or the diaphragm. Bright echogenic specks indicate residual air. Anechoic tubes may represent pulmonary vessels or fluid-filled bronchi (the latter have more echogenic walls). Differential diagnoses for alveolar filling are as in 6.14 and 6.15.

6.17 Single consolidated lung lobe

Increased opacity of the lobe with loss of visibility of the pulmonary vessels and border effacement of adjacent structures (Figure 6.8). Air bronchograms may be present (see 6.14 and Figure 6.6).
1. Lobar pneumonia – often the right middle lobe; best seen on the DV/VD view.
2. Neoplasia – primary tumour – lobe possibly enlarged, with convex borders possible and mediastinal shift away from the lobe.
3. Atelectasis (collapse) – smaller lobe, possibly with concave borders; mediastinal shift towards the lobe.
4. Lung lobe torsion – most commonly the right middle lobe followed by the cranial segment of the left cranial lobe; least likely to affect the caudal lobes. The lobe is initially enlarged, with air bronchograms or pulmonary vasculature, if visible, running in an abnormal direction. The bronchus may seem to end abruptly. Usually there is concurrent pleural effusion. The diagnosis may be confirmed by means of bronchoscopy, thoracotomy or diagnostic pneumothorax

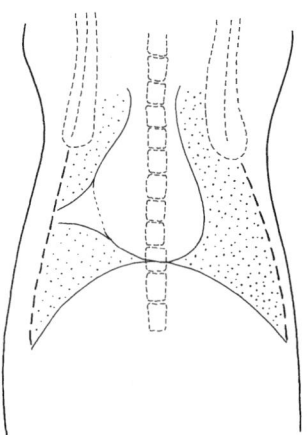

Figure 6.8 A single consolidated or collapsed lung lobe seen on the DV view; the right middle lobe is most often affected. Atelectasis (collapse) results in reduction in size of the lobe.

a. Spontaneous – deep-chested large breeds
b. Predisposed to by pleural effusion. Usually impossible to determine whether the effusion is primary or secondary. Cats often have a severe bloody effusion
c. Acute traumatic impact – rare; small breeds.

6.18 Ultrasonography of consolidated lung lobes

Consolidated lung lobes are usually seen as moderately echoic, well-demarcated structures which can be followed to the perihilar region. The main lobar blood vessels may be seen within the solid lung tissue in the perihilar region. Echogenic-walled, tubular structures with anechoic contents are fluid-filled bronchi. Hyperechoic foci within the lobe, with or without acoustic shadowing, usually indicate areas of residual aeration.
1. Uniformly hypoechoic lung lobe, smoothly marginated with pointed tips; echotexture similar to that of liver
   a. Atelectasis due to
      * adjacent thoracic mass
      * pleural effusion
      * airway obstruction
   b. Lobar pneumonia
   c. Lobar haemorrhage
   d. Lung lobe torsion (usually associated with pleural fluid).
2. Variable echogenicity with loss of normal shape and lacking internal liver-like structure
   a. Lobar neoplasia
   b. Abscessation.

6.19 Solitary pulmonary nodules or masses

A nodule is a well-marginated, evenly rounded lesion measuring up to 4 cm in diameter. A mass is well marginated and larger than a nodule; it may be smooth or irregular in outline. The larger the nodule or mass, the more radio-opaque it should be. Mineralised areas may be seen within larger masses.

Solitary lesions are easily missed if they are small or in the perihilar region, cranial thorax, costophrenic recesses or paraspinal gutters. A solitary lesion should be differentiated from a composite mass consisting of multiple small coalescing nodules. It is not possible to differentiate between causes radiologically but repeat radiographs after 3–4 weeks are indicated. If the nodule or mass has enlarged, then biopsy is advised. If no enlargement has occurred, repeat radiography should be performed after a further 3–4 months.

Nodules and masses may cavitate, especially if they are rapidly growing. In these cases a radiolucent, gas-filled centre to the lesion is seen. For a fuller description and list of causes see 6.27 and Figure 6.13.

1. Artefactual solitary pulmonary nodules or masses
   a. Overlying soft tissue structure (see 8.20.4)
   b. Costochondral junction
   c. Single blood vessel seen end on
   d. Healed rib fracture
   e. Adjacent pleural mass
   f. Small diaphragmatic rupture or hernia
   g. Diaphragmatic eventration (see 8.25.1).
2. Neoplasia
   a. Primary lung tumour. Often occurs in the perihilar region, tends to be large and may have partially irregular borders. Secondary changes include cavitation (becoming air filled), calcification, spread to regional lymph nodes, compression of adjacent bronchi or pleural effusion
      - adenocarcinoma
      - bronchogenic carcinoma
      - squamous cell carcinoma
      - malignant histiocytosis – middle-aged, large-breed dogs with male preponderance; mainly Bernese Mountain dog but also Rottweiler and Golden or Flatcoated retrievers
   b. Solitary lung metastasis – tend to involve the middle or periphery of the lung field and are usually nodular. Additional metastases usually develop quickly.
3. Granuloma (see 6.15.5) – may also cavitate
   a. Foreign body – especially working dogs aspirating grass awns
   b. Fungal – although more usually multiple, poorly defined and bizarrely shaped lesions; tend to be perihilar
   c. Bacterial
   d. Eosinophilic
   e. Parasitic
   f. Tuberculosis.
4. Abscess – often in younger patients; tends to occur in the perihilar or peripheral lung field; may cavitate.
5. Haematoma – history of trauma, resolves with time.
6. Cyst.
7. Fluid-filled bulla.
8. Exudate or mucus-filled bronchus or focal bronchiectasis.
9. Area of consolidation simulating a nodule (see 6.15).

6.20 Nodular lung pattern

Nodules have to be at least 3 mm in diameter to be visible unless either they are mineralised or multiple nodules are summated on each other (Figure 6.9). For differential diagnoses of cavitary nodules, see 6.27.

1. Superimposition of nipples, costochondral junctions in older dogs or thoracic wall nodules (see 8.20.4)
2. Normal blood vessels seen end on – these are more radio-opaque, perfectly circular and well marginated, decrease in size towards the periphery and are associated with adjacent longitudinal blood vessels.
3. Nodules associated with ageing (incidental findings)
   a. Pulmonary osteomata (heterotopic bone formation) in older, large breed dogs (see 6.4.6)

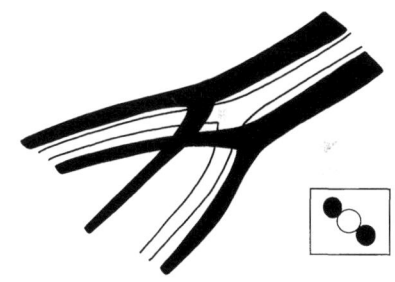

(a)

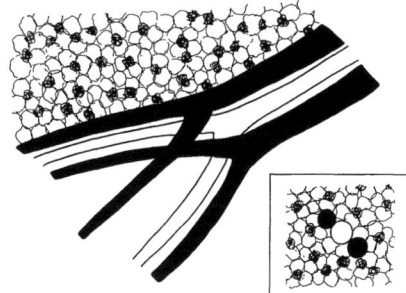

(b)

Figure 6.9 (a) Normal lung pattern – the bronchus runs between the artery and vein and is barely visible (inset shows cross-section). (b) Nodular lung pattern.

SMALL ANIMAL RADIOLOGICAL DIFFERENTIAL DIAGNOSIS

b. Calcified pleural plaques – appear identical to pulmonary osteomata (see 6.4.6)
c. Fibrotic nodules.
4. Multiple small lung nodules, 3–5 mm in diameter
   a. Miliary nodules – a large number of smaller, diffusely distributed nodules which may have summating opacities appearing to form larger conglomerates. They occur as result of widespread haematogenous and/or lymphatic dissemination of pathogens or neoplastic cells and may be accompanied by hilar lymphadenopathy
      - metastatic tumours (e.g. mammary and thyroid carcinoma and haemangiosarcoma)
      - pulmonary lymphosarcoma – usually with an interstitial lung pattern and mediastinal lymphadenopathy
      - haematogenous bacterial pneumonia
      - fungal pneumonia (see 6.15.5)
      - disseminated intravascular coagulation (DIC)
      - Mycobacterial pneumonia – rare
   b. Alveolar nodules due to aspiration/inhalation of radio-opaque material
      - aspirated barium
      - pneumoconiosis
   c. Pulmonary infiltrate with eosinophilia (PIE) – there may be an ill-defined nodular pattern superimposed over the interstitial pattern
   d. parasitic – usually fewer nodules; may calcify (see 6.15.5)
      - larval migrans
      - *Filaroides hirthi** and *F. milksi**
      - cats – aelurostrongylosis* (feline lungworm) – initial bronchoalveolar pattern although older cats with resolving disease tend to show a more nodular pattern
   e. Protozoal
      - toxoplasmosis*
   f. Idiopathic mineralisation (see 6.28.5)
   g. *Francisella* (*Pasteurella*) *tularensis** (tularaemia) – very rare, potential contact with rodents.
5. Multiple medium-sized lung nodules, 5–40 mm in diameter
   a. Metastatic tumours – often "cannonball" nodules; randomly distributed, well-defined and do not coalesce although may summate; especially from primary osteosarcoma. Rapidly growing metastases may cavitate and become air filled; main DDx cavitating abscesses or granulomata
   b. Pulmonary lymphosarcoma – usually with an interstitial lung pattern and mediastinal lymphadenopathy
   c. Fungal granulomata or abscesses (see 6.15.5)
      - Histoplasmosis nodules are often well circumscribed and may calcify
   d. Multicentric primary tumours
   e. Malignant histiocytosis – middle-aged large-breed dogs with male preponderance; mainly Bernese Mountain dog but also Rottweiler and Golden and Flatcoated retrievers
   f. Bacterial granulomata or abscesses
   g. Foreign body granulomata
      - multiple small nodules due to mineral or vegetable oil aspiration
   h. Enlarged blood vessels seen end on (see 6.24.1–4)
   i. Bronchi or bronchiectasis lesions filled with mucus or exudate
   j. Haematomata
   k. Fluid-filled cysts
      - congenital
      - hydatid
   l. Disseminated intravascular coagulation (DIC)
   m. Pulmonary lymphomatoid granulomatosis – rare neoplastic disorder; often with an interstitial/alveolar lung pattern and hilar lymphadenopathy too
   n. Parasitic
      - *Paragonimus kellicotti** (lung fluke); nodules are rare in the dog and cystic lesions are more common (see 6.27.4) but the nodular form is more common in the cat than the dog
      - cats – aelurostrongylosis* (feline lungworm – see 6.20.4)
   o. Feline infectious peritonitis (FIP).

6.21 Ultrasonography of pulmonary nodules or masses

Pulmonary nodules or masses are visible ultrasonographically only if they lie adjacent to the thoracic wall, heart or diaphragm or are outlined by free thoracic fluid.

1. Well-defined, thin-walled nodule or mass with anechoic or hypoechoic contents (the presence of gas may result in hyperechoic foci within the anechoic/hypoechoic contents)
   a. Cyst

b. Haematoma
   c. Abscess.
2. Variably well-defined, thick or irregular-walled nodule or mass with anechoic or hypoechoic contents (the presence of gas may result in hyperechoic foci within the anechoic/hypoechoic contents)
   a. Abscess
   b. Cavitating tumour
   c. Haematoma.
3. Solid, homogeneous nodule or mass
   a. Tumour of homogeneous cell type with little necrosis
   b. Alveolar consolidation or collapse simulating a mass (see 6.14–6.18 for lists of differential diagnoses).
4. Solid, heterogeneous nodule or mass
   a. Tumour of heterogeneous cell type and/or areas of necrosis, haemorrhage or calcification
   b. Haematoma
   c. Abscess
   d. Granuloma.

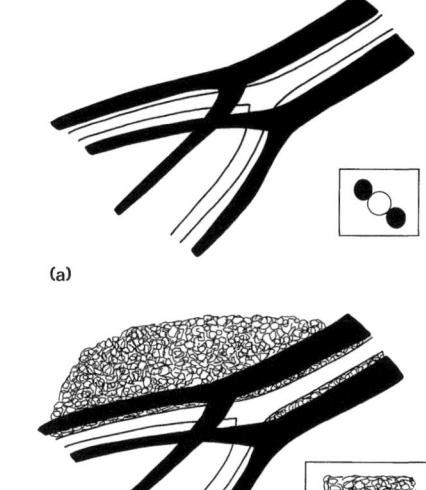

Figure 6.10 (a) Normal lung pattern – the bronchus runs between the artery and vein and is barely visible (inset shows cross-section). (b) Diffuse interstitial lung pattern – a hazy, diffuse increase in lung radio-opacity.

6.22 Diffuse, unstructured interstitial lung pattern

Changes occur primarily in the interstitial tissues and not the air spaces, although the air content of the affected lung may be secondarily reduced due to a decreased alveolar size. This results in a semi-opaque, diffuse or regional pulmonary background opacity with reduced visibility of the pulmonary vasculature (Figure 6.10). There is no border effacement but smudging or blurring of the outline of structures occurs. Other patterns may occur simultaneously; a bronchial component is often also present as is an alveolar pattern.
1. Artefactual interstitial lung pattern (see 6.13).
2. Age-related interstitial lung pattern
   a. In very young animals, due to increased water content of interstitial tissue
   b. In old animals, due to ageing changes in the lung.
3. Infectious causes – pneumonia
   a. Bacterial
   b. Viral (e.g. distemper) – often involves the caudodorsal lung lobes but the changes are minimal unless complicated by bacterial infection
   c. Fungal – often with mediastinal lymphadenopathy too
      • histoplasmosis*
      • cryptococcosis*
      • blastomycosis*
      • coccidioidomycosis*
      • *Pneumocystis carinii** – immune compromised patients, especially in younger Miniature Dachshunds and Cavalier King Charles Spaniels
   d. *Mycoplasma* infection
   e. Rocky Mountain spotted fever* (*Rickettsia rickettsii* infection)
   f. Babesiosis*
   g. Toxoplasmosis* – caudal lobes; especially cats
   h. Cats – aelurostrongylosis* (feline lungworm) – caudal lobes, often cats less than 1 year old; may also show a bronchoalveolar pattern progressing to a nodular pattern with time
   i. Cats – feline infectious peritonitis (FIP).
4. Oedema – interstitial oedema precedes alveolar oedema and the aetiologies are similar (see 6.14.1 and 6.14.7)
   a. Cardiogenic – in dogs symmetrically distributed in the perihilar region extending peripherally with progressing heart failure; in cats more perihilar or peripheral distribution, asymmetrical or right caudal lobe involvement

b. Non-cardiogenic – caudodorsal lobes, often asymmetrical.
5. Pulmonary haemorrhage
   a. Trauma – look for fractures and subcutaneous emphysema too
   b. Coagulopathy
      • DIC
      • anti-coagulant poisoning
      • haemophilia, von Willebrand's disease (especially Dobermann) and other inherited coagulopathies
      • immune-mediated diseases
      • bone marrow depression
   c. Metastatic haemangiosarcoma.
6. Neoplasia
   a. Primary
      • pulmonary lymphosarcoma; usually also with mediastinal lymphadenopathy
   b. Metastatic
      • pulmonary lymphatic metastasis due to anaplastic scirrhous mammary carcinoma – rare
   c. Pulmonary lymphomatoid granulomatosis – rare neoplastic disorder; with pulmonary nodules or masses and hilar lymphadenopathy too.
7. Allergic – PIE; ill-defined nodular pattern may also be present.
8. Parasitic
   a. Dirofilariasis* (heartworm) – plus hypervascular pattern (see 6.24.1)
   b. Angiostrongylosis* ("French" heartworm) – plus hypervascular pattern (see 6.24.1)
   c. *Filaroides hirthi** and *F. milksi**
   d. Cats – aelurostrongylosis* (feline lungworm – caudal lobes, often cats less than 1 year old; may also show a bronchoalveolar pattern progressing to a nodular pattern with time.
9. Pulmonary thromboembolism associated with immune-mediated haemolytic anaemia.
10. Pulmonary fibrosis
    a. Idiopathic – middle- to old-aged terriers, especially West Highland White; may also have a bronchial pattern
    b. Secondary to any chronic respiratory disease
    c. Pneumoconiosis – see below.
11. Inhalation – diffuse interstitial radio-opacity in acute cases and pulmonary fibrosis (pneumoconiosis) in chronic cases
    a. Smoke
    b. Dust
       • silica
       • asbestos.
12. Hyperadrenocorticism (Cushing's disease) or long-term corticosteroid administration – accompanied by calcification of the bronchial walls and possibly also the alveolar walls. Also hepatomegaly, osteopenia and soft tissue calcification.
13. Toxins – Paraquat poisoning; often with pneumomediastinum.
14. ARDS ("shock lung") – initial interstitial pattern progresses to a patchy alveolar pattern with reduced lung volume (see 6.14.7 for causes).
15. Uraemia – rare.
16. Pancreatitis.
17. Radiation – localised to the irradiated area of the lung.

6.23 Linear or reticular interstitial lung pattern

Similar to a diffuse, unstructured interstitial pattern but not all alveolar walls are affected. It consists of randomly arranged linear opacities which are more visible peripherally and may also be accompanied by small nodules to form a reticulonodular pattern (Figure 6.11).

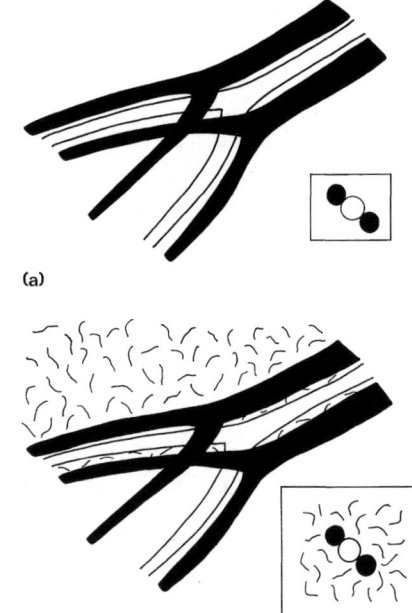

Figure 6.11 (a) Normal lung pattern – the bronchus runs between the artery and vein and is barely visible (inset shows cross-section).
(b) Reticular lung pattern (may be combined with a nodular pattern).

6 LOWER RESPIRATORY TRACT

1. Normal ageing due to interstitial fibrosis.
2. Lymphosarcoma – usually with mediastinal lymphadenopathy +/- fine nodular pattern.
3. Chronic fibrosing interstitial pneumonia.
4. Metastasis from anaplastic scirrhous mammary carcinoma.
5. Fungal pneumonia (see 6.15.5).

6.24 Vascular lung pattern

The visibility of blood vessels depends on the amount of air in the lungs. Arteries and veins run adjacent to and on opposite sides of the associated bronchi and can be distinguished from each other by their location. On the lateral view the cranial lobar arteries lie dorsal and parallel to the corresponding veins. In the cranial thorax the dorsal pair of vessels supply and drain the left cranial lung lobe and the ventral pair the right cranial lobe. On the DV/VD view the caudal lobe arteries arise more cranial and lateral to the corresponding bronchi and veins. The veins run to the left atrium, which lies in the bifurcation of the main-stem bronchi. Arteries are normally the same size as, or slightly larger than, veins. On lateral radiographs the arteries should be approximately 75% of the diameter of the proximal third of the fourth rib where they cross this rib. On DV/VD radiographs at the level of the tenth rib, the lobar artery width should not exceed that of that rib.

An abnormal vascular pattern is recognised by a change in number, size, shape or radio-opacity of pulmonary blood vessels (Figure 6.12).

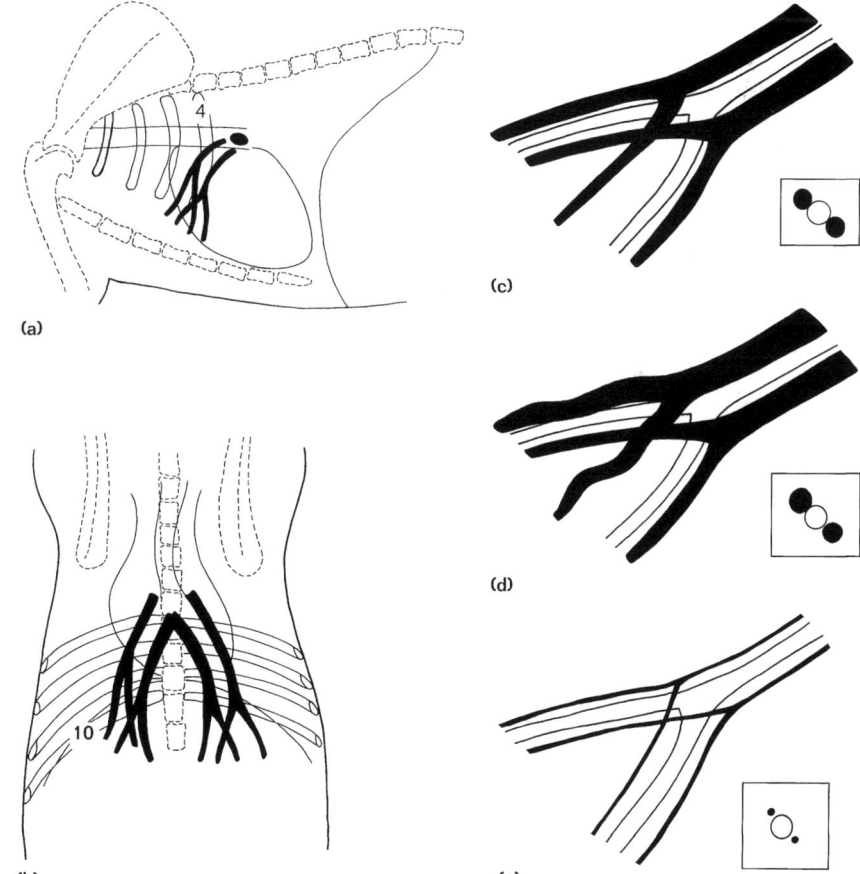

Figure 6.12 (a) Left cranial lobe blood vessels on the lateral view – approximately 75% of the diameter of the fourth rib. (b) Caudal lobe blood vessels on the DV view – no larger than the tenth rib. (c) Normal lung pattern – the bronchus runs between the artery and vein and is barely visible (inset shows cross-section). The blood vessels are easily seen and are equal in size. (d) Hypervascular lung pattern – the affected vessels (in this case the artery) are enlarged and may become tortuous. (e) Hypovascular lung pattern – the blood vessels are thin and thread-like.

SMALL ANIMAL RADIOLOGICAL DIFFERENTIAL DIAGNOSIS

1. Arteries larger than veins
   a. Dirofilariasis* (heartworm) – the dilated arteries are often truncated and tortuous. May be accompanied by right heart enlargement and prominence of the main pulmonary artery with possible bronchopneumonia or PIE
   b. Large left-to-right shunts
      - patent ductus arteriosus (PDA)
      - ventricular and atrial septal defect (VSD and ASD)
      - endocardial cushion defect
   c. Pulmonary thromboembolism – large perihilar artery with disproportionate reduction in its diameter in the middle or peripheral lung field, peripheral hypoperfusion and small or absent returning vein. There may also be a small pleural effusion. Clinical signs are often marked in the absence of radiographic changes
      - autoimmune haemolytic anaemia
      - renal amyloidosis
      - hyperadrenocorticism (Cushing's disease) or long-term corticosteroid administration
      - postoperative thromboembolism
   d. Pulmonary hypertension – may be accompanied by right heart enlargement
   e. Peripheral arteriovenous fistula
   f. Angiostrongylosis* (French heartworm) – changes are similar to, but usually less dramatic than, those caused by dirofilariasis
   g. Cats – aelurostrongylosis* (feline lungworm); also an initial bronchoalveolar pattern becoming more nodular with time.
2. Veins larger than arteries
   a. Left heart failure
   b. Right-to-left shunts, due to relatively smaller arteries (e.g. tetralogy of Fallot)
   c. Left-to-right shunts – in some cases the thin-walled veins show greater dilation than the arteries (e.g. VSD and ASD).
3. Generalised increased pulmonary vascularity – increased number and diameter of vessels, extending further to the periphery
   a. Passive pulmonary congestion – left heart failure
   b. Active pulmonary congestion – precedes pneumonia
   c. Left-to-right shunts
      - PDA
      - VSD and ASD
      - endocardial cushion defect
   d. Iatrogenic overhydration.
4. Increased vascular radio-opacity
   a. Left heart failure – the dilated veins may be more radio-opaque than the arteries
   b. Vessel wall mineralisation – rare and of uncertain aetiology
      - hyperadrenocorticism (Cushing's disease) or long-term corticosteroid administration
      - chronic renal failure
      - cats – secondary to hypertension.
5. Generalised decreased pulmonary vascularity – the lungs have an empty appearance with thinner peripheral vessels, which appear fewer in number and which do not reach the periphery
   a. Forced manual overinflation during anaesthesia
   b. Pulmonary hypoperfusion (may be accompanied by microcardia, small caudal vena cava and compensatory hyperinflation)
      - shock
      - severe dehydration
      - hypoadrenocorticism (Addison's disease)
      - localised hypoperfusion due to pulmonary thromboembolism – caudal lobes more likely to be affected
   c. Other causes of pulmonary overinflation (see 6.26.4–6)
   d. Pericardial disease, reducing right heart output
      - pericardial effusion with tamponade
      - restrictive pericarditis
   e. Right heart failure
   f. Congenital cardiac disease with right-to-left shunts
      - tetralogy of Fallot
      - reverse-shunting PDA
      - VSD and ASD
   g. Severe pulmonic stenosis.
6. Localised decreased pulmonary vascular pattern
   a. Pulmonary thromboembolism (see 6.24.1)
   b. Lobar emphysema compressing blood vessels.

6.25 Mixed lung pattern

Many abnormal lung patterns consist of a combination of two, three or even four constituent patterns. Usually, however, one pattern is dominant and will help to elucidate the aetiology. The alveolar and interstitial patterns may be hard to distinguish, and often co-exist. The hypovascular pattern is often an incidental finding in a sick or dehydrated

animal. Some examples of common mixed patterns are given here.
1. Dominant pattern bronchial
   a. Bronchial pattern due to ageing changes, with an ageing interstitial pattern and/or other disease process superimposed
   b. Bronchial and alveolar +/- interstitial
      • various pneumonias, especially as they resolve
   c. Bronchial pattern due to hyperadrenocorticism (Cushing's disease) or long-term corticosteroid administration, with other disease process superimposed – the bronchial pattern is clearly calcified.
2. Dominant pattern alveolar
   a. Alveolar and bronchial +/- interstitial
      • various pneumonias
      • cardiogenic oedema
      • pulmonary haemorrhage.
3. Dominant pattern hypervascular
   a. Hypervascular and alveolar
      • cardiogenic oedema (congenital or acquired heart disease)
   b. Hypervascular, alveolar +/- bronchial and interstitial
      • dirofilariasis* (heartworm) and to a lesser extent, angiostrongylosis* ("French" heartworm).
4. Dominant pattern interstitial
   a. Severe ageing interstitial pattern with other disease process superimposed
   b. Interstitial and bronchial
      • severe chronic bronchitis
      • PIE
      • lymphosarcoma; usually with mediastinal lymphadenopathy
      • Paraquat poisoning; usually with pneumomediastinum.

6.26 Generalised pulmonary hyperlucency

Two or more lung lobes are involved.
1. Artefactual pulmonary hyperlucency
   a. Overexposure, overdevelopment or fogging of the film
   b. Forced manual overinflation during anaesthesia
   c. Deep inspiration
   d. Emaciation
   e. Unilateral, due to thoracic rotation on DV or VD views.
2. Extrapulmonary hyperlucent areas that mimic increased pulmonary radiolucency
   a. Pneumothorax
   b. Air-filled megaoesophagus
   c. Diaphragmatic rupture with distended, gas-filled gastrointestinal tract within the thoracic cavity
   d. Subcutaneous emphysema
   e. Pneumomediastinum.
3. Pulmonary hypoperfusion (hypovascular pattern, undercirculation – see 6.24.5)
   a. Shock
   b. Severe dehydration
   c. Hypoadrenocorticism (Addison's disease)
   d. Cardiac tamponade
   e. Congenital cardiac disease with right-to-left shunts
      • tetralogy of Fallot
      • reverse-shunting PDA
      • VSD and ASD
   f. Severe pulmonic stenosis.
4. Overinflation by air-trapping due to expiratory obstruction
   a. Tracheal or bronchial foreign body
   b. Chronic bronchitis
   c. Allergic bronchitis, especially bronchial asthma in cats
   d. Upper respiratory tract obstruction (e.g. nasopharyngeal polyp).
5. Compensatory overinflation
   a. Following lobectomy
   b. Secondary to atelectasis of another lobe or lobes
   c. Secondary to congenital lobar atresia or agenesis.
6. Emphysema – the diaphragm may be caudally displaced and flattened, showing its costal attachments, the ribs positioned transversely and the cardiac silhouette small. Full inspiratory and expiratory radiographs should be made and if there is little difference in pulmonary radio-opacity and diaphragmatic position the diagnosis of emphysema is confirmed. Alternatively, a DV/VD view using a horizontal beam and the animal in lateral recumbency with the affected lobe down will show that the affected lung does not collapse
   a. Acquired primary emphysema – rare
   b. Congenital lobar emphysema – may involve one or more lobes; ipsilateral lobes may be compressed and mediastinal shift may occur. Shih Tzu and Jack Russell – usually recognised in puppyhood.

6.27 Focal areas of pulmonary hyperlucency (including cavitary lesions)

Improved visualisation of focal areas of pulmonary hyperlucency occurs on expiratory

SMALL ANIMAL RADIOLOGICAL DIFFERENTIAL DIAGNOSIS

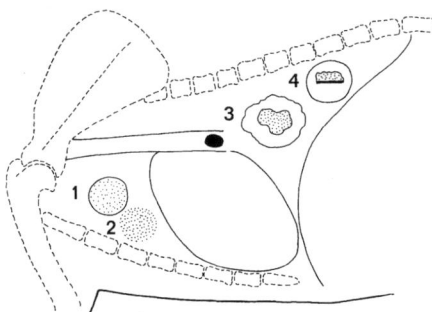

Figure 6.13 Focal pulmonary hyperlucent areas: 1 = cyst; 2 = bulla; 3 = cavitary lesion; 4 = cavitary lesion with fluid contents seen using horizontal beam radiography.

radiographs, as the surrounding lung becomes more radio-opaque (Figure 6.13). Fluid levels and wall thickness may be demonstrated in cysts and cavitated lesions by means of horizontal beam radiography.

1. Artefactual focal areas of pulmonary hyperlucency
   a. Intrapulmonary ring shadows may be mimicked by curved bronchial walls and pulmonary vessels and by lobar fissure lines, especially on DV/VD views
   b. Extrapulmonary ring shadows
      - superimposed subcutaneous gas
      - gas-filled stomach or intestinal loop herniated into thorax or paracostally
      - localised pneumomediastinum
      - oesophageal air
      - expansile rib osteolysis
      - foamy pneumothorax (concurrent pneumothorax and hydrothorax)
      - pleural adhesions accompanied by pneumothorax.
2. Normal – the tip of the left cranial lung lobe may be outlined just above the sternum on the lateral view, and may appear more radiolucent than surrounding lung.
3. Bronchial structures seen end-on
   a. Prominent bronchi due to age
   b. Chronic bronchitis
   c. Bronchiectasis.
4. Radiolucent structure with a thin wall – cysts and cyst-like structures; may rupture and cause spontaneous and recurrent pneumothorax
   a. Bronchogenic cyst – smooth, thin walled; young animals
   b. Pulmonary cyst

- *Paragonimus kellicotti** (lung fluke) – septated, with a thin smooth wall in dogs; cats are more likely to have a solid nodular form
- thin-walled, healed abscess
- hydatid cyst
- pneumatocoele (secondary to pneumonia or traumatised lung tissue).

5. Radiolucent structure with absent or barely perceptible wall
   a. Bulla – localised areas of emphysema, which are usually small and multiple with insignificant walls; sometimes large – may be accompanied by pneumothorax. Usually traumatic in origin but can be congenital
   b. Bleb – a subpleural bulla whose peripheral location makes it difficult to see unless it has resulted in pneumothorax.
6. Cavitary lesion – an air-filled region developing within abnormal lung tissue. Thick and irregular walls. Rare in cats. May develop from an apparently solid nodule or mass (see 6.19 for causes)
   a. Abscess/granuloma
      - bacterial
      - fungal – often thin walls and associated hilar lymphadenopathy
      - foreign body, especially aspirated grass awns in working dogs
      - tuberculosis
   b. Neoplasia
      - primary – cavitated primary lung tumours tend to have irregular, thick walls, and may be multilocular (e.g. various carcinomata)
      - metastatic – rapidly growing metastases (e.g. secondary to mammary tumour and thyroid adenocarcinoma)
   c. Cavitary infarct – rare.
7. Lobar emphysema.
8. Focal hyperlucent area peripheral to a pulmonary thromboembolism.

6.28 Intrathoracic mineralised opacities

1. Artefactual superimposed opacities (see 8.20 and 8.21).
2. Incidental mineralisation seen as an ageing change in dogs
   a. Pulmonary osteomata (heterotopic bone formation) in older, larger breed dogs (see 6.4.6)
   b. Calcified pleural plaques – appear identical to pulmonary osteomata (see 6.4.6)
   c. Calcified tracheal rings and bronchi, especially in chondrodystrophic breeds.

3. Oesophageal foreign body.
4. Aspirated contrast medium (barium) in alveoli or in hilar lymph nodes.
5. Pathological pulmonary mineralisation
   a. Healed fungal disease
      - histoplasmosis* – multiple small calcified nodules similar to pulmonary osteomata, accompanied by hilar lymph node calcification
   b. Metastatic tumours
      - from osteosarcoma
      - from chondrosarcoma
      - from bone-forming mammary tumours
   c. Parasitic nodules
   d. Primary tumours
   e. Chronic infectious disease
   f. Metastatic calcification
      - hyperadrenocorticism (Cushing's disease) or long-term corticosteroid administration – mainly of bronchial walls
      - primary and secondary hyperparathyroidism
      - hypervitaminosis D
      - chronic uraemia
   g. Idiopathic mineralisation – tends to be diffuse and extensive
      - alveolar or bronchial microlithiasis
      - pulmonary calcification
      - pulmonary ossification.
6. Pathological mediastinal mineralisation
   a. Lymph nodes
      - histoplasmosis*, especially during healing phase
      - tuberculosis
   b. Osteosarcoma transformation of oesophageal *Spirocerca lupi** granuloma
   c. Thymic tumours
   d. Metastatic mediastinal tumours.
7. Cardiovascular mineralisation
   a. Aorta (see 7.10.4)
   b. Coronary vessels (incidental finding) – tend to run caudoventrally from the aortic arch. Best seen on lateral views, as short, wavy lines of mineralisation
   c. Heart valves
      - idiopathic
      - bacterial endocarditis.

6.29 Hilar masses

Hilar masses usually result in poorly defined radio-opacities near the base of the heart. The increased thickness of the lungs at this level means that diffuse pulmonary pathology may create a false impression of a hilar mass. Genuine hilar masses are usually within the mediastinum – see 8.11.3 for details.

6.30 Increased visibility of lung or lobar edges

The lungs normally extend to the periphery of the thoracic cavity and individual lobe or lung edges are not seen except in two locations:
- in the cranioventral thorax where the mediastinum runs obliquely and outlines the cranial segment of the left cranial lung lobe on a lateral radiograph (see 8.7 and Figure 8.6);
- along the ventral margins of the lungs, which may appear "scalloped" in some dogs on the lateral radiograph due to intrathoracic fat.

Increased visibility of the lung or lobar edges may be due to intrapulmonary disease, thickening of the pleura or diseases of the pleural space. See 8.2, 8.3 and 8.6 for further details.

FURTHER READING

Barr, F., Gruffydd-Jones, T.J., Brown, P.J., Gibbs, C. (1987) Primary lung tumours in the cat. *Journal of Small Animal Practice* **28** 1115–1125.

Berry, C.R., Gallaway, A., Thrall, D.E. and Carlisle, C. (1993) Thoracic radiographic features of anticoagulant rodenticide toxicity in fourteen dogs. *Veterinary Radiology and Ultrasound* **34** 391–396.

Bolt, G., Monrad, J., Koch, J. and Jensen, A.L. (1994) Canine angiostrongylosis: a review. *Veterinary Record* **135** 447–452.

Burk, R.L., Corley, E.A., Corwin, A. (1978) The radiographic appearance of pulmonary histoplasmosis in the dog and cat; A review of 37 case histories. *Journal of the American Veterinary Radiological Society* **9** 2–6.

Coyne, B.E., Fingland, R.B. (1992) Hypoplasia of the trachea in dogs: 103 cases (1974–1990). *Journal of the American Veterinary Medical Association* **201** 768–772.

Forrest, L.J. and Graybush, C.A. (1998) Radiographic patterns of pulmonary metastasis in 25 cats. *Veterinary Radiology and Ultrasound* **39** 4–8.

Godshalk, C.P. (1994) Common pitfalls in radiographic interpretation of the thorax. *Compendium of Continuing Education for the*

Practicing Veterinarian (Small Animal) **16** 731–738.

Kirberger, R.M. and Lobetti, R.G. (1998) Radiographic aspects of *Pneumocystis carinii* pneumonia in the miniature dachshund. *Veterinary Radiology and Ultrasound* **39** 313–317.

Koblik, P.D. (1986) Radiographic appearance of primary lung tumours in cats: a review of 41 cases. *Veterinary Radiology* **27** 66–73.

Kramer, R.W. (1992) Radiology corner: The nodular pulmonary opacity – is it real? *Veterinary Radiology and Ultrasound* **33** 187–188.

Lord, P.F. and Gomez, J.A. (1985) Lung lobe collapse: pathophysiology and radiologic significance. *Veterinary Radiology* **26** 187–195.

Miles, K.G. (1988) A review of primary lung tumors in the dog and cat. *Veterinary Radiology* **29** 122–128.

Millman, T.M., O'Brien, T.R., Suter, P.F., Wolf, A.M. (1979) Coccidioidomycosis in the dog: its radiographic diagnosis. *Journal of the American Veterinary Radiological Society* **20** 50–65.

Myer, W. and Burt, J.K. (1973) Bronchiectasis in the dog: its radiographic appearance. *Journal of the American Veterinary Radiological Society* **14** 3–12.

Myer, W. (1979) Radiography review: the alveolar pattern of pulmonary disease. *Journal of the American Veterinary Radiological Society* **20** 10–14.

Myer, C.W. (1980) Radiography review: the vascular and bronchial patterns of pulmonary disease. *Veterinary Radiology* **21** 156–160.

Myer, W. (1980) Radiography review: the interstitial pattern of pulmonary disease. *Veterinary Radiology* **21** 18–23.

Park, R.D. (1984) Bronchoesophageal fistula in the dog: literature survey, case presentations, and radiographic manifestations. *Compendium of Continuing Education for the Practicing Veterinarian (Small Animal)* **6** 669–677.

Pechman, R.D. (1987) Effect of dependency versus nondependency on lung lesion visualisation. *Veterinary Radiology* **28** 185–190.

Rudorf, H., Herrtage, M.E., White, R.A.S. (1997) Use of ultrasonography in the diagnosis of tracheal collapse. *Journal of Small Animal Practice* **38** 513–518.

Schmidt, M. and Wolvekamp, P. (1991) Radiographic findings in ten dogs with thoracic actinomycosis. *Veterinary Radiology* **32** 301–306.

Shaiken, L.C., Evans, S.M., Goldschmidt, M.H. (1991) Radiographic findings in canine malignant histiocytosis. *Veterinary Radiology* **32** 237–242.

Silverman, S., Poulos, P.W., Suter, P.F. (1976) Cavitary pulmonary lesions in animals. *Journal of the American Veterinary Radiological Society* **17** 134–146.

Thrall, D.E. (1979) Radiographic diagnosis of metastatic pulmonary tumours. *Compendium of Continuing Education for the Practicing Veterinarian (Small Animal)* **1** 131–139.

Walker, M.A. (1981) Thoracic blastomycosis: A review of its radiographic manifestations in 40 dogs. *Veterinary Radiology* **22** 22–26.

7

Cardiovascular system

7.1 Normal radiographic appearance of the heart
7.2 Normal cardiac silhouette with cardiac pathology
7.3 Cardiac malposition
7.4 Reduction in heart size – microcardia
7.5 Generalised enlargement of the cardiac silhouette
7.6 Pericardial disease
7.7 Ultrasonography of pericardial disease
7.8 Left atrial enlargement
7.9 Left ventricular enlargement
7.10 Aortic abnormalities
7.11 Right atrial enlargement
7.12 Right ventricular enlargement
7.13 Pulmonary artery trunk abnormalities
7.14 Changes in pulmonary arteries and veins
7.15 Caudal vena cava abnormalities
7.16 Cardiac neoplasia

ANGIOGRAPHY

7.17 Angiography – left heart
7.18 Angiography – right heart

CARDIAC ULTRASONOGRAPHY

7.19 Left heart two-dimensional and M-mode echocardiography
7.20 Right heart two-dimensional and M-mode echocardiography
7.21 Contrast echocardiography – right heart
7.22 Doppler flow abnormalities – mitral valve
7.23 Doppler flow abnormalities – aortic valve
7.24 Doppler flow abnormalities – tricuspid valve
7.25 Doppler flow abnormalities – pulmonic valve

7.1 Normal radiographic appearance of the heart

The cardiac silhouette consists of pericardium, pericardial fluid, myocardium (including epicardium and endocardium), the origins of the major vessels and blood. Its size may change with the cardiac cycle and it may be slightly larger during expiration than inspiration. Its appearance is slightly different between right and left lateral recumbency and between sternal and dorsal recumbency and so a consistent technique should be adopted. Radiographic signs of heart disease include change in size or shape of the heart and evidence of right- or left-sided heart failure. Alteration in size or shape of the cardiac silhouette may be due to enlargement of any of its components and can often be distinguished only by angiography or ultrasonography. Conformation is the single most important cause for apparent cardiomegaly in barrel-chested dogs such as the Bulldog, Yorkshire Terrier and Dachshund, which have a relatively large heart with elevated trachea on lateral radiographs. The Golden Retriever also has an apparently large and square-shaped heart on the lateral radiograph. Generalised cardiomegaly may be evaluated in dogs by means of the *vertebral heart size measurement* (Figure 7.1a); on the lateral recumbent radiograph the distance between the ventral aspect of the carina and the cardiac apex is taken as a length value and the maximum width of the heart perpendicular to the length line is taken as the width of the heart. Starting at the cranial aspect of the fourth thoracic vertebra the number of vertebral lengths is determined for each measurement. Cardiomegaly is usually considered present when the combined measurement exceeds 10.6 thoracic vertebrae, although in some breeds (e.g. Labrador, Golden Retriever and Cavalier King Charles Spaniel) this value is commonly exceeded in normal dogs. In cats, generalised cardiomegaly is present when the maximum width of the heart perpendicular to the apicobasilar distance on

SMALL ANIMAL RADIOLOGICAL DIFFERENTIAL DIAGNOSIS

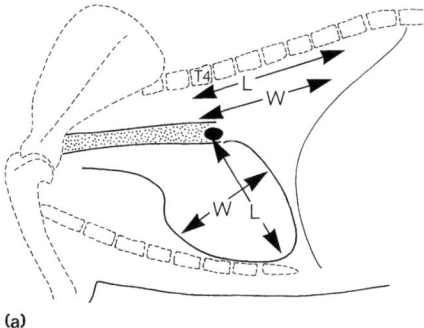

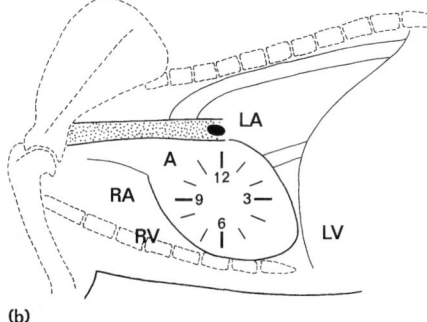

Their locations are:
A   = 11 to 1 o'clock
PA   = 1 to 2
LAA = 2 to 3
LV   = 3 to 5
RV   = 5 to 9
RA   = 9 to 11

Figure 7.1 (a) Method of vertebral heart scale measurement (T4 = fourth thoracic vertebra; L = maximum length of heart; W = maximum width of heart). (b) Clock-face analogy of cardiac anatomy (lateral view). (c) Clock-face analogy of cardiac anatomy (DV view) (A = aorta; LA = left atrium; LAA = left auricular appendage; PA = pulmonary artery; RA = right atrium; RV = right ventricle).

the lateral recumbent radiograph is greater than the distance from the cranial aspect of rib 5 to the caudal aspect of rib 7. Localised cardiac enlargement in both cats and dogs may be described according to the clock-face analogy (Figure 7.1b and c).

7.2 Normal cardiac silhouette with cardiac pathology

A normal cardiac silhouette may be present in spite of severe cardiac disease. Echocardiography and an ECG are essential diagnostic components of the cardiac examination for complete cardiac evaluation.

1. Conduction disturbances and arrhythmias.
2. Over-treated heart disease (e.g. excessive use of diuretics).
3. Concentric ventricular hypertrophy
   a. Secondary to congenital heart disease
      • aortic stenosis (left ventricular hypertrophy)
      • pulmonic stenosis (right ventricular hypertrophy)
   b. Acquired
      • idiopathic hypertrophic cardiomyopathy in cats and dogs
      • hypertrophic cardiomyopathy secondary to hyperthyroidism in older cats.
4. Small shunting lesions
   a. Small atrial and ventricular septal defects (ASD and VSD)
   b. Small patent ductus arteriosus (PDA).
5. Endocarditis.
6. Acute myocardial failure.
7. Pericardial disease
   a. Constrictive pericarditis
   b. Acute traumatic haemopericardium.
8. Acute ruptured chordae tendineae.
9. Myocardial neoplasia.
10. Early or mild myocarditis.

7.3 Cardiac malposition

Terminology

Levocardia   Heart lies in a normal left-sided position (Figure 7.2a)
Dextrocardia Heart lying predominantly in the right thorax with the cardiac apex pointing to the right (Figure 7.2b)
Situs solitus Normal position of thoracic and abdominal organs
Situs inversus Reversal of the normal thoracic and abdominal organs – mirror image (Figure 7.2c)

Dextrocardia

1. Artefact – incorrectly labelled DV/VD radiograph; check the position of the gastric air bubble and spleen in the cranial abdomen.

7 CARDIOVASCULAR SYSTEM

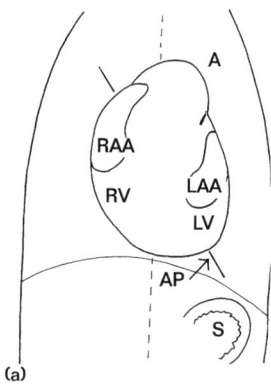

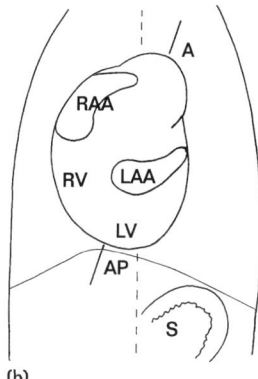

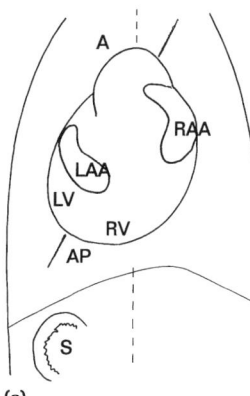

Figure 7.2 (a) Normal location of the heart (DV view); (b) dextrocardia; (c) dextrocardia with situs inversus. (A = aorta; Ap = apex; LAA = left auricular appendage; RAA = right auricular appendage; S = stomach; LV = left ventricle; RV = right ventricle)

2. Normal variant in wide-chested dogs and occasionally in the cat.
3. Acquired causes of dextrocardia
   a. Cardiac disease with left heart enlargement
   b. Mediastinal shift (see 8.8).
4. Congenital extracardiac abnormalities
   a. Pectus excavatum (see 8.22.1)
   b. Vertebral abnormalities resulting in an abnormally wide and shallow thorax.
5. Congenital cardiac abnormalities
   a. Primary dextrocardia with situs inversus – the cardiac apex, left ventricle, aortic arch and gastric air bubble all lie on the right side
      • part of Kartagener's syndrome (also includes rhinitis and bronchiectasis due to ciliary dyskinesia)
   b. Dextrocardia with situs solitus – cardiac chambers normal but apex to right of mid line
   c. Levocardia with partial abdominal situs inversus has also been described.

Dorsal displacement of the heart

6. Fat in the pericardium or ventral mediastinum.
7. Sternal abnormalities (see 8.22).
8. Pneumothorax on a lateral recumbent radiograph (see 8.2.2).
9. Mediastinal shift (see 8.8).
10. Cranioventral thoracic masses (see 8.11.1).

The heart may also be displaced cranially, caudally, ventrally or further to the left by herniated abdominal viscera or by a variety of mass lesions or bony abnormalities.

7.4 Reduction in heart size – microcardia

The heart silhouette is abnormally small and pointed, the ventricles appear narrower and the apex loses contact with the sternum. Thoracic blood vessels may appear smaller and the lungs hyperlucent (see hypovascular pattern; 6.24.5). The caudal vena cava is also reduced in size (Figure 7.3).

1. Artefactual reduction in heart size
   a. Deep-chested dogs – narrow, upright heart with straight caudal border
   b. Deep inspiration
   c. Pulmonary overinflation (see 6.26.4–6)
   d. Heart displaced from the sternum
      • pneumothorax
      • mediastinal shift.
2. Hypovolaemia
   a. Shock
   b. Dehydration

SMALL ANIMAL RADIOLOGICAL DIFFERENTIAL DIAGNOSIS

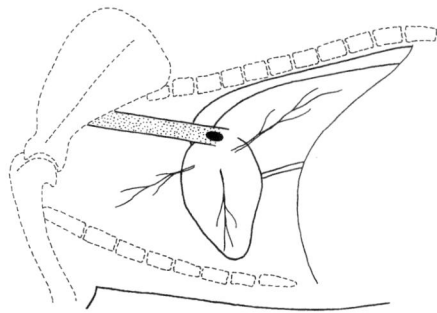

Figure 7.3 Microcardia, pulmonary hypoperfusion and small caudal vena cava.

   c. Hypoadrenocorticism (Addison's disease) – may be accompanied by megaoesophagus.
3. Muscle mass loss
   a. Emaciation
      • chronic systemic disease
      • malnutrition
   b. Hypoadrenocorticism (Addison's disease)
   c. Atrophic myopathies.
4. Constrictive pericarditis.
5. Post-thoracotomy.

7.5 Generalised enlargement of the cardiac silhouette

Some of the following diseases may cause only mild cardiomegaly or cardiomegaly only in advanced stages of the condition. Chamber dilation and heart wall hypertrophy cannot be distinguished radiographically and myocardial pathology is much more readily diagnosed by means of two-dimensional and M-mode echocardiography.
1. Normal in athletic breeds (e.g. Greyhound).
2. Artefactual, due to intrapericardial and mediastinal fat (see 7.6.1).
3. Fluid overload.
4. Bradycardia (e.g. due to sedation), allowing increased diastolic filling.
5. End-stage, left-heart failure due to mitral valve insufficiency
   a. Endocardiosis
   b. Valvular dysplasia
   c. Bacterial endocarditis.
6. Congenital cardiac disease (see 7.8, 7.9, 7.11 and 7.12).
7. Non-inflammatory myocardial disease
   a. Unknown aetiology
      • idiopathic dilated cardiomyopathy – large and giant breed, mainly male dogs, 2–7 years old – especially Dobermann, Great Dane, Irish Wolfhound, Scottish Deerhound, Boxer, Dalmatian and Spaniels
      • hypertrophic cardiomyopathy – rare in dogs; more common in adult male cats
      • restrictive cardiomyopathy – younger cats, rare; DDx endocardial fibroelastosis, a congenital condition in Siamese and Burmese kittens and cats under 1 year old
   b. Secondary to a known aetiology
      • end-stage mitral valve insufficiency
      • nutritional deficiency (e.g. carnitine)
      • toxic (e.g. cytotoxic drugs, such as doxorubicin), heavy metals and toxaemia
      • metabolic disorders such as hyperthyroidism (especially in older cats) and hyperadrenocorticism
      • cats – nutritional deficiency such as lack of taurine (dilated cardiomyopathy) – now rare due to dietary supplementation
      • cats – acromegaly (hypersomatotropism)
      • neuromuscular disorders
      • amyloidosis
      • lipidosis
      • mucopolysaccharidosis
      • infiltrative disease (e.g. neoplasia and glycogen storage diseases)
      • physical agents (e.g. heat and trauma)
      • old age.
8. Concurrent left and right heart valvular insufficiency
   a. Endocardiosis
   b. Valvular dysplasia
   c. Bacterial endocarditis.
9. Pericardial disease (see 7.6).
10. Inflammatory myocardial disease
    a. Infectious
       • viral (e.g. parvovirus in puppies)
       • bacterial
       • mycoplasma
       • protozoal (e.g. trypanosomiasis*)
       • parasitic
       • fungal
    b. Non-infectious
       • immune-mediated (e.g. rheumatoid arthritis).
11. Ischaemic myocardial disease
    a. Arteriosclerosis and thrombosis of large coronary artery branches

7 CARDIOVASCULAR SYSTEM

b. Arteriosclerosis, amyloidosis or hyalinosis of intramural coronary arteries
c. Angiopathies secondary to congenital heart disease.
12. Chronic anaemia.

7.6 Pericardial disease

Pericardial disease may be difficult to distinguish radiographically from generalised cardiomegaly. The main difference is that most cases of cardiomegaly have left atrial enlargement whereas pericardial effusion produces an enlarged, globular "cardiac silhouette" lacking specific chamber enlargement (Figure 7.4). Its margins may be sharp due to reduced movement blur. Pericardial effusion may also often be differentiated from generalised cardiomegaly by the type of failure that results, which is right-sided; left-sided or generalised failure is seen with the most common cause of generalised cardiomegaly, cardiomyopathy.

Ultrasonography is the imaging modality of choice to evaluate pericardial pathology and has replaced positive and negative contrast pericardiography and non-selective angiography as a further imaging procedure in cases of suspected pericardial effusion.

1. Artefactual appearance of pericardial effusion – obese dogs may have large amounts of intrapericardial and mediastinal fat, mimicking an enlarged cardiac silhouette and possible pericardial effusion. Fat is less radio-opaque than soft tissue such as the myocardium and on good-quality radiographs the pericardial fat can be distinguished from the myocardium.
2. Pericardial effusion – usually male dogs over 6 years old and weighing more than 20 kg

a. Non-inflammatory pericardial effusions
   - idiopathic benign effusion, especially in the St Bernard and Golden Retriever
   - hypoalbuminaemia
   - congestive heart failure
   - toxaemia
   - uraemia
   - trauma
   - neoplastic obstruction of lymph and blood vessels at the heart base
   - associated with a peritoneopericardial diaphragmatic hernia
b. Inflammatory pericardial effusions
   - idiopathic benign effusion
   - sterile foreign body
   - septic purulent process sometimes secondary to perforating wounds
   - tuberculosis
   - coccidioidomycosis*
   - steatitis
   - cats – feline infectious peritonitis (FIP)
c. Neoplastic pericardial effusions – usually haemorrhagic (rare in the cat)
   - right atrial haemangiosarcoma, especially the German Shepherd dog and often associated with pulmonary, splenic or hepatic haemangiosarcoma
   - heart base tumours (see 7.16.2)
   - mesothelioma
   - metastatic neoplasia
   - lymphosarcoma, especially cats
   - rhabdomyosarcoma
d. Haemopericardium
   - trauma (e.g. gun shot, bite wound, sequel to pericardiocentesis)
   - rupture of the left atrium by a severe jet lesion secondary to mitral valve insufficiency – espe-

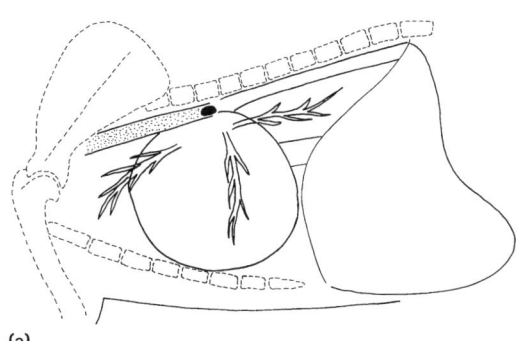
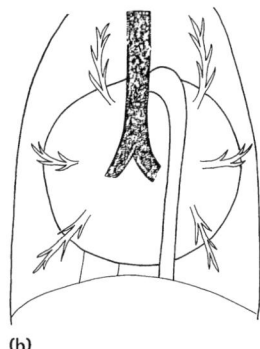

Figure 7.4 Pericardial effusion – the heart is enlarged and very rounded in shape. (a) Lateral view; (b) DV view.

SMALL ANIMAL RADIOLOGICAL DIFFERENTIAL DIAGNOSIS

cially Dachshund, Poodle and Cocker Spaniel
- coagulopathy
  e. Chylous pericardial effusion – very rare and of unknown aetiology.
3. Congenital peritoneopericardial diaphragmatic hernia – may be accompanied by sternal abnormalities and an umbilical hernia. Gas-filled intestinal loops or faecal material may be seen within the "cardiac" silhouette. Often only diagnosed later in life.
4. Pneumopericardium – rare, usually due to trauma.
5. Pericardial cyst – rare. If large, mimics a pericardial effusion. Young animals; may be associated with a peritoneopericardial diaphragmatic hernia.

7.7 Ultrasonography of pericardial disease

1. Pericardial fluid (see 7.6.2). Usually anechoic or hypoechoic fluid. Swirling echoes within the fluid are suggestive of large numbers of cells, debris or gas bubbles. It is important to check for the presence of cardiac tamponade secondary to the fluid accumulation; in the early stages this is indicated by collapse of the right atrial wall during systole and in more advanced cases by abnormal motion of the right ventricular free wall also.
2. Intrapericardial mass
   a Neoplasia
     - right atrial haemangiosarcoma
     - heart base tumour
   b. Thrombus
   c. Abdominal organs in a peritoneopericardial diaphragmatic hernia
   d. Pericardial cyst.
3. Thickening of the epicardium or pericardium – may lead to a restrictive state, in which complete filling of the cardiac chambers is prevented.
   a. Mesothelioma
   b. Reactive or inflammatory changes.

7.8 Left atrial enlargement

The lateral view shows bulging of the cardiac silhouette at 12–2 o'clock, with elevation and compression of the left main-stem bronchus. The caudal border of the heart is abnormally straight and upright or even slopes caudodorsally and the caudal cardiac waist is lost (see Fig 7.5a). On the DV view atrial enlargement may push the main stem bronchi further apart (to >60°) and the enlarged left auricular appendage creates a bulge at 2–3 o'clock (see Fig 7.5b). The increased opacity of the dilated left atrium may be mistaken as lymphadenopathy or a lung mass on either view. Secondary pulmonary changes in the form of vascular congestion or pulmonary oedema may be present (see 6.24 and 6.14).

Volume overload

1. Mitral valve insufficiency
   a. Endocardiosis – older, small-breed dogs
   b. Secondary to left ventricular failure when the enlarging ventricle results in dilation of the annular ring (e.g. dilated cardiomyopathy)
   c. Bacterial endocarditis
   d. Ruptured left ventricular chordae tendineae
   e. Congenital valvular dysplasia – especially Great Dane, German Shepherd dog, Bull Terrier and cats
   f. Ruptured papillary muscle.
2. Diastolic dysfunction of the left ventricle resulting in pooling of blood in the left atrium.
3. PDA with left-to-right shunting – especially Spaniel, Collie, German Shepherd dog, Keeshond, Pomeranian, Miniature Poodle and Irish Setter.
4. VSD with left-to-right shunting – especially Beagle, Bulldog, German Shepherd dog, Keeshond, Mastiff, Siberian Husky and cats.
5. Aorticopulmonary septal defect with left-to-right shunting.
6. Endocardial fibroelastosis – Siamese and Burmese kittens.

Pressure overload

7. Left ventricular hypertrophy leading to mitral insufficiency
   a. Aortic stenosis – especially German Shepherd dog, Boxer, Newfoundland, Pointer and Golden Retriever
   b. Hypertrophic cardiomyopathy – rare in dogs; in cats a "valentine-shaped" heart is seen on the DV view due to atrial enlargement
     - idiopathic hypertrophic cardiomyopathy; cats and dogs
     - hypertrophic cardiomyopathy secondary to hyperthyroidism in older cats
   c. Cats – restrictive cardiomyopathy – "valentine" heart on the DV view.
8. Congenital mitral valve stenosis – especially Newfoundland, Bull Terrier and cats – rare.

9. Atrial or ventricular neoplasia interfering with transvalvular flow – rare.

7.9 Left ventricular enlargement

On the lateral view cardiac enlargement is seen at 2–5/6 o'clock with increased height of the heart and elevation of the trachea (Figure 7.5a). Left atrial enlargement is usually also present. On the DV view (Figure 7.5b) the heart may appear elongated and enlargement is seen at 3–5 o'clock (right heart enlargement due to e.g. pulmonic stenosis may displace the cardiac apex further to the left on the DV radiograph mimicking left ventricular enlargement).

Volume overload

1. Mitral valve insufficiency (see 7.8.1).
2. Aortic insufficiency.

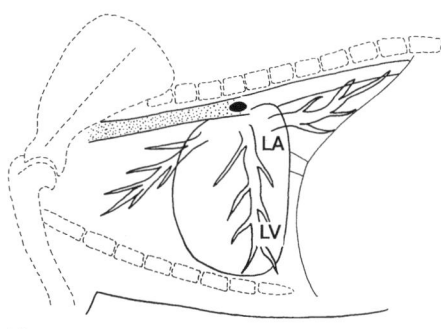

(a)

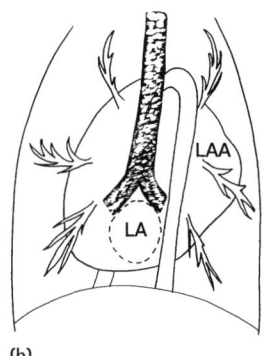

(b)

Figure 7.5 Left-sided cardiomegaly. (a) Lateral view, showing a tall heart and an enlarged left atrium; (b) DV view, showing the enlarged left auricular appendage at 2–3 o'clock and the left atrium as a mass between the main stem bronchi. Signs of left-sided heart failure (pulmonary hyperperfusion and oedema) may also be present. (LA = left atrium; LAA = left auricular appendage; LV = left ventricle.)

3. PDA with left-to-right shunting – the most common congenital cardiac condition in the dog but far less common in cats.
4. VSD with left-to-right shunting.
5. Endocardial cushion defects (persistent atrioventricular canal).

Pressure overload

Results in concentric hypertrophy and often does not cause ventricular silhouette enlargement.

6. Aortic stenosis.
7. Systemic hypertension.
8. Hypertrophic cardiomyopathy – rare in dogs. In cats a "valentine-shaped" heart is seen on the DV view due to atrial enlargement
   a. Idiopathic hypertrophic cardiomyopathy; cats and dogs
   b. Hypertrophic cardiomyopathy secondary to hyperthyroidism in older cats.
9. Coarctation (narrowing) of the aorta – very rare.

Myocardial failure [see 7.5]

10. Dilated cardiomyopathy.
11. Myocarditis.
12. Myocardial neoplasia (see 7.16).

Miscellaneous

13. Ventricular aneurysm – localised protrusion of the left ventricle.

7.10 Aortic abnormalities

1. Enlargement of the aortic arch or descending aorta. On the lateral view enlargement of the aortic arch may be seen at 11–12 o'clock with reduction or possibly obliteration of the cranial cardiac waist (Figure 7.6a). On the DV view an aortic "knuckle" is seen at 11–1 o'clock with mediastinal widening, and there is an apparent increase in the craniocaudal length of the heart (Figure 7.6b).
   a. Post-aortic stenosis dilation
   b. Large left-to-right shunting PDA, due to increase in aortic circulating blood volume and inherent aortic wall weakness
   c. Aneurysm secondary to *Spirocerca lupi** migration or granuloma
   d. Aortic body tumour (chemodectoma)
   e. Coarctation (narrowing) of the aorta with post-stenotic dilation.
2. Redundant (tortuous or bulging) aorta
   a. Brachycephalic breeds, especially the Bulldog

SMALL ANIMAL RADIOLOGICAL DIFFERENTIAL DIAGNOSIS

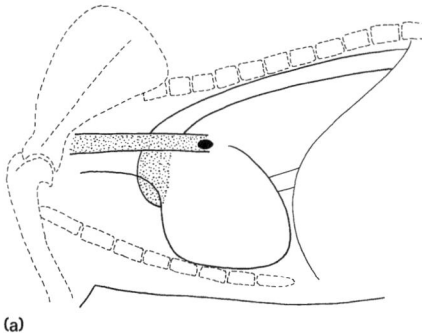

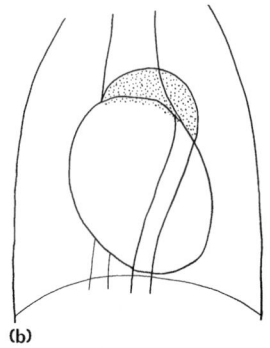

Figure 7.6 Location of an enlarged aortic arch. (a) Lateral view; (b) DV view.

  b. Some older dogs
  c. Congenital hypothyroidism
  d. Common in old cats accompanied by a more horizontal heart – aorta bulges cranially and to the left.
3. Right-sided aorta – congenital persistent right aortic arch (PRAA); a vascular ring anomaly with secondary oesophageal dilation (see 8.16.2).
4. Calcification or mineralisation of the aorta – rare
  a. Lymphosarcoma
  b. Renal failure
  c. Primary or secondary hyperparathyroidism
  d. Arteriosclerosis
  e. Hyperadrenocorticism (Cushing's disease)
  f. *Spirocerca lupi** larval migration
  g. Idiopathic
  h. Hypervitaminosis D
  i. Coronary artery calcification – short, wavy lines originating at the aortic arch.

7.11 Right atrial enlargement

On the lateral view bulging of the cardiac silhouette occurs at 10–11 o'clock, with increased craniocaudal dimension of the heart and elevation of the terminal trachea and/or loss of the cranial cardiac waist in severe cases. There may be a widened caudal vena cava as result of venous congestion (see Fig 7.7a). On the DV view, bulging is seen at 9–11 o'clock (see Fig 7.7b).

Volume overload

1. Tricuspid valve insufficiency
  a. Endocardiosis
  b. Congenital tricuspid valve dysplasia – more common in cats
  c. Secondary to right ventricular failure when the enlarging ventricle results in dilation of the annular ring
  d. Ebstein's anomaly – the valve leaflets are deformed and the valvular insertions are displaced distally into the right ventricle
  e. Bacterial endocarditis
  f. Ruptured right ventricular chordae tendineae
  g. Anomalous pulmonary venous drainage.
2. ASD with left-to-right shunting.
3. Arteriovenous fistula elsewhere in the body.

Pressure overload

4. Right ventricular hypertrophy leading to tricuspid insufficiency
  a. Pulmonic stenosis – may result in secondary tricuspid valve insufficiency, especially Bulldog, Fox Terrier, Chihuahua, Miniature Schnauzer, Beagle and Keeshond
  b. Tetralogy of Fallot – especially the Keeshond.
5. Atrial or ventricular neoplasia interfering with transvalvular flow (see 7.16).
6. Cor pulmonale (see 7.12.9).
7. Congenital tricuspid valve stenosis – rare.

Miscellaneous

8. Right atrial neoplasia – haemangiosarcoma, especially the German Shepherd dog, and often associated with pulmonary, splenic or hepatic haemangiosarcoma.

7.12 Right ventricular enlargement

Artefactual right ventricular enlargement may be seen on left lateral recumbent radiographs, in which there is increased sternal contact, rounding of the heart outline and elevation of the cardiac apex from the sternum. On the DV view, tilting of the chest with the sternum to the right may also create the false

7 CARDIOVASCULAR SYSTEM

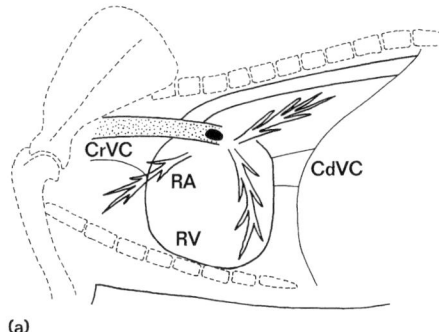

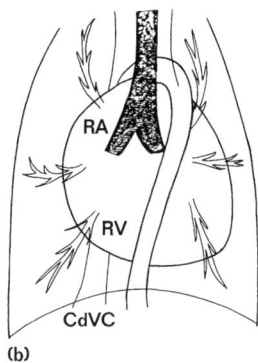

Figure 7.7 Right-sided cardiomegaly. (a) Lateral view, showing rounding of the cranial heart margin and increase in sternal contact; (b) DV view, in which the heart has an "inverted D" shape due to rounding of the right heart border. Signs of right-sided heart failure (vena cava engorgement, hepatomegaly and ascites) may also be present. (CdVC = caudal vena cava; CrVC = cranial vena cava; RA = right atrium; RV = right ventricle.)

appearance of right-sided bulging. On the lateral view right ventricular enlargement creates cardiac bulging at 5/6–9/10 o'clock with increased craniocaudal dimension and increased sternal contact of more than 2.5 sternebrae in deep-chested dogs and 3.5 in broad-chested dogs. Accentuation of the cranial cardiac waist may occur (Figure 7.7a). On the DV view enlargement is at 5–9 o'clock, with excessive rounding of the right ventricle producing an "inverted D"-shaped heart (Figure 7.7b). Signs of right-sided failure include caudal vena cava engorgement, hepatomegaly and ascites (pleural effusion is common in cats).

Volume overload

1. Tricuspid valve insufficiency (see 7.11.1).
2. Pulmonic valve insufficiency.
3. VSD.
4. ASD.
5. Endocardial cushion defects (persistent atrioventricular canal) – more common in cats.
6. Arteriovenous fistula elsewhere in the body.

Pressure overload

Results in concentric hypertrophy and therefore may cause less cardiac silhouette enlargement than with volume overload.

7. Secondary to left heart failure or mitral valve disease (see 7.8).
8. Pulmonic stenosis.
9. Pulmonary hypertension (cor pulmonale)
   a. Dirofilariasis* (heartworm) or angiostrongylosis* ("French" heartworm) – with hypervascular lung pattern and secondary bronchopneumonia
   b. Severe lung pathology; examples include:
      - thromboembolism
      - primary pulmonary hypertension
      - chronic obstructive pulmonary disease (COPD)
      - high-altitude disease
      - pulmonary arteriovenous fistula.
10. Eisenmenger's syndrome – pulmonary blood flow obstruction or pulmonary hypertension results in right-to-left shunting through a congenital shunt (e.g. PDA or septal defect) and therefore cyanosis
    a. Defects combined with pulmonic stenosis
       - tetralogy of Fallot – the most common cyanotic heart disease of dogs (especially the Keeshond) and cats
       - trilogy or pentalogy of Fallot
       - double outlet right ventricle – may be difficult to distinguish from tetralogy of Fallot
       - cats – persistent truncus arteriosus.
11. Single right coronary artery resulting in secondary constrictive pulmonic stenosis.

Myocardial failure

12. Dilated cardiomyopathy
    a. Generalised together with left ventricular involvement
    b. Arrhythmogenic right ventricular cardiomyopathy.
13. Myocarditis.
14. Myocardial neoplasia (see 7.16).

Miscellaneous

15. Ventricular aneurysm – localised protrusion of the right ventricle.

133

SMALL ANIMAL RADIOLOGICAL DIFFERENTIAL DIAGNOSIS

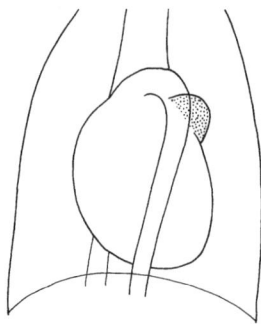

Figure 7.8 Location of an enlarged pulmonary artery segment; a knuckle is seen at 1–2 o'clock on the DV view.

7.13 Pulmonary artery trunk abnormalities

On the lateral view enlargement may be difficult to see unless it is very large, as the bulge may be superimposed over the terminal trachea. On the DV view a pulmonary artery knuckle is seen at 1–2 o'clock (Figure 7.8). On the VD view, a pulmonary artery knuckle is commonly seen in normal animals due to lateral tilting of the heart.
1. Artefactual
   a. Radiograph made at the end of ventricular systole, especially in deep-chested dogs
   b. Rotation of the chest
   c. Dorsal recumbency for VD view.
2. Post-pulmonic stenosis dilation.
3. Increased circulating blood volume with large left-to-right shunts
   a. PDA
   b. ASD
   c. VSD.
4. Elevated pulmonary artery pressure secondary to pulmonary hypertension (cor pulmonale) (see 7.12.9).
5. Large collections of Dirofilaria* and Angiostrongylus* worms.

7.14 Changes in pulmonary arteries and veins

See 6.24 – Vascular lung pattern.

7.15 Caudal vena cava abnormalities

Temporary changes in the diameter of the caudal vena cava are common incidental findings and may be due to thoracic and abdominal pressure changes and to differences in the cardiac or respiratory cycle. The ratio of the greatest caudal vena cava diameter to the aortic diameter at the same intercostal space may be calculated. A ratio of <1.0 indicates a normal caudal vena cava; a ratio of >1.5 indicates an abnormally widened caudal vena cava.

Persistent widening of the caudal vena cava
1. Right heart failure.
2. Tricuspid valve insufficiency.
3. Cardiac tamponade due to pericardial effusion.
4. Constrictive pericarditis.
5. Obstruction of the right atrium or ventricle
   a. Tumours (see 7.16)
   b. Thrombi.
6. Tumours infiltrating the caudal vena cava
   a. Phaeochromocytoma
   b. Other invasive tumours from the right atrium, liver and kidney.
7. Large collections of Dirofilaria* worms.
8. Pulmonary hypertension (see 7.12.9).
9. Cor triatriatum dexter – septal membrane in the right atrium.
10. Idiopathic caudal vena cava stenosis.
11. Caudal vena cava thrombi.

Narrowed caudal vena cava
Often accompanied by microcardia, pulmonary undercirculation and in extreme cases a small aorta.
12. Shock.
13. Severe dehydration.
14. Pulmonary overinflation (see 6.26.4–6).
15. Hypoadrenocorticism (Addison's disease).

Absent caudal vena cava
16. Very rare congenital anomaly – abdominal blood flow returns via a greatly distended azygos vein.

7.16 Cardiac neoplasia

Uncommon; often there is little visible change to the cardiac silhouette unless the tumour is large or a pericardial effusion results (see 7.6). Heart base tumours may elevate the terminal trachea. Most clinically significant tumours are visible ultrasonographically.

Right atrial wall tumours
1. Haemangiosarcoma – especially the German Shepherd dog (primary or metastatic). May be accompanied by pericardial effusion and/or pulmonary, splenic or hepatic haemangiosarcoma.

Heart base tumours
2. Aortic body tumour (chemodectoma) – more common in older, male, brachycephalic dogs; very rare in the cat.

7 CARDIOVASCULAR SYSTEM

3. Ectopic thyroid tumour.
4. Ectopic parathyroid tumour.

Right chamber tumours
5. Myxoma.
6. Haemangiosarcoma – pericardial effusion common.
7. Fibroma.
8. Ectopic thyroid carcinoma.
9. Fibrosarcoma.
10. Myxosarcoma.
11. Chondrosarcoma.
12. Infiltrative chemodectoma.

Myocardial tumours
13. Metastatic tumours.

14. Haemangiosarcoma.
15. Rhabdomyosarcoma.
16. Lymphosarcoma – especially cat.

Left chamber tumours
Very rare in dogs and cats.
17. Metastatic tumours.
18. As for right chamber tumours.

Epicardial tumours
Pericardial effusion is common
19. Mesothelioma.
20. Metastatic neoplasia.

ANGIOGRAPHY

Many of the diagnoses previously made angiographically can now be made using echocardiography. *Selective angiography* is generally reserved for veterinary schools and specialist referral centres as it requires high-pressure injectors and rapid cassette changers. *Non-selective angiography* can readily be performed in private practice. The largest possible catheter is placed in a peripheral vein or passed to the right atrium or terminal cranial or caudal vena cava. A water-soluble iodinated contrast medium is injected rapidly at a dose rate of 1–2 ml/kg and 2–6 radiographs are made immediately in lateral recumbency at 1–2 second intervals using a cassette tunnel. Sedation or general anaesthesia is necessary to prevent motion and avoid the need for manual restraint. Radiographs made within the first 4–5 seconds will generally demonstrate the right heart chambers and those made after 5–6 seconds the left heart chambers.

7.17 Angiography – left heart

Selective angiography with the catheter tip in the ascending aorta – abnormalities

1. Dilated aorta
   a. Ascending aorta dilated
      - post stenotic dilation
   b. Proximal descending aorta dilated
      - PDA
      - PDA ductus diverticulum post surgically
      - dilation distal to coarctation (narrowing) of the aorta
   c. Distal descending aorta dilated
      - *Spirocerca lupi**

2. Contrast crossing into the pulmonary vasculature – PDA with left-to-right shunting (usual).
3. Contrast refluxing into the left ventricle – aortic insufficiency.
4. Valvular defects.
5. Supravalvular stenosis.
6. Aortic interruption – absent initial descending aorta with a collateral vertebral artery supplying the caudal descending aorta.
7. Anomalous branching of the aortic arch.
8. Coronary artery anomalies.

Selective angiography with the catheter tip in the left ventricle – abnormalities

9. Contrast refluxing into the left atrium
   a. Mitral valve insufficiency
   b. Mechanical effect of the catheter
   c. Premature ventricular contractions during the contrast injection.
10. Small left ventricular lumen with thick walls
    a. Pressure overload – (see 7.9.6–9)
    b. Hypertrophic cardiomyopathy
       - idiopathic hypertrophic cardiomyopathy; rare in dogs, more common in cats
       - hypertrophic cardiomyopathy secondary to hyperthyroidism in older cats.
11. Large left ventricular lumen with thin walls – volume overload (see 7.9.1–5).
12. Aortic stenosis.
13. Filling defects in the left ventricle
    a. Thrombi

SMALL ANIMAL RADIOLOGICAL DIFFERENTIAL DIAGNOSIS

   b. Papillary muscle hypertrophy in pressure overload (see 7.9.6–9)
   c. Tumours – rare.
14. Poor filling of the aorta – poor myocardial contractility
15. Simultaneous filling of the right ventricle and pulmonary artery
    a. VSD with left-to-right shunting
    b. Tetralogy of Fallot.

Selective angiography with the catheter tip in the left atrium – abnormalities

16. Enlarged left atrium (see 7.8).
17. Simultaneous filling of the right atrium – ASD with left-to-right shunting.
18. Filling defects in the left atrium
    a. Thrombi
    b. Tumours – rare.
19. Mitral valve defects.

7.18 Angiography – right heart

Non-selective angiography with the catheter in a vein, or selective angiography with the catheter in the right atrium, ventricle or pulmonary artery – abnormalities

1. Filling defects in the right atrium, ventricle or pulmonary artery
   a. Papillary muscle hypertrophy in pressure overload (see 7.12.7–11)
   b. *Dirofilaria** or *Angiostrongylus** worms
   c. Thrombi
   d. Lobar pulmonary artery thromboembolism
   e. Tumours (see 7.16).
2. Small right ventricular lumen with thick walls – pressure overload (see 7.12.7–11).
3. Large right ventricular chamber with thin walls – volume overload (see 7.12.1–6).
4. Simultaneous filling of the left atrium – ASD with right-to-left shunting.
5. Simultaneous filling of the left ventricle
   a. VSD with right-to-left shunting
   b. Tetralogy of Fallot.
6. Contrast in the right atrium with ventricular catheter tip placement
   a. Tricuspid insufficiency
   b. Mechanical effect of the catheter
   c. Premature ventricular contractions during the contrast injection.
7. Tricuspid and pulmonic valve defects.
8. Pulmonic stenosis.
9. Apparent thick atrial wall – restrictive pericarditis.
10. Eisenmenger's syndrome (see 7.12.10).
11. Dilated pulmonary arch – post-stenotic dilation.
12. Simultaneous filling of the pulmonary artery and aorta – PDA with right-to-left shunting (unusual).
13. Contrast in the right ventricle with pulmonary artery catheter tip placement
    a. Pulmonic valve insufficiency
    b. Mechanical effect of the catheter.

CARDIAC ULTRASONOGRAPHY

Two-dimensional-echocardiography is the ideal diagnostic imaging modality for evaluation of the internal structure of the heart. The best images are obtained by scanning from the dependent side through a hole in a special table or platform. The heart falls to the dependent side and displaces the adjacent lung away from the heart creating an acoustic window. Cardiac chamber and wall size are more accurately measured by means of M-mode echocardiography. Flow abnormalities may be detected using Doppler echocardiography or by identifying abnormalities of valvular motion in M-mode.

7.19 Left heart two-dimensional and M-mode echocardiography

In the normal animal the left heart chamber dimensions and ventricular wall thickness should be approximately 2–3 times those of the right ventricle, as seen from a right parasternal long axis view.

Left atrial abnormalities on echocardiography

Atrial enlargement is present in the dog when the left atrium to aortic diameter ratio is >0.95 on a right parasternal long axis view.

1. Left atrial enlargement – volume overload (see 7.8.1–6)
   a. Mitral valve insufficiency – valvular abnormalities
      - incomplete closure during systole
      - valvular growths or nodules: endocardiosis and bacterial endocarditis
      - congenital valve deformity – mitral dysplasia

7 CARDIOVASCULAR SYSTEM

- reverse doming (valve prolapses into the atrium) due to weak chordae tendineae
- flail valve (valve prolapses into the atrium) due to chordae tendineae or papillary muscle rupture
  b. ASD; the adjacent edges of the septal walls are often thickened.
2. Left atrial enlargement – pressure overload (see 7.8.7–9)
   a. Mitral valve stenosis
      - doming of the valve leaflets
      - thickening of the valve leaflets
      - incomplete separation of the valve leaflets.
3. Left atrial lumen abnormalities
   a. Thrombi – hypoechoic; may float freely or be attached to the wall, particularly in the auricular appendage; may act as a ball valve
   b. Tumours – very rare, hypo- to hyperechoic (see 7.16)
   c. Ruptured chordae tendineae – thin, linear streak in the region of the valve.

Mitral valve M-mode abnormalities (Figure 7.9)

4. Increased E point to septal separation (EPSS)
   a. With normal mitral valve movement
      - myocardial failure (e.g. dilated cardiomyopathy), due to decreased fractional shortening

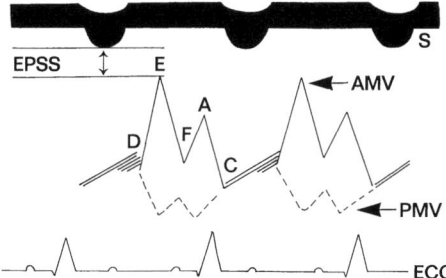

Figure 7.9 Schematic representation of normal M-mode mitral valve motion seen from the right parasternal long axis view. EPSS = E point to septal separation; AMV = anterior mitral valve; PMV = posterior mitral valve; D = end of ventricular systole; E = peak opening of mitral valve during early diastolic flow; F = nadir of initial diastolic closing; A = peak mitral valve opening during atrial contraction; C = complete closure of valve at the start of ventricular systole; S = interventricular septum; ECG = electrocardiogram trace.

- volume overload (e.g. PDA) (see 7.8.1–6 and 7.9.1–5)
  b. Restricted mitral valve motion
     - aortic insufficiency
     - mitral valve stenosis.
5. Decreased E point to septal separation (EPSS)
   a. Increased fractional shortening
      - mitral valve insufficiency
      - aortic insufficiency
      - sympathetic over-stimulation
   b. Mitral valve growths
      - endocardiosis
      - bacterial endocarditis
   c. Pathological septal thickening
      - subaortic stenosis
      - hypertrophic cardiomyopathy
      - hyperthyroidism
      - infiltrative cardiac disease
      - systemic hypertension
   d. Physiological septal thickening
      - athletic dogs.
6. Thickened mitral valve leaflets
   a. Endocardiosis
   b. Bacterial endocarditis
   c. Mitral valve dysplasia
   d. Mitral valve stenosis.
7. Lack of late diastolic (A peak) opening – atrial fibrillation.
8. Diastolic anterior mitral valve flutter – aortic valve insufficiency.
9. Systolic anterior motion of the anterior mitral valve
   a. Subaortic stenosis
   b. Hypertrophic cardiomyopathy
   c. Left ventricular hypertrophy
   d. Hyperkinesis.
10. Decreased EF slope
    a. Mitral valve stenosis (will include concordant anterior diastolic motion of the anterior and posterior mitral valve leaflets)
    b. Left ventricular diastolic dysfunction (e.g. hypertrophic cardiomyopathy)
    c. Decreased transmitral flow.
11. Normal E and A peaks followed by one or more A peaks only – second- and third-degree atrioventricular block.

Left ventricular abnormalities on echocardiography

12. Left ventricular chamber enlargement (see 7.9)
    a. Mitral valve insufficiency – valvular abnormalities
       - see 7.19.1 and 2
       - displaced papillary muscles and chordae tendineae

SMALL ANIMAL RADIOLOGICAL DIFFERENTIAL DIAGNOSIS

    b. Aortic valve insufficiency – valvular abnormalities
- incomplete closure during systole
- valvular growths or nodules: endocardiosis and bacterial endocarditis
- abnormally positioned valve

    c. VSD seen in the proximal part of the septum.

13. Thickened left ventricular wall
    a. Pressure overload with prominent papillary muscles and a small chamber (see 7.9.6–9)
    b. Hypertrophic cardiomyopathy
       - idiopathic hypertrophic cardiomyopathy; rare in dogs, more common in cats
       - hypertrophic cardiomyopathy secondary to hyperthyroidism in older cats
    c. Boxer cardiomyopathy
    d. Myocardial tumours (see 7.16)
    e. Hyperthyroidism
    f. Cats – mild restrictive cardiomyopathy
    g. Cats – hypertrophic muscular dystrophy.

14. Altered fractional shortening of the left ventricle
    a. Increased
       - mitral valve insufficiency
       - aortic stenosis and/or insufficiency
       - ventricular septal defect
    b. Decreased
       - with myocardial failure (see 7.5)
       - end-stage left heart failure
       - drugs, including general anaesthesia.

Aortic valve M-mode abnormalities

15. Systolic fluttering – aortic stenosis.
16. Doming of the valve – aortic stenosis.
17. Decreased aortic excursion
    a. Advanced myocardial failure
    b. Reduced cardiac output.

7.20 Right heart two-dimensional and M-mode echocardiography

In the normal dog, the right heart chamber dimensions and ventricular wall thickness should be approximately one-third to one-half those of the left ventricle, as seen from a right parasternal long axis view.

Right atrial abnormalities on echocardiography

1. Right atrial enlargement – volume overload (see 7.11.1–3)
   a. Tricuspid valve insufficiency – valvular abnormalities
      - incomplete closure during systole
      - valvular growths or nodules: endocardiosis and bacterial endocarditis
      - congenital valve deformity – tricuspid dysplasia
      - reverse doming (valve prolapses into the atrium) due to weak chordae tendineae
      - flail valve (valve prolapses into the atrium) due to chordae tendineae or papillary muscle rupture
      - abnormally positioned valves: Ebstein's anomaly
      - interference by *Dirofilaria** or *Angiostrongylus** worms
   b. Atrial septal defect; the adjacent edges of the septal walls are often thickened.

2. Right atrial enlargement – pressure overload (see 7.11.4–7)
   a. Tricuspid valve stenosis – rare
      - doming of the valve
      - thickening of the valve
      - incomplete separation of the valve leaflets.

3. Right atrial wall abnormalities
   a. Abnormal flapping motion of the right atrial wall – cardiac tamponade due to pericardial effusion; collapses inwards during diastole
   b. Hypoechoic mass – haemangiosarcoma.

4. Right atrial lumen abnormalities
   a. Thrombi – hypoechoic masses; may float freely or be attached to the wall, particularly in the auricular appendage
   b. Tumours – hypo- to hyperechoic (see 7.16)
   c. Short, parallel echogenic lines 2 mm apart – *Dirofilaria* or *Angiostrongylus* worms
   d. Septal membrane in the atrium – cor triatriatum dexter
   e. Thin linear streak in the region of the valve – ruptured chordae tendineae.

Tricuspid valve M-mode abnormalities

5. Thickened tricuspid valves
   a. Endocardiosis
   b. Bacterial endocarditis
   c. Tricuspid valve dysplasia
   d. Tricuspid valve stenosis.

6. Diastolic tricuspid valve flutter – pulmonic valve insufficiency.
7. Additional hyperechoic lines – *Dirofilaria** or *Angiostrongylus** worms.

Right ventricular abnormalities on echocardiography

8. Right ventricular chamber enlargement (see 7.12)
   a. Tricuspid valve insufficiency – valvular abnormalities
      - see right atrium (7.20.1 and 2)
      - displaced papillary muscle and chordae tendineae
      - abnormally positioned tricuspid valve: Ebstein's anomaly
   b. Pulmonic valve insufficiency – valvular abnormalities
      - incomplete closure during systole
      - valvular growths or nodules: endocardiosis and bacterial endocarditis
      - abnormally positioned valve
   c. VSD seen in the proximal part of the septum.
9. Thickened right ventricular wall with smaller chamber – pressure overload (see 7.12.7–11)
   a. Pulmonic stenosis
      - thickening of the valve leaflets
      - doming of the valve leaflets
   b. Myocardial tumours (see 7.16).
10. Abnormal flapping motion of the right ventricular wall – cardiac tamponade due to pericardial effusion.
11. Right ventricular lumen abnormalities (see right atrium. 7.20.4).
12. Transposed aorta – tetralogy of Fallot.

7.21 Contrast echocardiography – right heart

The anechoic blood may be temporarily replaced by multiple small echogenic specks. These are created by rapid injections of specific contrast agents, gases or agitated saline into a peripheral vein. The echogenic specks should pass rapidly through the right heart and be absorbed in the pulmonary vasculature.

1. Pulsating filling defects within the echogenic cloud in the right atrium or ventricle adjacent to the septum – left-to-right shunting ASD or VSD, respectively.
2. Simultaneous specks in the left atrium or ventricle – right-to-left shunting (rare) ASD or VSD, respectively.
3. Persistence of echogenic specks in the right atrium and ventricle – tricuspid valve insufficiency.
4. Persistence of echogenic specks in the right ventricle – pulmonic valve insufficiency.
5. Echogenic specks in the abdominal aorta with normoechoic left heart and ascending aorta – PDA with right-to-left shunting (unusual).
6. Echogenic specks in the ascending aorta with normoechoic left heart – tetralogy of Fallot (overriding aortic arch).

7.22 Doppler flow abnormalities – mitral valve

1. Ventricular side increased forward diastolic flow
   a. Laminar flow due to increased blood volume
      - mitral valve insufficiency
      - left-to-right shunting PDA
      - right-to-left shunting ASD
   b. Turbulent flow – mitral stenosis – rare.
2. Ventricular side decreased forward diastolic flow
   a. Left-to-right shunting ASD
   b. Hypovolaemia
      - shock
      - dehydration
   c. Drugs resulting in decreased blood pressure
   d. Poor cardiac output
   e. Left ventricular diastolic dysfunction; second diastolic flow peak likely to be higher than the first diastolic peak
      - aortic stenosis
      - hypertrophic cardiomyopathy
      - systemic hypertension
      - restrictive cardiomyopathy.
3. Atrial side increased forward diastolic flow – laminar flow due to increased blood volume (see 7.22.1).
4. Atrial side turbulent, high-velocity, reversed systolic flow – mitral insufficiency
   a. Mild, detectable just behind the valve – physiological
   b. Endocardiosis
   c. Bacterial endocarditis
   d. Dilated left ventricle with secondary dilation of the annular ring
   e. Mitral valve dysplasia.
5. Atrial side turbulent, low-velocity reversed diastolic flow – second- and third-degree atrioventricular block.

7.23 Doppler flow abnormalities – aortic valve

1. Aortic side increased forward systolic flow

SMALL ANIMAL RADIOLOGICAL DIFFERENTIAL DIAGNOSIS

   a. Laminar flow due to increased blood volume
      - left-to-right shunting PDA
      - right-to-left shunting ASD or VSD
      - severe aortic insufficiency
   b. Turbulent, high velocity – stenosis, usually subvalvular.
2. Aortic side decreased forward systolic flow
   a. Left-to-right shunting ASD or VSD
   b. Hypovolaemia
      - shock
      - dehydration
   c. Drugs resulting in decreased blood pressure
   d. Poor cardiac output.
3. Ventricular side increased forward systolic flow – laminar flow due to increased blood volume (see 7.23.1).
4. Ventricular side reversed turbulent diastolic flow – aortic insufficiency
   a. Mild, just behind the valve – physiological
   b. Accompanying valvular stenosis
   c. Bacterial endocarditis
   d. Idiopathic
   e. Flail aortic valve.

7.24 Doppler flow abnormalities – tricuspid valve

1. Ventricular side increased forward diastolic flow
   a. Laminar flow due to increased blood volume
      - tricuspid valve insufficiency
      - left-to-right shunting ASD
   b. Turbulent flow – tricuspid stenosis – rare.
2. Ventricular side decreased forward diastolic flow
   a. Right-to-left shunting ASD (rare)
   b. Hypovolaemia
      - shock
      - dehydration
   c. Drugs resulting in decreased blood pressure
   d. Poor cardiac output
   e. Right ventricular diastolic dysfunction; second diastolic flow peak likely to be higher than the first diastolic peak
      - pulmonic stenosis
      - pulmonary hypertension.
3. Atrial side increased forward diastolic flow – laminar flow due to increased blood volume (see 7.24.1).
4. Atrial side turbulent, high-velocity, reversed systolic flow – tricuspid insufficiency

   a. Mild, detectable just behind the valve – physiological
   b. Endocardiosis
   c. Bacterial endocarditis
   d. Dilated right ventricle with secondary dilation of the annular ring
   e. Secondary to pulmonic stenosis
   f. Tricuspid valve dysplasia.

7.25 Doppler flow abnormalities – pulmonic valve

1. Pulmonary artery side increased forward systolic flow
   a. Laminar flow due to increased blood volume
      - left-to-right shunting ASD or VSD
      - severe pulmonic valve insufficiency
   b. Turbulent, high velocity
      - adjacent to the valve due to valvular stenosis
      - starting further distally due to pulmonary artery atresia.
2. Pulmonary artery side increased forward or reversed (depending on cursor location) diastolic flow of turbulent, low to medium velocity – left-to-right shunting PDA.
3. Pulmonary artery side decreased forward systolic flow
   a. Right-to-left shunting ASD or VSD – rare
   b. Hypovolaemia
      - shock
      - dehydration
   c. Drugs resulting in decreased blood pressure
   d. Poor cardiac output
   e. Pulmonary hypertension.
4. Ventricular side increased forward systolic flow – laminar flow due to increased blood volume (see 7.25.1).
5. Ventricular side reversed, turbulent diastolic flow – pulmonic valve insufficiency
   a. Mild, just behind the valve – physiological
   b. Idiopathic
   c. Accompanying valvular stenosis.
6. Pulmonary peak systolic velocity reached within the first third of flow time (peak velocity is normally reached close to the middle of flow time)
   a. Pulmonary hypertension
   b. *Dirofilaria** or *Angiostrongylus** worms in the right heart.

FURTHER READING

Bonagura, J.D. and Pipers, F.S. (1981) Echocardiographic features of pericardial effusion in dogs. *Journal of the American Veterinary Medical Association* **179** 49–56.

Bonagura, J.D. (1983) M-mode echocardiography: basic principles. *Veterinary Clinics of North America; Small Animal Practice* **13** 299–319.

Bonagura, J.D., O'Grady, M.R. and Herring, D.S. (1985) Echocardiography: principles of interpretation. *Veterinary Clinics of North America; Small Animal Practice* **15** 1177–1194.

Bonagura, J.D. and Herring, D.S. (1985) Echocardiography: congenital heart disease. *Veterinary Clinics of North America; Small Animal Practice* **15** 1195–1208.

Bonagura, J.D. and Herring, D.S. (1985) Echocardiography: acquired heart disease. *Veterinary Clinics of North America; Small Animal Practice* **15** 1209–1224.

van den Broek, A.H.M. and Darke, P.G.G. (1987) Cardiac measurements on thoracic radiographs of cats. *Journal of Small Animal Practice* **28** 125–135.

Buchanan, J.W. and Bucheler, J. (1995) Vertebral scale system to measure canine heart size in radiographs. *Journal of the American Veterinary Medical Association* **206** 194–199.

Buchanan, J.W. (2000) Vertebral scale system to measure heart size in radiographs. *Veterinary Clinics of North America; Small Animal Practice* **30** 379–394.

Cobb, M.A. and Brownlie, S.E. (1992) Intrapericardial neoplasia in 14 dogs. *Journal of Small Animal Practice* **33** 309–316.

Darke, P.G.G. (1992) Doppler echocardiography. *Journal of Small Animal Practice* **33** 104–112.

Darke, P.G.G. (1993) Transducer orientation for Doppler echocardiography in dogs. *Journal of Small Animal Practice* **34** 208.

Godshalk, C.P. (1994) Common pitfalls in radiographic interpretation of the thorax. *Compendium of Continuing Education for the Practicing Veterinarian (Small Animal)* **16** 731–738.

Jacobs, G. and Knight, D.H. (1985) M-mode echocardiographic measurements in nonanesthetized healthy cats: effect of body weight, heart rate, and other variables. *American Journal of Veterinary Research* **46** 1705–1711.

Kirberger, R.M. (1991) Mitral valve E point to septal separation in the dog. *Journal of the South African Veterinary Association* **62** 163–166.

Kirberger, R.M., Bland-van den Berg, P. and Daraz, B. (1992) Doppler echocardiography in the normal dog. Part I, velocity findings and flow patterns. *Veterinary Radiology and Ultrasound* **33** 370–379.

Kirberger, R.M., Bland-van den Berg, P. and Grimbeek, R.J. (1992) Doppler echocardiography in the normal dog. Part II, factors influencing blood flow velocities and a comparison between left and right heart blood flow. *Veterinary Radiology and Ultrasound* **33** 380–386.

Lehmkuhl, L.B., Bonagura, J.D., Biller, D.S. and Hartman, W.M. (1997) Radiographic evaluation of caudal vena cava size in dogs. *Veterinary Radiology and Ultrasound* **38** 94–100.

Litster, A.L. and Buchanan, J.W. (2000) Vertebral scale system to measure heart size in radiographs of cats. *Journal of the American Veterinary Medical Association* **216** 210–214.

Lombard, C.W. (1984) Echocardiographic and clinical signs of canine dilated cardiomyopathy. *Journal of Small Animal Practice* **25** 59–70.

Luis Fuentes, V. (1992) Feline heart disease: an update. *Journal of Small Animal Practice* **33** 130–137.

Luis Fuentes, V. (1993) Cardiomyopathy in cats. *In Practice* **15** 301–308.

Lusk, R.H. and Ettinger, S.J. (1990) Echocardiographic techniques in the dog and cat. *Journal of the American Animal Hospital Association* **26** 473–488.

Martin, M. (1999) Pericardial disease in the dog. *In Practice* **21** 378–385.

Miller, M.W., Knauer, K.W. and Herring, D.S. (1989) Echocardiography: Principles of interpretation. *Seminars in Veterinary Medicine and Surgery (Small Animals)* **4** 58–76.

Moise, N.S. (1989) Doppler echocardiographic evaluation of congenital heart disease. *Journal of Veterinary Internal Medicine* **3** 195–207.

Moon, M.L., Keene, B.W., Lessard, P. and Lee, J. (1993) Age related changes in the feline cardiac silhouette. *Veterinary Radiology and Ultrasound* **34** 315–320.

Myer, C.W. and Bonagura, J.D. (1982) Survey radiography of the heart. *Veterinary Clinics of North America; Small Animal Practice* **12** 213–237.

O'Grady, M.R., Bonagura, J.D., Powers, J.D. and Herring, D.S. (1986) Quantitative cross-sectional echocardiography in the normal dog. *Veterinary Radiology* **27** 34–49.

Rishniw, M. (2000) Radiography of feline cardiac disease. *Veterinary Clinics of North America; Small Animal Practice* **30** 395–426.

Soderberg, S.F., Boon, J.A., Wingfield, W.E. and Miller, C.W. (1983) M-mode echocardiography as a diagnostic aid for feline cardiomyopathy. *Veterinary Radiology* **24** 66–73.

Thomas, W.P., Sisson, D., Bauer, T.G. and Reed, J.R. (1984) Detection of cardiac masses in dogs by two-dimensional echocardiography. *Veterinary Radiology* **25** 65–72.

Thomas, W.P. (1984) Two-dimensional, real-time echocardiography in the dog: technique and anatomic validation. *Veterinary Radiology* **25** 50–64.

Thomas, W.P., Gaber, C.E., Jacobs, G.J, Kaplan, P.M., Lombard, C.W., Moise, N.S. and Moses, B.L. (1993) Recommendation for standards in transthoracic two-dimensional echocardiography in the dog and cat. *Journal of Veterinary Medicine* **7** 247–252.

Thrall, D.E. and Losonsky, J.M. (1979) Dyspnoea in the cat: Part 3 – radiographic aspects of intrathoracic causes involving the heart. *Feline Practice* **9** 36–49.

Tilley, L.P., Bond, B., Patnaik, A.K. and Liu, S-K. (1981) Cardiovascular tumors in the cat. *Journal of the American Animal Hospital Association* **17** 1009–1021.

8

Other thoracic structures – pleural cavity, mediastinum, thoracic oesophagus, thoracic wall

PLEURAL CAVITY

8.1 Anatomy and radiography of the pleural cavity
8.2 Increased radiolucency of the pleural cavity
8.3 Increased radio-opacity of the pleural cavity
8.4 Pleural and extrapleural nodules and masses
8.5 Ultrasonography of pleural and extrapleural lesions
8.6 Pleural thickening – increased visibility of lung or lobar edges

MEDIASTINUM

8.7 Anatomy and radiography of the mediastinum
8.8 Mediastinal shift
8.9 Variations in mediastinal radio-opacity
8.10 Mediastinal widening
8.11 Mediastinal masses
8.12 Mediastinal lymphadenopathy
8.13 Ultrasonography of the mediastinum

THORACIC OESOPHAGUS

8.14 Normal radiographic appearance of the oesophagus
8.15 Oesophageal contrast studies – technique and normal appearance
8.16 Oesophageal dilation
8.17 Variations in radio-opacity of the oesophagus
8.18 Oesophageal masses
8.19 Oesophageal foreign bodies

THORACIC WALL

8.20 Variations in soft tissue components of the thoracic wall
8.21 Variations in the ribs
8.22 Variations in the sternum
8.23 Variations in thoracic vertebrae
8.24 Ultrasonography of the thoracic wall
8.25 Variations in the appearance of the diaphragm
8.26 Ultrasonography of the diaphragm

MISCELLANEOUS

8.27 Thoracic trauma
8.28 Ultrasonography of thoracic trauma

PLEURAL CAVITY

8.1 Anatomy and radiography of the pleural cavity

The pleural cavity is a potential space between visceral and parietal pleura and surrounding each lung (Fig. 8.1). It contains only a small amount of serous fluid and is normally not visible. Visceral pleura is adherent to the lung surfaces; parietal pleura lines the thoracic wall and forms the mediastinum. In the dog the caudoventral mediastinal pleura has fenestrations connecting the right and left pleural cavities, making bilateral pleural disease more likely. In the cat the mediastinal pleura is more often intact and unilateral pleural disease is more common. Unilateral or asymmetric pleural pathology may result in a mediastinal shift with the heart and associated structures moving to the opposite side (see 8.8). Often the cause of pleural pathology can be determined only after removal of pleural fluid or air, and follow-up radiographs should therefore always be made after thoracocentesis. Positional radiography is

SMALL ANIMAL RADIOLOGICAL DIFFERENTIAL DIAGNOSIS

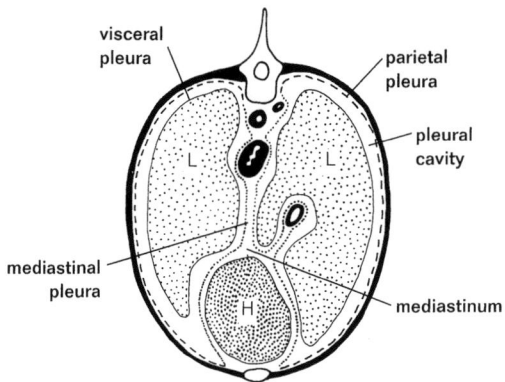

Figure 8.1 Schematic representation of the thorax in cross-section, showing the pleural and mediastinal spaces (H = heart; L = lung).

often beneficial to distinguish pleural pathology from other thoracic pathology. Pleurography, lymphangiography, positive contrast peritoneography and gastrointestinal contrast studies may be of value in making a specific diagnosis. If diagnostic ultrasound is available, it should be performed before draining any pleural fluid (see 8.5).

8.2 Increased radiolucency of the pleural cavity

Increased radiolucency results from air within the pleural cavity. The adjacent lung will collapse to a variable degree making lung edges visible because free air is more radiolucent

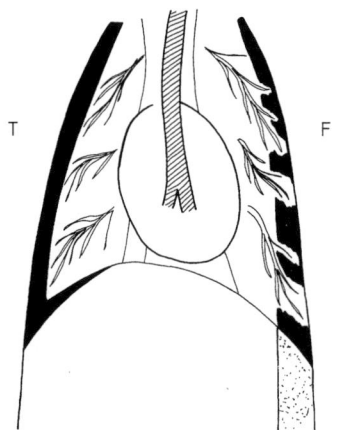

Figure 8.2 "False" (F) and true (T) pneumothorax seen on the DV view. With false pneumothorax the vascular markings are seen to extend to the periphery on hot light examination, and the skin folds continue beyond the thorax.

than the air/interstitium content of the lung. The lungs show an increased radio-opacity due to reduced air content.

1. Artefactual increased radiolucency of the pleural cavity – on careful examination, often requiring a hot light, pulmonary blood vessels will be seen in the area suspected of containing free air.
    a. Overexposure, overdevelopment or fogging of the film
    b. Lateral to superimposed axillary folds on the DV view especially in deep-chested dogs; these can usually be followed outside the thoracic cavity (so-called "false pneumothorax" – Figure 8.2)
    c. Overinflation of the lungs (see 6.26)
    d. Deep inspiration
    e. Hypovolaemia and pulmonary undercirculation
    f. Subcutaneous emphysema
    g. Lobar emphysema.
2. Pneumothorax – the cardiac apex will be displaced from the sternum on lateral recumbent radiographs (differentiate from microcardia in which the heart apex may also be raised – see 7.4). Expiratory radiographs and left lateral recumbent views are more sensitive for the detection of small amounts of free air; alternatively a standing lateral radiograph or a VD radiograph using a horizontal beam with the patient in lateral recumbency can be used; free air will collect beneath the uppermost part of the spine or ribcage respectively. Pneumothorax is usually bilateral and symmetrical; focal areas of gas accumulation suggest underlying lung lobe pathology. Flattening and caudal displacement of the diaphragm suggests tension pneumothorax and prompt treatment is required.
    a. Trauma, with perforation of
        - lung and visceral pleura
        - thoracic wall and parietal pleura
    b. Spontaneous pneumothorax; tends to be recurring and occurs with rupture of
        - congenital or acquired bulla, bleb, pulmonary cyst or bullous emphysema; often only diagnosed post mortem
        - bacterial pneumonia
        - tumours
        - pleural adhesions
        - parasitic lesions (*Paragonimus**, *Oslerus** and *Dirofilaria**)
    c. Perforations of
        - oesophagus
        - trachea

8 OTHER THORACIC STRUCTURES

- bronchi
- cavitary mass
  d. Iatrogenic
  - lung aspirates
  - thoracotomy
  - thoracocentesis
  - neck surgery
  - vigorous cardiac massage
  e. Extension of pneumomediastinum (see 8.9.1–6).
3. Diaphragmatic rupture – displaced, gas-filled gastrointestinal tract may result in localised areas of increased radiolucency in the pleural cavity. The wall of the stomach or intestine is usually clearly seen because of enteric gas inside and pulmonic air outside the wall and mineralised fragments in ingesta may also be visible
   a. Large radiolucency on the left side of the thorax – herniated and dilated stomach
   b. Small tubular radiolucencies – herniated small intestine; may enlarge with obstruction or incarceration.
4. Hydropneumothorax – VD radiographs made with a horizontal beam and the patient in lateral recumbency may be required – usually more fluid than air is present
   a. Pyopneumothorax – most common
   - ruptured pulmonary abscess with bronchopleural fistula
   - perforating oesophageal foreign body
   b. Haemopneumothorax
   - following trauma
   - iatrogenic following thoracocentesis.

8.3 Increased radio-opacity of the pleural cavity

Lung edges are displaced from the thoracic wall and become visible due to the difference in soft tissue opacity peripherally and the air-filled lung centrally (see Fig. 8.3).
1. Fat opacity – in obese patients a large sternal fat pad and a thinner layer of pleural fat may be seen.
2. Pleural effusion – small amounts of fluid create fissure lines (see 8.6.2 and Fig. 8.5), border effacement of the heart on DV views and rounded lung edges at the costophrenic angle on VD views, and are best seen on expiratory radiographs or horizontal beam VD views with the affected side down and the beam centred on the lower ribcage. Increasing volumes of fluid result in greater border effacement of the heart and

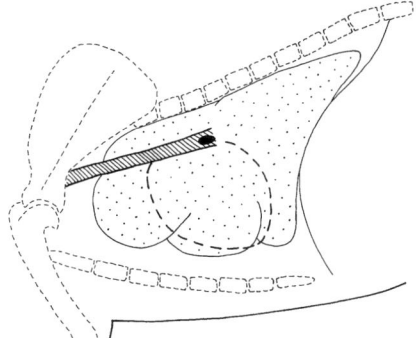

Figure 8.3 Pleural effusion – the heart outline is obscured and the lungs are partly collapsed, being surrounded by a diffuse soft tissue radio-opacity.

diaphragm with pulmonary opacity approaching that of the fluid as the lungs collapse and contain less air. Fluid may be free and move with gravity or may be encapsulated or trapped. Fluid collecting around a single lung lobe suggests underlying lobar pathology. All fluids have the same radiographic opacity and thoracocentesis is required to establish the type of fluid present. Repeat radiographic examinations should be made after draining the fluid to evaluate degree of success of fluid removal and to assess the lungs, mediastinum and chest wall more completely. The presence of simultaneous pleural and peritoneal effusions carries a worse prognosis.
   a. Artefactual increased radio-opacity of the pleural cavity
   - in obese dogs and cats fat accumulates along the sternum, sub-pleurally and in the pericardial sac, mimicking effusion. On careful examination the fat will be seen to be less radio-opaque than the adjacent cardiac and diaphragmatic silhouettes and no fissure lines will be visible
   - in chondrodystrophic breeds the costochondral junctions are indented medially which may mimic pleural effusion on the DV/VD radiograph
   b. Transudate or modified transudate; likely to be bilateral
   - heart failure (especially in cats)
   - neoplasia, especially lymphosarcoma
   - liver lobe incarcerated in a diaphragmatic rupture
   - idiopathic effusion
   - sterile foreign body
   - pneumonia

SMALL ANIMAL RADIOLOGICAL DIFFERENTIAL DIAGNOSIS

- hypoproteinaemia
- hepatic disorders
- lung lobe torsion
- glomerulonephritis
- thromboembolism – mild
- cats – hyperthyroidism with or without heart failure
- cats – secondary to perinephric pseudocyst

c. Exudate; more likely to be unilateral or asymmetrical as often inflammatory
- pyothorax
- foreign body
- nocardiosis*
- tuberculosis
- pneumonia
- fungal effusions
- autoimmune disorders (e.g. systemic lupus erythematosus and rheumatoid arthritis) – usually small volumes
- neoplasia; mesothelioma most likely
- chyle – in cats often accompanied by right heart failure and may result in constrictive pleuritis
- cats – feline infectious peritonitis (FIP)

d. Haemorrhage
- trauma
- coagulopathy
- bleeding haemangiosarcoma
- autoimmune disorders.

3. Diaphragmatic rupture – herniation of liver, spleen, fluid-filled gastrointestinal tract or uterus all result in increased pleural opacity.

8.4 Pleural and extrapleural nodules and masses

1. Artefactual lesions due to overlying soft tissue or osseous changes (see 8.20 and 8.21)
2. Extrapleural masses – these bulge into the pleural cavity from the parietal side of the chest wall, creating an "extrapleural sign" characterised by a well-demarcated, convex contour with tapering cranial and caudal edges (Figure 8.4). Such lesions have a tendency to grow inwards rather than outwards and may widen the adjacent intercostal spaces and involve the ribs. They do not move with respiratory motion of the lung on fluoroscopy. There is no (or minimal) pleural effusion unless the disease process has extended into the pleural cavity. Special oblique radiographs may be required to skyline the pathology.
   a. Rib tumours (see 8.21.5)
   b. Inflammatory conditions

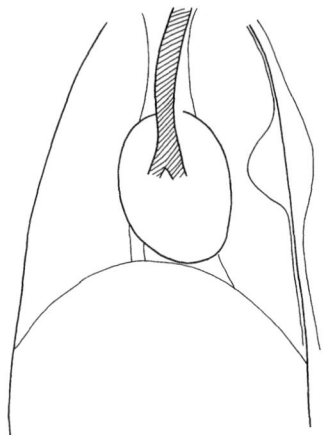

Figure 8.4 The "extra-pleural sign" seen on the DV view, indicative of a mass lesion arising outside the pleura and not within the lung. See also Figure 8.13.

- osteomyelitis of the osseous thoracic wall structures
- abscess
- granuloma
- foreign body reaction

c. Soft tissue tumours
- lipoma – fat radio-opacity usually obvious
- haemangiosarcoma
- fibrosarcoma
- rhabdomyosarcoma

d. Sternal lymphadenopathy (see 8.12.7–10)
e. Haematoma – as result of trauma and associated rib fractures.

2. Small diaphragmatic ruptures, hernias and eventration – sometimes incidental findings (see 8.25.1).
3. Pleural tumours – visible only after pleural drainage and if large enough
   a. Mesothelioma
   b. Metastatic carcinomatosis.
4. Pleural abscess or granuloma (e.g. secondary to foreign body).
5. Encapsulated or loculated pleural fluid – does not move with gravity.
6. Pleural fluid collecting around a diseased lung lobe.
7. Fibrin remnants after pleural drainage.

8.5 Ultrasonography of pleural and extrapleural lesions

1. Pleural effusion – the ultrasonographic appearance of pleural fluid is variable, but is usually anechoic to hypoechoic. Many echoes within the fluid usually signify the

presence of clumps of cells, debris and/or gas bubbles. However, thoracocentesis is required to determine the nature of the fluid. Fluid surrounds and separates the lung lobes from each other and the thoracic wall. It also facilitates imaging of intrathoracic structures that are not usually seen, such as the great vessels in the cranial mediastinum. The identification of echogenic tags and deposits on pleural surfaces is suggestive of the presence of an exudate, blood or chyle or a diffuse tumour such as mesothelioma. For possible causes of pleural effusion, see 8.3.2.

2 Hypoechoic/anechoic, well circumscribed areas
   a. Encapsulated or trapped fluid
   b. Pleural abscess
   c. Haematoma
   d. Sternal lymphadenopathy
   e. Soft tissue tumour of homogenous cellularity and with little haemorrhage or necrosis
   f. Ectopic liver or a small portion of liver prolapsed through a diaphragmatic tear.
3. Heterogeneous area
   a. Rib or sternal tumour
   b. Soft tissue tumour of heterogeneous cellularity and/or fibrosis, calcification, necrosis or haemorrhage
   c. Inflammatory conditions
      • abscess
      • granuloma
      • foreign body reaction.
4. Viscera within the thorax – the identification of abdominal viscera (e.g. liver, spleen, gastrointestinal tract) within the thoracic cavity is a more certain ultrasonographic indicator of diaphragmatic rupture than identification of the diaphragmatic defect. Variable quantities of thoracic fluid may also be seen
   a. Artefactual, due to "mirror image artefact" giving the impression of liver tissue within the thorax when scanning transhepatically
   b. Viscera not contained within the pericardium – traumatic diaphragmatic rupture
   c. Viscera apparently contained within the pericardium – congenital peritoneopericardial diaphragmatic hernia.

8.6 Pleural thickening – increased visibility of lung or lobar edges

Lungs normally extend to the periphery of the thoracic cavity, and individual lobe or lung edges are not seen except in two locations:

a. in the cranioventral thorax, where the mediastinum runs obliquely and outlines the cranial segment of the left cranial lobe on a lateral radiograph (see 8.7 and Fig. 8.6);
b. along the ventral margins of the lungs, which may appear "scalloped" in some dogs on the lateral radiograph due to intrathoracic fat.

1. Retracted lung borders making the edges visible
   a. Artefactual
      • axillary skin folds or skin folds created by a foam wedge placed under the sternum – the line extends beyond the thorax and pulmonary vasculature is visible peripheral to the line
      • inwardly displaced costochondral junctions in chondrodystrophic breeds, especially the Dachshund and Bassett Hound, creating a false impression of pleural fluid on the DV view
   b. Incidental intrathoracic fat
   c. Pneumothorax
   d. Pleural effusion
   e. Constrictive pleuritis secondary to pyo- or chylothorax ("cortication")
   f. Atelectasis.

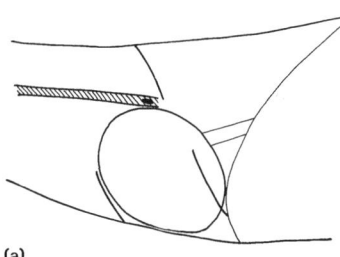

(a)

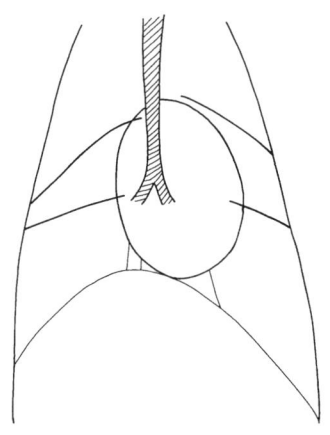

(b)

Figure 8.5 Location of pleural fissure lines on (a) right lateral and (b) DV view.

2. Fissure lines – thin, radio-opaque lines along the lobar borders (Figure 8.5)
   a. Artefactual
      - thin, mineralised costal cartilages (on the DV view these tend to be concave cranially whereas fissure lines are concave caudally)
      - scapular spine or edges
   b. Incidental – a fine fissure line is occasionally seen over the heart on left lateral radiographs of larger dogs
   c. Mild pleural effusion – fissure lines are wider peripherally than centrally
   d. Fibrinous pleuritis ("cortication") secondary to pyo- or chylothorax – especially in cats. Rounded lung borders outlined by fine, radio-opaque lines are seen as the lungs fail to re-expand fully after thoracocentesis
   e. Pleural fibrosis or scarring – fine lines of uniform width
      - old age and healed disease
      - fungal disease (e.g. coccidioidomycosis* and nocardiosis*)
      - parasitic disease (e.g. *Filaroides hirthi* and *F. milksi**)
   f. Pleural oedema in left heart failure
   g. Dry pleuritis
   h. Mediastinal fluid accumulation – reverse fissure lines are seen on the DV/VD view and are wider centrally than peripherally (see 8.10 and Figure 8.8).
3. Peripheral lobar consolidation or collapse highlighting interfaces with adjacent lobes.

MEDIASTINUM

8.7 Anatomy and radiography of the mediastinum

The mediastinum consists of two layers of mediastinal pleura separating the thorax into two pleural cavities, and accommodates a large number of structures including the heart, large blood vessels, oesophagus and lymph nodes lying roughly in the midline (see Figs 8.1 and 8.6). It communicates cranially with fascial planes of the neck and caudally with the retroperitoneal space via the aortic hiatus. Cranial to the heart the large dorsal and central soft tissue radio-opacity is formed from the cranial thoracic blood vessels, oesophagus, trachea and lymph nodes. On DV/VD radiographs of dogs the width of the cranial mediastinum should not normally exceed twice the width of the vertebral bodies. Ventrally, the cranial mediastinum forms a thin soft tissue fold running obliquely from craniodorsal to caudoventral on the lateral view. On DV/VD radiographs it extends from craniomedial in a caudolateral direction to the left side, separating the right and left cranial lung lobes. This fold contains the sternal lymph node ventrally and the thymus in young animals. Caudally, the ventral mediastinum is seen on DV/VD radiographs as a fold displaced into the left hemithorax by the accessory lung lobe. In cats the width of the craniodorsal mediastinum is less than the width of the superimposed thoracic vertebrae on the DV/VD view and the cranioventral fold is difficult to see.

The DV/VD view is usually more informative than the lateral view for the investigation

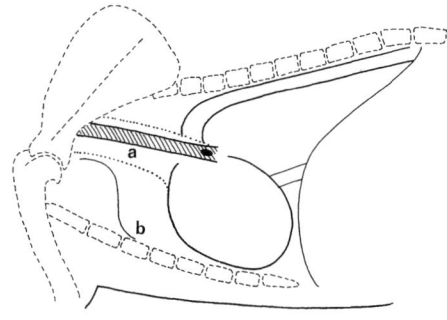

(a)

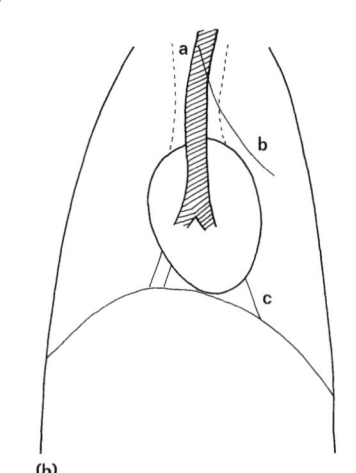

(b)

Figure 8.6 Location of the mediastinum on (a) lateral and (b) DV/VD views (a = cranial mediastinal structures – blood vessels, oesophagus, trachea and lymph nodes; b = cranioventral fold of the mediastinum; c = caudoventral fold of the mediastinum).

of mediastinal disease, although both views should be obtained.

8.8 Mediastinal shift

Mediastinal shift is diagnosed by evaluating the position of the heart, trachea, main-stem bronchi, aortic arch, and vena cava on true DV/VD views.
1. Artefactual
   a. Oblique DV/VD views.
2. Uneven inflation of the two hemithoraces due to unilateral pathology

Mediastinal movement towards the affected hemithorax
   a. Hypostatic congestion
      • general anaesthesia and lateral recumbency (may occur within a few minutes of induction – especially in large dogs)
      • prolonged lateral recumbency with severe illness
      • faulty intubation – endotracheal tube in one bronchus
   b. Atelectasis
      • mass or foreign body obstructing a bronchus
      • cats – feline bronchial asthma with lobar bronchus obstruction
   c. Lung lobe torsion
   d. Lobectomy
   e. Lobar agenesis/hypoplasia
   f. Radiation induced fibrosis and atelectasis
   g. Unilateral phrenic nerve paralysis

Mediastinal movement away from the affected hemithorax
   h. Unilateral or asymmetric pneumothorax and tension pneumothorax
   i. Unilateral or asymmetric pleural effusion
   j. Diaphragmatic rupture or hernia
   k. Large solitary lung or pleural mass
   l. Lobar emphysema.
3. Chronic pleural disease with adhesions.
4. Contralateral thoracic wall pathology (see 8.20 and 8.21).
5. Sternal and vertebral deformities (see 8.22 and 8.23).

8.9 Variations in mediastinal radio-opacity

Most mediastinal changes have a soft tissue opacity but the mediastinum may be less radio-opaque, due to the presence of fat or air, or more radio-opaque, due to mineralisation.

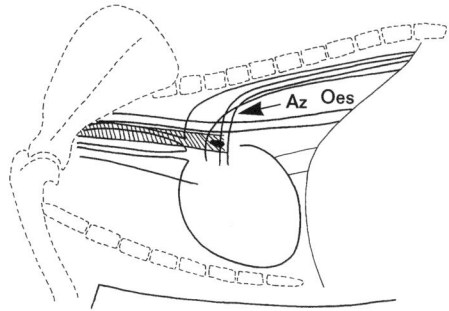

Figure 8.7 Pneumomediastinum – increased visibility of mediastinal structures (Az = azygos vein and Oes = oesophagus, which are not normally visible. Cranial mediastinal blood vessels are also apparent and the tracheal walls are more obvious than normal.)

Reduced mediastinal radio-opacity due to air – pneumomediastinum

Generalised pneumomediastinum with dissecting radiolucencies results in increased visibility of mediastinal structures such as blood vessels, tracheal walls and oesophagus (Figure 8.7). Air may extend into the fascial planes of the neck, retroperitoneum and pericardium (rare). Occasionally localised pneumomediastinum is seen as pockets of mediastinal air. An air-filled megaoesophagus will also produce mediastinal widening of air lucency (see 8.16). Pneumomediastinum may lead to pneumothorax, but the reverse does not occur.
1. Iatrogenic pneumomediastinum
   a. Post-transtracheal aspiration
   b. Post-lung aspirate
   c. Overinflation of the lungs during positive pressure ventilation.
2. Extension of air from the neck
   a. Soft tissue trauma with an open wound
   b. Tracheal perforation
   c. Oesophageal perforation
   d. Pharyngeal perforation
   e. Soft tissue infection with gas formation.
3. Extension of air from the bronchi or lungs – predisposed to by pulmonary bulla, bleb, cyst or bronchial parasitism
   a. Rupture of the bronchi or lungs
      • compressive trauma
      • lung lobe torsion
   b. Spontaneous pneumomediastinum – racing Greyhounds.
4. Secondary to severe dyspnoea – especially Paraquat poisoning (see also 6.22).

5. Emphysematous mediastinitis.
6. Extension from pneumoretroperitoneum

Reduced mediastinal radio-opacity – fat

7. Obesity – especially in chondrodystrophic dogs.

Increased mediastinal radio-opacity, greater than soft tissue

8. Iatrogenic
   a. Intravenous or intra-arterial catheter
   b. Endotracheal tube
   c. Feeding tube
   d. Oesophageal stethoscope.
9. Mineralisation
   a. Neoplastic mass
      - osteosarcoma transformation of *Spirocerca lupi** granuloma
      - thymic tumour
      - metastatic mediastinal tumour
   b. Chronic infectious lymph node involvement (see 8.12) e.g. histoplasmosis* or tuberculosis
   c. Mineralised oesophageal foreign bodies (see 8.19)
   d. Cardiovascular mineralisation – aorta, coronary vessels and heart valves (see 6.28.7).
10. Metal
    a. Bullets and other metallic foreign bodies
    b. Contrast media.

8.10 Mediastinal widening

Generalised mediastinal widening may be caused by accumulation of fat or fluid.

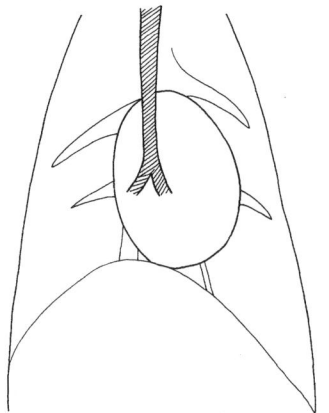

Figure 8.8 Reverse fissure lines due to mediastinal fluid, seen on the DV view.

Mediastinal fluid may result in reverse fissure lines as fluid dissects into the interlobar fissures from the hilar region. The reverse fissure lines are wide centrally and narrow peripherally (Figure 8.8) and should not be confused with atelectatic lung lobes, especially a collapsed right middle lobe which may appear small and triangular (see 6.17.3 and Fig. 6.8). Localised or walled-off accumulations of fluid mimic mediastinal masses (see 8.11).

1. Incidental mediastinal widening
   a. A widened cranial mediastinum is routinely seen on DV/VD radiographs of Bulldogs. The trachea is in its normal position, slightly to the right of the midline
   b. In obese patients, especially in small and miniature breeds, large fat deposits result in a widened, smoothly marginated cranial mediastinum. The trachea is in its normal position, slightly to the right of the mid line
   c. Thymic "sail" on the DV/VD view in young animals, between the right and left cranial lung lobes.
2. Mediastinal masses (see 8.11).
3. Generalised megaoesophagus (see 8.16).
4. Haemorrhage.
   a. Trauma with rupture of a blood vessel, often with cranial rib fractures
   b. Neoplastic erosion of a blood vessel
   c. Coagulopathies.
5. Mediastinitis or mediastinal abscess secondary to
   a. Oesophageal or tracheal perforation
   b. Extension of lymphadenitis, pleuritis, pneumonia, or a deep neck wound
   c. Cats – mediastinal feline infectious peritonitis (FIP).
6. Oedema or transudate (often with pleural fluid too)
   a. Acute systemic disease
   b. Trauma
   c. Hypoproteinaemia
   d. Right heart failure
   e. Neoplasia, especially with cranial mediastinal masses in cats.
7. Chylomediastinum.

8.11 Mediastinal masses

Mediastinal masses will displace adjacent structures, particularly the trachea. Oesophageal contrast studies, angiography, horizontal beam radiography, pleurography and ultrasonography may provide additional information about the location and nature of the mass (Figure 8.9). Mediastinal masses may

8 OTHER THORACIC STRUCTURES

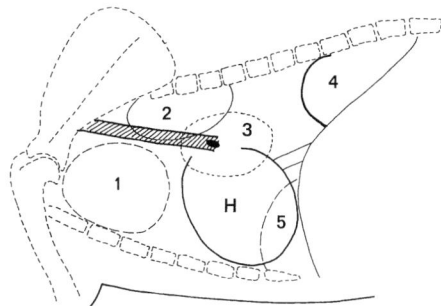

Figure 8.9 Location of mediastinal masses on the lateral view (H = heart). 1 = cranioventral masses, 2 = craniodorsal masses, 3 = hilar and perihilar masses, 4 = caudodorsal masses and 5 = caudoventral masses.

be mimicked by localised fluid accumulations (see 8.10). Cranial mediastinal masses may cause secondary oesophageal obstruction.

1. Cranioventral mediastinal masses (precardiac)
   a. Artefactual
      - masses in the tip of the cranial lung lobe may be in contact with the mediastinum and the resultant border effacement may mimic a cranial mediastinal mass
      - pleural fluid often collects around the cranial lung lobes, mimicking a mediastinal mass, especially in cats
   b. Normal thymus – in immature animals a thymic "sail" is seen in the cranioventral mediastinal fold pointing caudolaterally to the left on the DV/VD view and should not be confused with a reverse fissure line
   c. Neoplasia – often accompanied by a pleural effusion
      - lymphosarcoma; the most common cause in cats
      - thymoma – often accompanied by myasthenia gravis and megaoesophagus
      - malignant histiocytosis – middle-aged, large-breed dogs; male preponderance; mainly Bernese Mountain dog but also Rottweiler and Golden and Flatcoated retrievers
      - ectopic thyroid/parathyroid tumour
      - rib tumour – look for bony changes too (see 8.21.5 and Fig. 8.13)
      - other tumours (e.g. lipoma and fibrosarcoma)
   d. Oesophageal dilation secondary to a vascular ring anomaly (see 8.16.6 and Fig. 8.11)
   e. Sternal lymphadenopathy (see 8.12.7–10)
   f. Mediastinal abscess or granuloma
      - foreign body reaction (e.g. sharp object penetrating via sternum)
      - nocardiosis*
      - actinomycosis*
   g. Mediastinal haematoma
   h. Mediastinal cyst (e.g. branchial cysts).

2. Craniodorsal mediastinal masses (precardiac) – an oesophagram may be indicated to evaluate the degree of oesophageal involvement or displacement
   a. Oesophageal
      - dilation (see 8.16)
      - foreign bodies (see 8.19)
      - oesophageal neoplasia – rare (see 8.18.6)
   b. Aortic aneurysm
   c. Heart base tumours (see 7.16.2)
   d. Associated with vertebral lesions
      - neoplasia
      - severe spondylosis
      - osteomyelitis
   e. Mediastinal abscess or granuloma
      - foreign body reaction
      - nocardiosis*
      - actinomycosis*
   f. Haematoma
      - aortic haemorrhage secondary to aberrant *Spirocerca lupi** migration
      - coagulopathy.

3. Hilar and perihilar masses – usually poorly defined masses at the base of the heart; may be mimicked by localised pulmonary oedema. The adjacent trachea and mainstem bronchi may be displaced or compressed (see Figure 6.4b and d)
   a. Lymphadenopathy – usually with associated pulmonary or pleural pathology and other systemic signs (see 8.12.1–6)
      - tracheobronchial lymph nodes
      - bronchial lymph nodes
      - mediastinal lymph nodes
   b. Oesophageal pathology
      - foreign bodies (see 8.19)
      - *Spirocerca lupi** granuloma
      - oesophageal neoplasia, often secondary to *Spirocerca lupi** granuloma
   c. Heart base tumours (see 7.16.2)
   d. Cardiovascular structures mimicking masses (see 7.8, 7.10, 7.11 and 7.13)
      - left or right atrial enlargement
      - post-stenotic dilation of the aorta or pulmonary artery

151

SMALL ANIMAL RADIOLOGICAL DIFFERENTIAL DIAGNOSIS

- pulmonary artery enlargement
- aortic aneurysm
e. Adjacent pulmonary or bronchial mass
f. Ectopic thyroid mass.
4. Caudal mediastinal masses (postcardiac)
a. Artefactual – accessory lung lobe mass; mid to dorsal thorax
b. Oesophageal masses (see 8.18 and 8.19); mid to dorsal thorax
  - foreign body
  - *Spirocerca lupi** granuloma
  - oesophageal neoplasia (e.g. osteosarcoma or fibrosarcoma secondary to *Spirocerca lupi** granuloma, leiomyoma or leiomyosarcoma)
  - hiatal hernia or gastro-oesophageal intussusception
  - oesophageal diverticulum
c. Peritoneopericardial diaphragmatic hernia; ventral thorax
d. Diaphragmatic eventration (see 8.25.1)
e. Diaphragmatic abscess or granuloma – foreign body
f. Mediastinal cyst.

8.12 Mediastinal lymphadenopathy

Enlargement of the tracheobronchial (hilar), bronchial and mediastinal lymph nodes results in poorly defined hilar masses (Figure 8.9). These are often associated with pulmonary and pleural pathology and other systemic signs. Sternal lymphadenopathy results in a subpleural enlargement at the insertion point of the cranial ventral mediastinal fold.

Hilar region lymphadenopathy

1. Fungal infections
   a. Coccidioidomycosis* – younger dogs; rare in cats
   b. Histoplasmosis* – mainly dogs and rare in cats; may calcify on recovery
   c. Blastomycosis* – mainly dogs, rare in cats
   d. Cryptococcosis* – more often in cats; uncommon in dogs.
2. Neoplasia
   a. Lymphosarcoma – often with an interstitial lung pattern too (see 6.22 and 6.23)
   b. Malignant histiocytosis – middle-aged, large-breed dogs with male preponderance; mainly Bernese Mountain dog but also Rottweiler and Golden and Flatcoated retrievers
   c. Metastatic neoplasia from the lungs and other body regions.
3. Bacterial infection/granuloma
   a. Tuberculosis
   b. Nocardiosis* – mainly younger dogs
   c. Actinomycosis*.
4. Eosinophilic pulmonary granulomatosis.
5. Pulmonary lymphomatoid granulomatosis – with alveolar lung pattern and pulmonary nodules or masses too.
6. After resolved pleural or pulmonary infections.

Sternal lymphadenopathy

7. Neoplasia
   a. Lymphosarcoma – often with an interstitial lung pattern too (see 6.22 and 6.23)
   b. Malignant histiocytosis (see 8.12.2)
   c. Metastatic neoplasia from
      - mammary tumour
      - cranial abdominal tumour.
8. Bacterial infection (see 8.12.3).
9. Fungal infection (see 8.12.1); especially cryptococcosis* in cats.
10. After resolved pleural or pulmonary infections.

8.13 Ultrasonography of the mediastinum

1. Cranial mediastinal mass – evaluation of the cranial mediastinum may be carried out from either a right or a left cranial intercostal approach, from the thoracic inlet, or via a transoesophageal approach if endoscopic ultrasonography is available
   a. Hypoechoic to anechoic; homogeneous
      - mediastinal fluid
      - abscess or granuloma
      - cyst
      - haematoma
      - lymphadenopathy
      - tumour of homogenous cellularity (e.g. lymphosarcoma)
      - ectopic thyroid tissue
   b. Heterogeneous in echogenicity or echotexture
      - abscess or granuloma
      - haematoma
      - tumour of heterogeneous cellularity and/or fibrosis, calcification, necrosis or haemorrhage.
2. Caudal mediastinal mass – the caudal mediastinum is often most clearly imaged from a cranial abdominal approach, through the liver. If the lungs are well aerated and there is no pleural or medi-

8 OTHER THORACIC STRUCTURES

astinal fluid, small mediastinal masses may, however, be difficult to image
   a. Hypoechoic to anechoic, homogeneous
      - mediastinal fluid
      - abscess or granuloma
      - cyst
      - haematoma
      - tumour of homogeneous cellularity
      - liver within a peritoneopericardial hernia
      - ectopic liver
   b. Heterogeneous in echogenicity and echotexture
      - abscess or granuloma
      - haematoma
      - tumour of heterogeneous cellularity and/or fibrosis, calcification, necrosis or haemorrhage
      - abdominal viscera (within a peritoneopericardial diaphragmatic hernia or via a traumatic rupture of the diaphragm)
      - oesophageal mass (see 8.18).
3. Hilar and perihilar masses – if transoesophageal ultrasonography is not available, hilar masses are often best imaged through the heart. The heart is imaged in a short axis view and the transducer angled dorsally to image the heart base. The heart is then imaged in a long axis view, paying particular attention to the great vessels as they enter and exit the heart and atria
   a. Enlargement of cardiac chambers or great vessels
      - left atrial enlargement (see 7.19.1 and 7.19.2)
      - post-stenotic dilation of the aorta or pulmonary artery
      - right atrial enlargement (see 7.20.1 and 7.20.2)
   b. Solid mass involving the cardiac chambers or great vessels (may be associated with pericardial effusions)
      - heart base tumour – a hypo- to hyperechoic mass usually adjacent to, or surrounding, the aortic outflow tract
      - haemangiosarcoma – usually a hypoechoic mass involving the wall of the right atrium
   c. Solid mass dorsal to the heart base (imaged either using the heart as a window, or via the transoesophageal route)
      - lymphadenopathy (see 8.12)
      - pulmonary mass (see 6.21)
      - oesophageal mass (see 8.18)
      - oesophageal foreign body (see 8.19).

THORACIC OESOPHAGUS

8.14 Normal radiographic appearance of the thoracic oesophagus

A normal empty oesophagus is rarely visible on survey radiographs. Occasionally in dogs and cats it is seen caudally as a poorly defined, linear, faint soft tissue opacity dorsal to the caudal vena cava on a left lateral radiograph. A small amount of lumenal air may often be observed cranial to the heart in conscious dogs, especially if they are dyspnoeic or struggling, and generalised oesophageal dilation is a common finding under anaesthesia. The oesophagus may also become visible in animals with pneumomediastinum or pneumothorax.

8.15 Oesophageal contrast studies – technique and normal appearance

No specific preparation is required for contrast studies of the oesophagus. The patient must be conscious, although light sedation may be needed in fractious patients. Barium sulphate liquid or paste is usually indicated but a "barium burger" is required for cases of suspected oesophageal dilation or stricture, in which paste or liquid may give false negative results. Lateral radiographs are usually more informative than DV/VD views and fluoroscopic screening with videotape facility is required for assessment of functional disorders.

Barium paste or liquid oesophagram

If only a small quantity is required it can be administered with a syringe to which a short piece of stout rubber tubing is attached. The contrast medium is deposited between the molar teeth and the cheek and the patient is given sufficient time to swallow between squirts. Aspiration of the barium should be avoided. Alternatively a stomach tube or catheter can be passed through the opening in a spacer gag positioned transversely

SMALL ANIMAL RADIOLOGICAL DIFFERENTIAL DIAGNOSIS

across the mouth just behind the canine teeth, so that its tip reaches the mid-cervical oesophagus. The barium liquid is then injected slowly via the tube or catheter.

Barium burger

One part of barium liquid is mixed with three parts of meat, which the patient is required to eat, although hand-feeding may be necessary. Fortunately, many dogs in need of such studies are hungry because of persistent regurgitation. Cats will not usually eat barium burgers.

Iodine oesophagram

If there is a possibility that the oesophagus may be ruptured (e.g. after removal of an oesophageal foreign body) 5–10 ml of a low-osmolarity water-soluble iodine preparation must be given to avoid complications arising from barium leaking into the pleural cavity (adhesions and granuloma formation).

The canine oesophagus consists of striated muscle and after barium administration will be visible as a longitudinal linear pattern of barium trapped between the mucosal folds. In the cat the terminal third of the oesophagus is smooth muscle and has a striated herringbone appearance on positive-contrast studies.

8.16 Oesophageal dilation

A dilated oesophagus may be filled with food, fluid or (most commonly) air (Figure 8.10). When air filled, the oesophageal wall becomes visible due to the presence of air inside the oesophagus and air outside the wall in the adjacent lungs or trachea. With the latter, the combined visibility of the tracheal and oesophageal wall is known as a *tracheo-oesophageal stripe sign*. The trachea may be displaced ventrally by the weight of the distended oesophagus. Chronic oesophageal dilation with regurgitation may lead to aspiration bronchopneumonia (see 6.14.2).

Generalised oesophageal dilation

Megaoesophagus results from a motility disorder due to central nervous system disease or neuromuscular disorders. Megaoesophagus is rare in cats.
1. Transient megaoesophagus
   a. Heavy sedation or general anaesthesia
   b. Severe respiratory infections (e.g. acute tracheobronchitis)
   c. Sliding hiatal hernia.

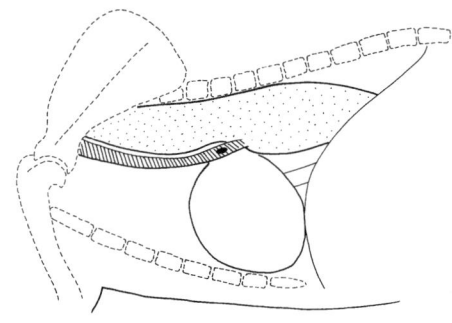

Figure 8.10 Air-filled megaoesophagus, on (a) lateral and (b) DV/VD views. On the lateral view, the oesophageal and tracheal walls summate, producing the "tracheo-oesophageal stripe sign". The trachea is displaced ventrally.

2. Congenital or hereditary megaoesophagus
   a. Vascular ring anomaly (mainly persistent right aortic arch) – results in localised dilation cranial to the constriction but a small percentage of these cases also have oesophageal dilation caudal to the constriction, resulting in generalised dilation. If air-filled, the constriction may be seen.
   b. Hereditary megaoesophagus – Wirehaired Fox Terriers and Miniature Schnauzers
   c. Familial predisposition – German Shepherd dog, Great Dane, Newfoundland Retriever and Shar-Pei
   d. Canine glycogen storage disease – young Lapland dogs
   e. Hereditary myopathy – young Labrador Retrievers

8 OTHER THORACIC STRUCTURES

   f. Canine giant axonal neuropathy – young German Shepherd dogs.
3. Acquired megaoesophagus
   a. Idiopathic
   b. Immune-mediated myopathies
      - polymyositis – large breeds
      - acquired myasthenia gravis – may be associated with thymoma
      - acute polyradiculoneuritis
      - systemic lupus erythematosus
      - cats – feline dysautonomia (Key–Gaskell syndrome); now rare
   c. Metabolic neuropathies and myelopathies
      - hypoadrenocorticism (Addison's disease) – often accompanied by microcardia
      - hypothyroidism
      - corticosteroid-induced polymyopathy
      - diabetes mellitus
      - hyperinsulinism
      - uraemia
   d. Toxic neuropathies
      - organophosphates
      - heavy metals, particularly lead but also zinc, cadmium and thallium
      - chlorinated hydrocarbons
      - herbicides
      - botulism
   e. Secondary to
      - reflux oesophagitis, particularly as result of axial oesophageal hiatal hernias (see 8.18.3)
      - distal oesophageal foreign body
      - acute gastric dilation/volvulus syndrome (GDV)
      - snake bite
   f. Hypertrophic muscular dystrophy
   g. Thiamine deficiency.

Localised oesophageal dilation

4. Transient, localised oesophageal dilation
   a. Dyspnoea
   b. Aerophagia
   c. Normal swallowing.
5. Redundant oesophagus, seen particularly on contrast studies as a ventral oesophageal deviation at the thoracic inlet. Mainly brachycephalic breeds (e.g. Bulldog) but also described in the cat. Usually clinically insignificant.
6. Congenital localised oesophageal dilation
   a. Usually a vascular ring anomaly (Figure 8.11) with oesophageal dilation cranial to the heart; uncommon in cats

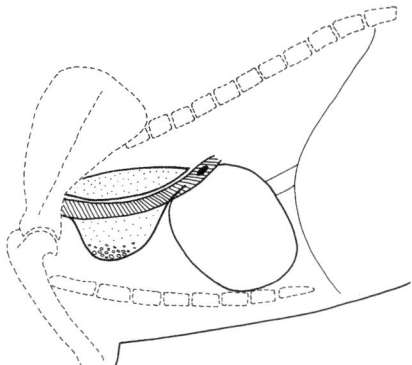

Figure 8.11 Vascular ring anomaly – localised oesophageal dilation cranial to the heart base, within which fragments of retained ingesta are often seen. The distal oesophagus may also be dilated.

   - 95% are due to a persistent right aortic arch (PRAA) – particularly German Shepherd dog, Boston Terrier and Irish Setter; main type in cats
   - double aortic arch – often accompanied by tracheal compression and coughing
   - right aortic arch with aberrant right subclavian artery
   - normal aorta with aberrant right subclavian artery
   - persistent right ductus arteriosus
   b. Dilation cranial to a congenital focal stenosis
   c. Segmental oesophageal hypomotility – may be congenital; Shar-Pei and Newfoundland Retriever
   d. Congenital oesophageal diverticulum.
7. Dilation cranial to an oesophageal hiatal hernia or gastro-oesophageal intussusception.
8. Dilation adjacent to an oesophageal foreign body.
9. Iatrogenic segmental stenosis (peptic oesophageal stricture) following general anaesthesia; dilation forms cranial to the stenosis.
10. Cranial to a stricture or narrowing caused by
    a. Compression of the oesophagus by a large external mass (e.g. a cranial mediastinal tumour)
    b. Scar tissue (e.g. after foreign body removal or ingestion of hot or caustic substances)
    c. Granuloma
    d. Mucosal adhesion

e. Congenital focal stenosis
   f. Oesophageal neoplasia.
11. Oesophagitis.
12. Oesophageal diverticulum – often medium to small-breed dogs
   a. Pulsion diverticulum – usually with motility disturbances
   b. Traction diverticulum – usually secondary to perioesophageal inflammation.

8.17 Variations in radio-opacity of the oesophagus

1. Reduced oesophageal radio-opacity – air
   a. Small amounts
      • normal swallowed air
      • localised dilation
      • redundant oesophagus at the thoracic inlet
   b. Large amounts – megaoesophagus (see 8.16).
2. Soft tissue oesophageal radio-opacity
   a. Non-distended soft tissue opacity of the caudal oesophagus or superimposing on cervicothoracic trachea – normal variants
   b. Small amounts on single radiograph and absent on follow up radiographs – normal, transient fluid in oesophagus
   c. Large amounts – fluid and food in a megaoesophagus (see 8.16)
   d. Non-mineralised foreign body (see 8.19)
   e. Oesophageal soft tissue mass (see 8.18).
3. Mineralised oesophageal radio-opacity
   a. Bone – oesophageal foreign body (see 8.19)
   b. Osteosarcoma transformation of *Spirocerca lupi* granuloma
   c. Precardiac ingesta accumulation in an amotile distended oesophagus with vascular ring anomaly; usually cranial to the heart (see 8.18.6 and Fig. 8.11)
   d. Delayed transit of solid medicaments given per os (e.g. tablets).

8.18 Oesophageal masses

Oesophageal masses may be intraluminal, intramural or extraluminal.

Intraluminal oesophageal masses

1. Intraluminal foreign body (see 8.19).
2. Gastro-oesophageal intussusception – the stomach and possibly other abdominal organs invaginate into the oesophagus

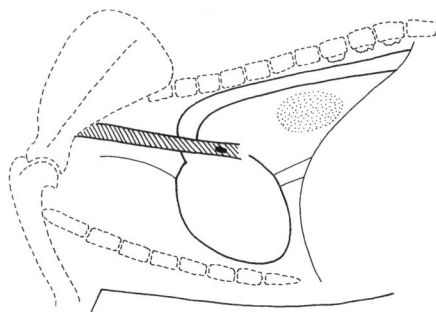

Figure 8.12 *Spirocerca lupi* granuloma in the distal oesophagus. Typical vertebral changes are also present.

usually secondary to megaoesophagus; especially German Shepherd dog puppies.
3. Axial oesophageal hiatal hernia – may slide in and out, involving the distal oesophagus and part of the stomach with secondary reflux oesophagitis and megaoesophagus. Congenital in the Shar-Pei.
4. Oesophageal diverticulum containing fluid or food.

Intramural oesophageal masses

5. Oesophageal granuloma
   a. *Spirocerca lupi** – the granuloma arises out of the dorsal oesophageal wall and barium will thus only pass ventral to the mass (Figure 8.12). May contain ill-defined foci of mineralisation due to transformation to osteosarcoma, and pulmonary metastasis may be present; thoracic spondylitis is seen and hypertrophic osteopathy may also occur (see 1.14.6)
   b. Mural foreign body or infection.
6. Oesophageal neoplasia
   a. Secondary to *Spirocerca lupi** granuloma
      • osteosarcoma
      • fibrosarcoma
   b. Metastatic or infiltrative oesophageal tumour – rare
   c. Primary oesophageal tumour – rare
      • leiomyoma or leiomyosarcoma
      • squamous cell carcinoma.

Extraluminal oesophageal masses

7. Para-oesophageal hiatal hernia – the gastric fundus is displaced through a diaphragmatic defect adjacent to the oesophageal hiatus.
8. Para-oesophageal abscess (e.g. following oesophageal perforation).

8.19 Oesophageal foreign bodies

Oesophageal foreign bodies may be radio-opaque (such as bone and fishing hooks) or soft tissue opacity (such as gristle). Foreign bodies lodge most commonly at the thoracic inlet, over the base of the heart and just cranial to the diaphragm. The latter may mimic *Spirocerca lupi** granuloma, except that contrast medium will pass all around an intraluminal foreign body. Oesophageal foreign bodies may displace adjacent structures, particularly the trachea, and a small amount of air may be seen cranial or around them. In cats fish bones and needles with thread are commonly observed.

Complications usually occur in neglected cases
1. Aspiration pneumonia secondary to regurgitation.
2. Localised inflammatory reaction
    a. Oesophagitis
    b. Perioesophagitis
    c. Focal mediastinitis.
3. Oesophageal perforation – should be confirmed by administering small amounts of water-soluble iodine contrast agents and not barium, as barium causes granulomatous reactions if it enters the mediastinum. Leakage may not be evident on the oesophagram if the perforation has been partially or totally sealed by adhesions or fibrosis. Complications of oesophageal perforation include:
    a. Pneumothorax
    b. Pneumomediastinum
    c. Pleuritis and pleural effusion
    d. Oesophagobronchial fistula
    e. Oesophagotracheal fistula.
4. Subsequent oesophageal stricture
    a. Mucosal scarring and oesophageal stenosis
    b. Perioesophageal fibrosis resulting in stenosis.

THORACIC WALL

A thorough radiological examination of the thorax always includes evaluation of the extrathoracic structures. By examining both orthogonal views the extrathoracic location of the suspect pathology can usually be determined.

8.20 Variations in soft tissue components of the thoracic wall

1. Widened thoracic wall – soft tissue radio-opacity
    a. Diffuse widening
        * cellulitis
        * oedema
        * injected electrolyte solutions
    b. Localised widening
        * soft tissue neoplasia
        * rib lesion with bony changes subtle or overlooked
        * abscess or granuloma
        * cyst
        * haematoma
        * paracostal hernia
        * pleural and extrapleural nodules and masses (see 8.4).
2. Widened thoracic wall – fat radio-opacity. Fat in fascial planes should not be mistaken for subcutaneous emphysema; it is slightly less radio-opaque than soft tissue and highlights the muscles and fascial planes
    a. Obesity
    b. Chest wall lipoma.
3. Widened thoracic wall – gas radiolucency. Subcutaneous air due to:
    a. Trauma (e.g. bites and rib fractures)
    b. Infection
    c. Pneumomediastinum – extension via fascial planes
    d. Paracostal hernia with gas-filled bowel loops – more common in cats.
4. Nodular, linear and other localised radio-opacities
    a. Soft tissue opacities – these may easily be confused with intrapulmonary and pleural/extrapleural nodules. If there is doubt as to whether or not an apparent pulmonary nodule is due to a superficial structure such as a nipple, the radiograph should be repeated after painting the nipple with a small amount of barium
        * artefactual from dirty cassettes and intensifying screens or wet/dirty foam positioning wedges
        * muscle attachments to ribs – seen in obese animals on the DV/VD views, separated by fat; linear soft tissue radio-opacities that are symmetrical on the two sides of the chest

SMALL ANIMAL RADIOLOGICAL DIFFERENTIAL DIAGNOSIS

- nipples
- skin masses
- engorged female ticks
- wet hair, particularly in long-haired breeds, with matted blood
- skin folds running caudally from the axilla
- superimposed foot pads – poorly positioned hind limbs on DV radiographs
- superimposed fingers during manual restraint without adequate radiation safety procedures
- bandages, catheters, ECG pads

b. Mineralised opacities
- artefactual, from dirty cassettes and intensifying screens
- mineralisation around the costochondral junctions in older dogs
- wide costochondral junctions in chondrodystrophic breeds
- fractures of adjacent bony structures
- embedded tooth after dog fight
- sand, dirt or glass debris
- mineralised tumours (e.g. of ribs or mammary glands)
- calcification of nipples
- dystrophic calcification of soft tissue lesions
- paracostal hernias containing mineralised foetus or gastrointestinal contents
- calcified cyst walls – egg shell appearance
- calcinosis cutis with hyperadrenocorticism (Cushing's disease)

c. Heavy metal opacity
- microchip identification markers
- spilt contrast medium on patient or cassette
- bandage clips, ECG attachments
- bullets and pellets
- needles, pins, arrowheads, etc.

8.21 Variations in the ribs

Normal thoracic radiography may result in underexposure of bony structures and if pathology is suspected a further radiograph of the affected region should be made using appropriate exposures, positioning and centring.

1. Mineralisation of costal cartilages – normal from a few months of age onwards – starts caudally and often has a granular pattern in the young dog, becoming more sclerotic and irregular with age. Rosettes of mineralisation may form around the cos-

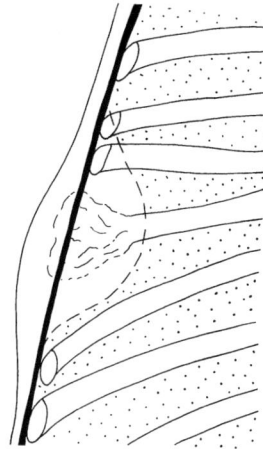

Figure 8.13 Rib tumour seen on a DV or lesion-oriented oblique view. There is a mixed, osteolytic and proliferative bone lesion with displacement of the adjacent ribs and associated soft tissue swelling. Internally, the "extra-pleural sign" is seen (see 8.4.2 and Figure 8.4).

tochondral junctions in older dogs. In older cats, the costal cartilages may be densely mineralised in short segments.

2. Transverse lucent or sclerotic lines in the costal cartilages
   a. Ageing changes, especially in cats
   b. Fractures.
3. Altered width of intercostal spaces
   a. Artefactual – poor positioning with a curved spine
   b. Rib or spinal fractures
   c. Rib or soft tissue tumours
   d. Intercostal muscle tearing
   e. Uneven pulmonary inflation
   f. Tension pneumothorax
   g. Thoracic wall pain
   h. Following thoracotomy
   i. Congenital rib or vertebral abnormalities, especially hemivertebrae, resulting in crowding of rib heads
   j. Pleural disease
   k. Large thoracic masses.
4. Barrel-chested conformation
   a. Breed characteristic – e.g. Basset, Bulldog, Boston Terrier
   b. Severe pleural disease
   c. Large intrathoracic tumours
   d. Tension pneumothorax
   e. Pulmonary overinflation.
5. Osteolysis +/– bone production affecting the ribs (Figure 8.13)
   a. Primary tumours – usually a mixed, aggressive bone lesion

- osteosarcoma – most common; usually distal rib
- chondrosarcoma
- haemangiosarcoma
- fibrosarcoma
- multiple myeloma – usually osteolytic, may be multiple
- osteochondroma (cartilaginous exostosis) – young dogs; may be single or multiple (see 1.15.2 and Fig. 1.19)
- osteoma
  b. Osteomyelitis
  c. Metastatic tumours – often smaller and multiple, and mainly osteolytic.
6. New bone on the ribs
  a. Healed fractures – new bone smooth and solid
  b. Hypertrophic non-union fractures – common, due to continual respiratory movement (see Fig. 1.14)
  c. Osteochondroma (cartilaginous exostosis) – young dogs; may be single or multiple (see 1.15.2 and Figure 1.19)
  d. Periosteal reaction stimulated by adjacent rib or soft tissue mass.
7. Congenital rib variants – unilateral or bilateral; on transitional vertebrae (see 5.3.2)
  a. Vestigial ribs
    - L1
    - C7
  b. Abnormal rib curvature due to pectus excavatum (see 8.22.1)
  c. Flared ribs 1 and/or 2
  d. Fusion of distal ribs 1 and 2.
8. Notching of the caudal borders of ribs 4–8 secondary to dilated intercostal arteries supplying collateral circulation in animals with coarctation of the aorta – very rare.

8.22 Variations in the sternum

1. Changes in sternebral alignment
  a. Malalignment of sternebrae is often seen and the xiphisternum especially may appear subluxated or luxated; usually of little clinical significance
  b. "Swimmers" ("flat pup" syndrome)
  c. Pectus excavatum (funnel chest, congenital chondrosternal depression) – the sternum deviates dorsally into the thorax, displacing the heart and ribs
  d. Pectus carinatum (pigeon breast) – the sternum is excessively angled caudoventrally – may be associated with cardiomegaly due to congenital cardiac pathology (e.g. patent ductus arteriosus)
  e. Sternebral absence, splitting (sternal dysraphism) or malformation may be associated with peritoneopericardial diaphragmatic hernia.
2. Mineralised intersternebral cartilages and "sternal spondylosis" – a normal ageing variant, especially in large dogs.
3. Osteolysis, expansile lesions and/or bone production affecting sternebrae
  a. Osteomyelitis – may have a similar appearance to discospondylitis (see 5.8.3); likely to be due to a penetrating foreign body
  b. Neoplasia
    - chondrosarcoma
    - osteosarcoma
    - fibrosarcoma.

8.23 Variations in thoracic vertebrae

See also Chapter 5. Only conditions that may affect the thorax are listed here.
1. Congenital vertebral malformations.
2. Vertebral fractures, luxations and subluxations associated with thoracic trauma.
3. Vertebral neoplasia with extension into the thorax or lung metastases.
4. Spondylitis of caudal thoracic vertebra – pathognomonic for *Spirocerca lupi** granuloma of the distal oesophagus.

8.24 Ultrasonography of the thoracic wall

1. Diffuse thickening of the thoracic wall on ultrasonography
  a. Increased echogenicity or poor image quality
    - obesity
    - subcutaneous emphysema
  b. Normal or decreased echogenicity
    - obesity
    - subcutaneous oedema
    - haemorrhage
    - cellulitis
    - electrolyte solutions injected subcutaneously and dispersed.
2. Localised swelling of the thoracic wall on ultrasonography
  a. Fluid accumulation (anechoic to hypoechoic)
    - abscess
    - haematoma
    - cyst
    - seroma following surgery
    - recently injected electrolyte solutions
  b. Soft tissue (hypoechoic to hyperechoic)

SMALL ANIMAL RADIOLOGICAL DIFFERENTIAL DIAGNOSIS

- abscess
- granuloma
- neoplasia.

3. Hyperechoic areas with acoustic shadowing
   a. Normal ribs – multiple, regularly spaced
   b. Subcutaneous emphysema
   c. Foreign body
   d. Paracostal hernia with gas-filled bowel loops
   e. Dystrophic calcification
   f. Rib tumour.

8.25 Variations in the appearance of the diaphragm

The diaphragm consists of a right and left crus dorsally and a cranioventral cupola. The caudal vena cava passes through the caval hiatus in the right crus. On recumbent lateral radiographs in dogs the dependent crus is pushed cranially by the abdominal contents (Figure 8.14). If the caudal vena cava passes through the cranial crus and the crura are parallel, then the dog is lying on its right side; if the caudal vena cava passes through the caudal crus and over the cranial crus and the crura diverge, the dog is lying on its left side. The heart outline is often more rounded on the left lateral view. On the DV and VD views the cupola and two crural silhouettes normally vary markedly due to X-ray beam direction and the pressure of abdominal contents influenced by gravity. On the DV view the cupola is clearly visualised as a single dome with the right hemidiaphragm normally more cranial than the left. On the VD view three bulges may be seen: a central cupola and two

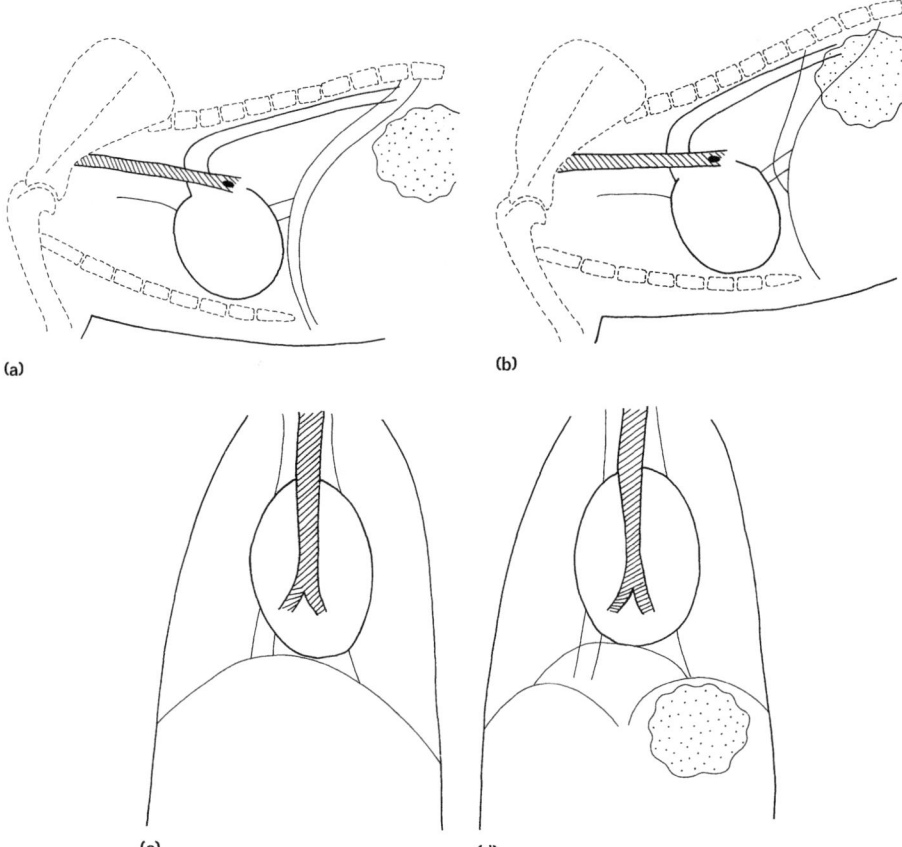

Figure 8.14 Diaphragm shape changes with posture. (a) Right lateral recumbency – the crura are parallel with the right crus lying more cranially; (b) left lateral recumbency – the crura diverge dorsally and the gas-filled gastric fundus may overlie the caudodorsal lung field; (c) sternal recumbency for the DV view – the diaphragm is smoothly curved with the apex to the right of the mid line; (d) dorsal recumbency for the VD view – the crura and cupola produce separate bulges.

8 OTHER THORACIC STRUCTURES

adjacent, more caudal, crura. The heart outline may show bulges on the VD view as the chambers and major vessels are thrown into profile by slight tilting of the heart. The variations in diaphragm shape with posture are less obvious in small dogs and in cats.

1. Cranially displaced diaphragm – unilateral or bilateral
   a. Abdominal causes
      - obesity
      - gastric distension with gas or food
      - severe ascites
      - severe hepatomegaly
      - severe splenomegaly
      - large abdominal mass
      - advanced pregnancy/pyometra
      - severe pain
      - severe pneumoperitoneum
   b. Thoracic causes
      - expiration
      - pulmonary fibrosis in aged patients
      - pleural adhesions
      - atelectasis
      - severe pain
      - radiation therapy induced fibrosis or atelectasis
      - lung lobectomy
      - diaphragmatic paralysis – confirm with fluoroscopy
      - diaphragm tumour
   c. Diaphragmatic rupture with a displaced, loose diaphragmatic flap
   d. Diaphragmatic eventration – thinning and weakening of one hemidiaphragm with absence or atrophy of the muscles and cranial protrusion into the thorax; DDx true diaphragmatic hernia, thoracic mass touching the diaphragm, diaphragmatic or liver mass, diaphragmatic paralysis. Usually no associated clinical signs.
2. Caudally displaced diaphragm – unilateral or bilateral
   a. Abdominal causes
      - emaciation
      - viscera displaced ventrally or caudally through a large body wall hernia or rupture
   b. Thoracic causes – may be accompanied by "tenting", which represents the diaphragmatic attachments to the thoracic wall and is seen on the DV/VD view as pointed projections emanating from the diaphragmatic silhouette
      - forced or deep inspiration
      - intrathoracic masses
      - pleural effusion
      - severe closed pneumothorax
      - tension pneumothorax
      - chronic bronchitis
      - chronic obstructive lung disease
      - acquired emphysema
      - congenital lobar emphysema
      - cats – feline bronchial asthma.
3. Diaphragm border effacement
   a. Pleural effusion
   b. Acquired diaphragmatic rupture – usually ventrally. Additional diagnostic studies include oral positive contrast agents, positive contrast peritoneography and ultrasonography
   c. Diaphragmatic hernia – displacement of viscera through an enlarged anatomical opening, usually the oesophageal hiatus
      - hiatal hernia, which includes sliding oesophageal hiatal, paraoesophageal, paravenous and para-aortic hernias; oral positive contrast studies are helpful in diagnosis
      - peritoneopericardial diaphragmatic hernia – continuous with an enlarged "cardiac" silhouette; additional studies as above may be useful
   d. Alveolar pattern of adjacent lung
   e. Caudal mediastinal masses (see 8.11.4)
   f. Extrapleural masses in contact with the diaphragm.
4. Irregular diaphragmatic contour
   a. Pleural and extrapleural nodules and masses (see also 8.4)
      - rhabdomyosarcoma
      - metastatic or invasive mediastinal or pleural tumours
      - granuloma
   b. Tenting of the diaphragm (see 8.25.2)
   c. Small diaphragmatic ruptures and hernias
   d. Hypertrophic muscular dystrophy (scalloped appearance) – also in cats.

8.26 Ultrasonography of the diaphragm

1. Enhanced visualisation of the diaphragm
   a. Fluid in the pleural cavity or mediastinum
   b. Fluid in the abdominal cavity
   c. Caudal thoracic mass enhancing sound passage
   d. Consolidation of caudal lung lobes enhancing sound passage.
2. Irregular diaphragmatic outline
   a. Nodular hepatic disease
   b. Irregular caudal thoracic mass
   c. Diaphragmatic inflammatory deposits (fibrin deposition, granulomata)

SMALL ANIMAL RADIOLOGICAL DIFFERENTIAL DIAGNOSIS

  d. Diaphragmatic neoplastic deposits (metastases, or mediastinal or pleural tumours).
3. Loss of integrity of the diaphragmatic outline
  a. Diaphragmatic rupture
  b. Congenital peritoneopericardial diaphragmatic hernia.

MISCELLANEOUS

8.27 Thoracic trauma

Multiple lesions may be present following thoracic trauma, and systematic radiographic evaluation is vital to recognise the cause and extent of possible life-threatening conditions and to prioritise them for treatment. Follow-up radiographs should be made to check the effectiveness of treatment and in patients that were initially radiologically normal but which fail to recover as expected or deteriorate. Refer to specific organ systems for more detail.

1. Soft tissues of the thoracic wall
   a. Gas accumulation – subcutaneous emphysema
   b. Swelling – oedema or haemorrhage
   c. Foreign bodies
   d. Paracostal hernia – more common in cats.
2. Skeletal structures
   a. Single or multiple rib fractures, often with associated pneumothorax, haematoma, pleural effusion or pulmonary contusion
   b. Widened intercostal spaces due to intercostal muscle tearing
   c. Sternal, vertebral, scapular and long bone fractures and/or luxations.
3. Cranial abdomen – organ trauma resulting from caudal thoracic injuries; clinical and radiographic changes may have a delayed onset (e.g. organs incarcerated in an diaphragmatic rupture).
4. Pleural cavity
   a. Pneumothorax
      - closed
      - open
      - tension; diaphragm caudally displaced and flattened
   b. Diaphragmatic rupture
   c. Haemothorax
   d. Subpleural haematoma
   e. Haemopneumothorax
   f. Pyothorax – delayed onset
   g. Chylothorax – delayed onset
   h. Bilothorax – very rare,
5. Lungs
   a. Contusions – poorly defined interstitial or alveolar infiltrates; resolve in a few days
   b. Haematomata – appear after contusions, rounded and take weeks to resolve
   c. Cysts and bullae
   d. Lacerations
   e. Atelectasis
   f. Oedema – post head trauma
   g. Pneumonia – delayed onset
   h. Acute respiratory distress syndrome (ARDS or " shock lung") – usually of delayed onset (see 6.14.7).
6. Cardiovascular system
   a. Evidence of shock
      - microcardia
      - hypovascular lung field
      - small caudal vena cava and aorta
   b. Haemopericardium with cardiac tamponade
      - acute, difficult to see radiologically if only a small volume change
      - may be delayed days or weeks, often after bullet or air-gun pellet wounds
   c. Pneumopericardium – auricles become visible; generally not clinically significant
   d. Traumatic cardiac displacement
      - rupture of cardiac ligaments
      - rupture of pericardium with heart displaced outside pericardium
      - secondary to mediastinal shift (see 8.8).
7. Mediastinum
   a. Pneumomediastinum
   b. Mediastinal haemorrhage
   c. Mediastinal oedema
   d. Chylomediastinum.

8.28 Ultrasonography of thoracic trauma

Ultrasonography is generally used to evaluate further abnormal or suspicious areas ident-

8 OTHER THORACIC STRUCTURES

ified on thoracic radiographs. Refer to specific organ systems for more detail.
1. Soft tissues of the thoracic wall
   a. Fluid accumulation (haematoma)
   b. Foreign bodies
   c. Subcutaneous location of abdominal viscera.
2. Pleural cavity
   a. Free fluid in thoracic cavity
   b. Diaphragmatic rupture.
3. Lungs – moderate or extensive areas of lung collapse or consolidation.
4. Heart
   a. Evidence of shock (tachycardia)
   b. Displacement of the heart (e.g. by abdominal viscera in diaphragmatic rupture)
   c. Pericardial haemorrhage +/– tamponade
   d. Dysfunctional myocardium (e.g. due to ischaemia, contusion).
5. Mediastinum – fluid accumulation.

FURTHER READING

General

Berry, C.R., Gallaway, A., Thrall, D.E. and Carlisle, C. (1993) Thoracic radiographic features of anticoagulant rodenticide toxicity in fourteen dogs. *Veterinary Radiology and Ultrasound* **34** 391–396.

Blackwood, L., Sullivan, M. and Lawson, H. (1997) Radiographic abnormalities in canine multicentric lymphoma: a review of 84 cases. *Journal of Small Animal Practice* **38** 62–69.

Godshalk, C.P. (1994) Common pitfalls in radiographic interpretation of the thorax. *Compendium of Continuing Education for the Practicing Veterinarian (Small Animal)* **16** 731–738.

Reichle, J.K. and Wisner, E.R. (2000) Non-cardiac thoracic ultrasound in 75 feline and canine patients. *Veterinary Radiology and Ultrasound* **41** 154–162.

Schmidt, M. and Wolvekamp, P. (1991) Radiographic findings in ten dogs with thoracic actinomycosis. *Veterinary Radiology* **32** 301–306.

Tidwell, A.S. (1998) Ultrasonography of the thorax (excluding the heart). *Veterinary Clinics of North America; Small Animal Practice* **28** number 4 993–1016.

Pleural cavity

Aronson, E. (1995) Radiology corner: Pneumothorax: ventrodorsal or dorsoventral view – does it make a difference? *Veterinary Radiology and Ultrasound* **36** 109–110.

Thrall, D.E. (1993) Radiology corner: Misidentification of a skin fold as pneumothorax. *Veterinary Radiology and Ultrasound* **34** 242–243.

Mediastinum

Myer, W. (1978) Radiography review: the mediastinum. *Journal of the American Veterinary Radiological Society* **19** 197–202.

Scrivani, P.V., Burt, J.K. and Bruns, D. (1996) Radiology corner: Sternal lymphadenopathy. *Veterinary Radiology and Ultrasound* **37** 183–184.

Oesophagus

Mears, E.A. and Jenkins, C.C. (1997) Canine and feline megaesophagus. *Compendium of Continuing Education for the Practicing Veterinarian (Small Animal)* **19** 313–326.

Sickle, R.L. and Love, N.E. (1989) Radiographic diagnosis of esophageal disease in dogs and cats. *Seminars in Veterinary Medicine and Surgery (Small Animals)* **4** 179–187.

van Gundy, T. (1989) Vascular ring anomalies. *Compendium of Continuing Education for the Practicing Veterinarian (Small Animal)* **11** 35–45.

Dvir, E. Kirberger, R.M. and Malleczek, D. (2000) Radiographic and computed tomographic changes and clinical presentation of spirocercosis in the dog. *Veterinary Radiology and Ultrasound* in press.

Thoracic wall

Berry, C.R., Koblik, P.D. and Ticer, J.W. (1990) Dorsal peritoneopericardial mesothelial remnant as an aid to the diagnosis of feline congenital peritoneopericardial diaphragmatic hernia. *Veterinary Radiology* **31** 239–245.

Dennis, R. (1993) Radiographic diagnosis of rib lesions in dogs and cats. *Veterinary Annual* **33** 173–192.

Fagin, B. (1989) Using radiography to diagnose diaphragmatic hernia. *Veterinary Medicine* **7** 662–672.

Williams, J., Leveille, R. and Myer, C.W. (1998) Imaging modalities used to confirm diaphragmatic hernia in small animals. *Compendium of Continuing Education for the Practicing Veterinarian (Small Animal)* **20** 1199–1208.

9

Gastrointestinal tract

STOMACH

9.1 Normal radiographic appearance of the stomach
9.2 Displacement of the stomach
9.3 Variations in stomach size
9.4 Variations in stomach contents
9.5 Variations in the stomach wall
9.6 Gastric contrast studies – technique and normal appearance
9.7 Technical errors on the gastrogram
9.8 Gastric luminal filling defects
9.9 Abnormal gastric mucosal pattern
9.10 Variations in stomach emptying time
9.11 Ultrasonographic examination of the stomach
9.12 Normal ultrasonographic appearance of the stomach
9.13 Variations in gastric contents on ultrasonography
9.14 Lack of visualisation of the normal gastric wall layered architecture on ultrasonography
9.15 Focal thickening of the gastric wall on ultrasonography
9.16 Diffuse thickening of the gastric wall on ultrasonography

SMALL INTESTINE

9.17 Normal radiographic appearance of the small intestine
9.18 Variations in the number of small intestinal loops visible
9.19 Displacement of the small intestine
9.20 Bunching of small intestinal loops
9.21 Increased width of small intestinal loops
9.22 Variations in small intestinal contents
9.23 Small intestinal contrast studies – technique and normal appearance
9.24 Technical errors with small intestinal contrast studies
9.25 Variations in small intestinal luminal diameter
9.26 Small intestinal luminal filling defects
9.27 Increased small intestinal wall thickness
9.28 Variations in small intestinal transit time
9.29 Ultrasonographic examination of the small intestine
9.30 Normal ultrasonographic appearance of the small intestine
9.31 Variations in small intestinal contents on ultrasonography
9.32 Dilation of the small intestinal lumen on ultrasonography
9.33 Lack of visualisation of the normal small intestinal wall layered architecture on ultrasonography
9.34 Abnormal arrangement of the small intestine on ultrasonography
9.35 Focal thickening of the small intestinal wall on ultrasonography
9.36 Diffuse thickening of the small intestinal wall on ultrasonography

LARGE INTESTINE

9.37 Normal radiographic appearance of the large intestine
9.38 Displacement of the large intestine
9.39 Large intestinal dilation
9.40 Variations in large intestinal contents
9.41 Variations in large intestinal wall opacity
9.42 Large intestinal contrast studies – technique and normal appearance
9.43 Technical errors with large intestinal contrast studies
9.44 Large intestinal luminal filling defects
9.45 Increased large intestinal wall thickness
9.46 Abnormal large intestinal mucosal pattern
9.47 Ultrasonographic examination of the large intestine
9.48 Normal ultrasonographic appearance of the large intestine
9.49 Ultrasonographic changes in large intestinal disease

STOMACH

9.1 Normal radiographic appearance of the stomach

The type and amount of ingesta present will affect the size and shape of the stomach. Variable amounts of swallowed food, liquid and air combined with normal gastric contractions result in a varying shape to the body of the stomach. Retention of food in the stomach for more than 12 hours after eating is abnormal. The position of the stomach differs between breeds of dogs and between dogs and cats. In cats and in most breeds of dog the stomach axis lies parallel to the caudal ribs on the lateral projection, against the liver, and so displacement of the stomach axis reflects a change in liver size (Figure 9.1a & b). In deep-chested breeds the stomach axis is perpendicular to the spine and this may mimic reduced liver size. The pylorus may lie slightly cranial to the rest of the stomach, and its position and appearance varies slightly between right and left lateral recumbency. In right lateral recumbency the pylorus is likely to be fluid-filled and appears as a round soft tissue mass; in left lateral recumbency it may contain a gas bubble. In deep-chested dog breeds on the ventrodorsal view the stomach axis lies transversely approximately at the level of the tenth intercostal space, with the fundus to the left and the pylorus to the right of the mid line (Figure 9.1c). In barrel-chested breeds the stomach is more curved, with the fundus lying more cranially and the pylorus towards the mid line. In cats on the ventrodorsal view an empty stomach is located with the pylorus in the midline and the remainder of the stomach to the left side (Figure 9.1d). Distension of the feline stomach results in displacement of the pylorus to the right side.

9.2 Displacement of the stomach

1. Cranial displacement of the stomach
   a. Reduced liver size (see 11.14.3 and Figure 11.6)
   b. Diaphragmatic hernia or rupture
   c. Peritoneopericardial diaphragmatic hernia (PPDH)
   d. Gastro-oesophageal intussusception
   e. Hiatal hernia
   f. Mesenteric masses (see 11.37.6)
   g. Colonic masses

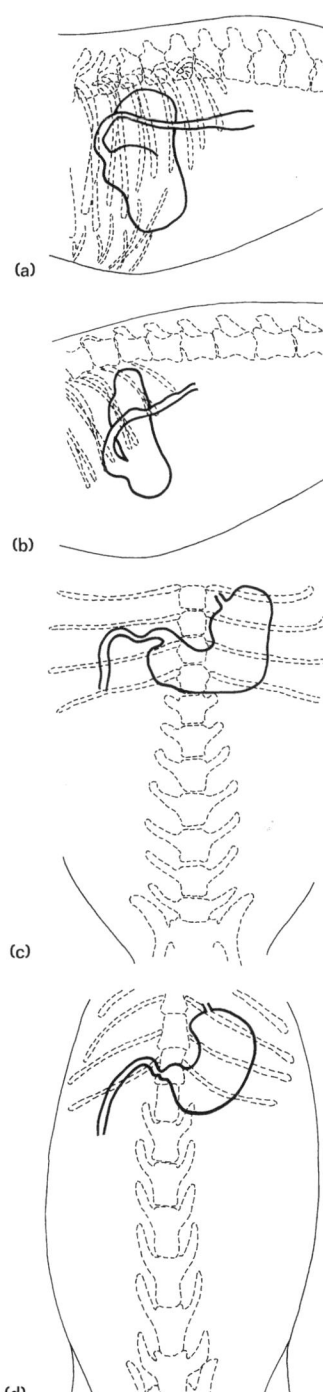

Figure 9.1 Normal stomach location: (a) lateral view, dog; (b) lateral view, cat; (c) VD view, dog; (d) VD view, cat.

h. Pancreatic masses, left limb (see 11.36.3)
   i. Other large abdominal masses including late pregnancy.
2. Caudal displacement of the stomach
   a. Enlarged liver (see 11.14.1 and Fig. 11.5)
   b. Thoracic expansion.
3. Stomach displaced towards the right
   a. Enlarged spleen
   b. Left-sided liver enlargement.
4. Stomach displaced towards the left
   a. Right-sided liver enlargement.
   b. Enlarged pancreas

9.3 Variations in stomach size

A small amount of gas and/or fluid is normally observed in the stomach after an 8-hour fast.
1. Stomach not visible
   a. Completely empty, collapsed
   b. Absence of abdominal fat
      • young animals
      • emaciation
   c. Peritoneal effusion.
2. Stomach visible but empty
   a. Fasted or anorexic (NB: this does not rule out obstruction if the animal has vomited recently).
3. Stomach normal shape and size; gas and/or fluid contents
   a. Normal with some aerophagia
   b. Recent drink
   c. Acute gastritis (no signs on plain radiographs).
4. Stomach distended but normal in shape
   a. Endotracheal tube in oesophagus not trachea
   b. Acute dilation by air and/or fluid
      • aerophagia due to dyspnoea
      • aerophagia secondary to any painful condition such as pancreatitis or blunt trauma
      • acute gastritis
      • outflow obstructed by a foreign body
      • post abdominal surgery
      • anticholinergic drugs
   c. Chronic dilation – likely to show a "gravel sign" (see 9.4.2 and Fig. 9.3)
      • chronic obstruction by foreign bodies in the stomach or duodenum
      • pyloric lesions: pylorospasm, muscular hypertrophy, mucosal hypertrophy, pyloric or duodenal neoplasia, pyloric or duodenal scar tissue, pyloric or duodenal ulceration, pyloric or duodenal granulomata
   d. Pancreatitis.
5. Stomach distended with an abnormal shape
   a. Gastric dilation/volvulus syndrome (GDV; Figure 9.2) – especially in large, deep-chested dogs. The stomach will be abnormally distended by food, liquid and gas, with compartmentalisation of the stomach lumen giving a double gas bubble appearance. Frequently the pylorus will be displaced dorsally and towards the left side; the fundus will be displaced ventrally and towards the right side unless the degree of rotation approaches 360°. It is helpful to perform both right and left lateral recumbent radiographs as gas will move around in the stomach and may help to identify the position of the pylorus.

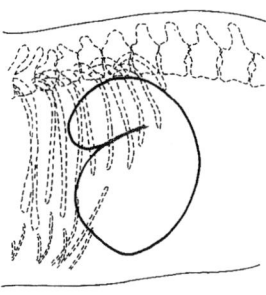

(a)

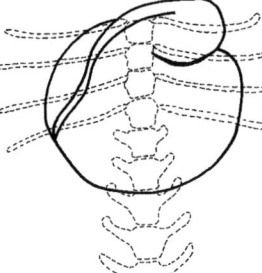

(b)

Figure 9.2 Gastric dilation and volvulus (GDV): (a) lateral view; (b) VD view. The stomach is markedly distended with gas +/– ingesta and shows compartmentalisation. It may be difficult to identify which is the pylorus and which the fundus unless gas is present in the duodenum (seen here on the VD view).

9 GASTROINTESTINAL TRACT

9.4 Variations in stomach contents

The animal should ideally be fasted for 12 hours before elective abdominal radiography. Retention of food in the stomach after 12 hours is abnormal; however, sometimes the animal eats unknown to the owner during the fast, so consider repeating the radiographs under a more controlled fasting situation.

1. Small amount of gas and/or fluid – normal.
2. Mineral opacity material
   a. Medications containing bismuth and kaolin
   b. "Gravel sign" – accumulation of small, mineralised fragments of ingesta which form proximal to chronic partial obstructions; in this case secondary to a pyloric outflow problem (Figure 9.3)
   c. Foreign bodies (sometimes incidental findings in dogs)
      - metallic materials
      - stones, pebbles, etc.
      - bones or bone fragments; DDx mineralisation of rugal folds secondary to chronic renal failure
      - dense rubber or glass
   c. Barium from a previous contrast study.
3. Soft tissue radio-opacity with interspersed small gas bubbles
   a. Food – normal if not fasted
   b. Abnormal retention of food if fasted for more than 12 hours (e.g. due to outflow obstruction to the pylorus and/or duodenum)
   c. Foreign bodies
      - plastic/cellophane
      - fabrics
      - string/carpet
      - phytobezoar such as grass
      - trichobezoar such as hairball.
4. Uniform soft tissue radio-opacity
   a. Recently ingested liquid
   b. Retained liquids due to acute gastric dilation
   c. Retained liquids due to outflow obstruction of the pylorus and duodenum
   d. Foreign bodies
      - plastic/cellophane
      - fabrics
      - string/carpet
      - phytobezoar such as grass
      - trichobezoar such as hairball
   e. Large gastric tumour or polyp
   f. Blood clot
   g. Gastrogastric intussusception.
5. Gas
   a. Aerophagia
   b. GDV.

9.5 Variations in the stomach wall

The gastric wall thickness can be evaluated accurately only when the stomach is moderately distended by gas or radio-opaque contrast medium. Rugal folds are predominantly located in the fundus and are smaller and more

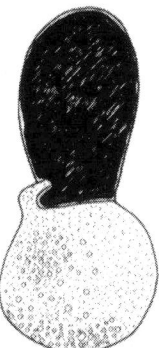

Figure 9.3 "Gravel sign" in the stomach due to a chronic, partial outflow obstruction. Small, radio-opaque fragments of ingesta accumulate in a distended pylorus.

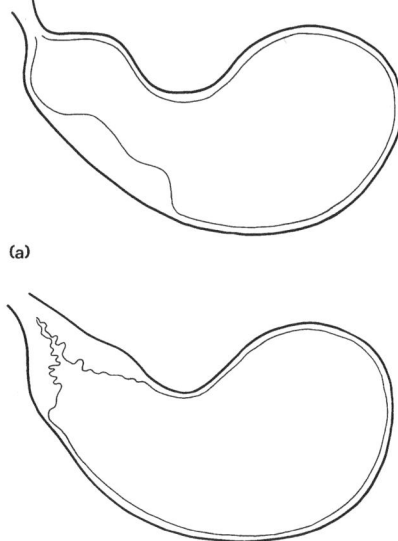

Figure 9.4 Gastric tumours (best seen on contrast radiography) (a) not affecting the pylorus – often seen as a smooth thickening of the stomach wall with raised edges; (b) around the pyloric outflow tract – often ragged and circumferential, producing an "apple core" appearance.

SMALL ANIMAL RADIOLOGICAL DIFFERENTIAL DIAGNOSIS

numerous in dogs than cats. Few rugal folds should be observed in the pyloric antral region.
1. Focally thickened stomach wall
   a. Pseudomass from transient wall contraction of an empty stomach
   b. Neoplasia (Figure 9.4)
      - adenocarcinoma
      - leiomyoma/leiomyosarcoma
      - lymphosarcoma (especially cats)
   c. Pyloric muscular or mucosal hypertrophy
   d. Focal chronic hyperplastic gastropathy
   e. Focal infiltrative gastritis
      - eosinophilic
      - granulomatous
      - fungal infections*, especially phycomycosis.
2. Diffusely thickened stomach wall
   a. Secondary to persistent vomiting
   b. Chronic gastritis
   c. Eosinophilic gastritis
   d. Lymphosarcoma (especially cats)
   e. Non-beta tumour of pancreas
   f. Chronic hyperplastic gastropathy.
3. Mineralisation of the rugal folds
   a. Artefactual due to the presence of linear gastric foreign bodies
   b. Chronic renal failure.
4. Gas in the stomach wall
   a. Gastric ulceration
   b. Partial gastric wall perforation
   c. Necrosis secondary to GDV
   d. Secondary to pancreatitis.

9.6 Gastric contrast studies – technique and normal appearance

If rupture of the stomach is suspected iodinated contrast medium rather than barium should be used. If the procedure is elective, preparation should involve a fast of at least 12 hours and appropriate chemical restraint. Radiographs should be taken in right lateral, left lateral, sternal and dorsal recumbency. The exposure factors used should be reduced following administration of air and increased with positive contrast media.

Pneumogastrogram

Pass a stomach tube and inflate the stomach with room air. Shows:
- stomach location
- radiolucent foreign bodies and intraluminal masses
- stomach wall thickness
- little or no information about the mucosal surface

Positive contrast gastrogram

a. Small volume barium sulphate or iodinated contrast medium: shows stomach location
b. Barium-impregnated polyethylene spheres (BIPS): gives some information about stomach emptying
c. Large volume (7–12 ml/kg) 30% w/v barium sulphate or 2–3 ml/kg isotonic iodinated contrast medium. Shows:
   - stomach size
   - stomach shape
   - contractility

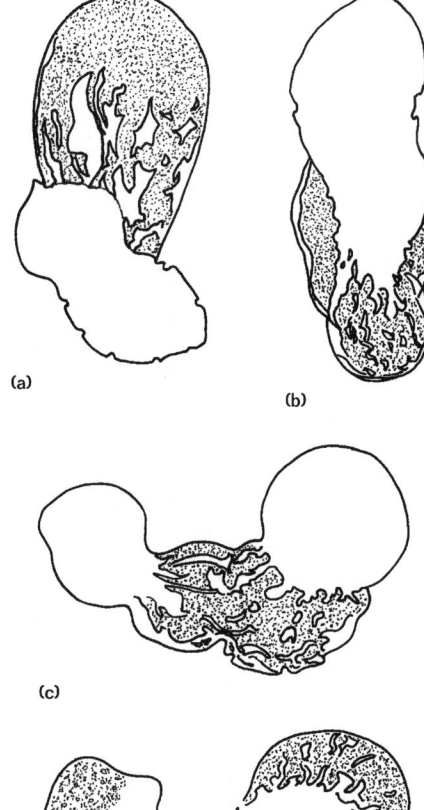

Figure 9.5 Normal double-contrast gastrogram. (a) Right lateral recumbency, with barium in the pylorus and gas in the fundus; (b) left lateral recumbency, with barium in the fundus and gas in the pylorus (+/– the duodenum); (c) dorsal recumbency for the VD view, with barium in the fundus and pylorus and gas in the body of the stomach; (d) sternal recumbency for the DV view, with barium in the body of the stomach and gas in the fundus and pylorus.

- contents (as filling defects)
- liquid phase of stomach emptying

d. Large volume food studies (barium or BIPS mixed in food). Shows the solid phase of stomach emptying.

Double contrast gastrogram

1 ml/kg barium 100% w/v given by stomach tube, then the stomach is distended with air. Shows:
- excellent mucosal detail
- stomach wall thickness
- radiolucent foreign bodies.

The normal gastrogram (Figure 9.5) shows positive contrast medium pooling in dependent areas and luminal gas rising. Positive contrast medium in the inter-rugal clefts creates gently-curving lines when seen *en face* and a serrated margin to the stomach when seen tangentially. On a correctly exposed radiograph of a patient in reasonable body condition the thickness of the stomach wall can be assessed. Peristaltic waves create symmetrical, smooth indentations to the shape of the stomach, varying from film to film.

9.7 Technical errors on the gastrogram

1. Lack of survey (plain) radiographs
   a. Radio-opaque foreign bodies overlooked
   b. Incorrect exposure factors used for the contrast study
   c. Patient not adequately fasted.
2. Inappropriate exposure factors – add 5–10 kVp to settings used to obtain survey radiographs for positive contrast studies
   a. Underexposed positive contrast studies will hinder detection of smaller radiolucent foreign bodies
   b. Overexposed pneumogastrogram will hinder detection of smaller radiolucent foreign bodies.
3. Inadequate distension of the stomach
   a. Precludes accurate evaluation of wall thickness and of masses
   b. Results in a longer gastric emptying time as inadequate distension fails to stimulate emptying reflexes.
4. Too much positive contrast used – small foreign bodies will be "drowned" and not visible on single positive contrast studies; later radiographs should be taken to look for residual contrast adhering to foreign material.
5. Inadequate number of images (in absence of fluoroscopic examination) – may preclude the detection of foreign bodies, soft tissue masses and ulceration.
6. Overdiagnosis based on single or few images – mural lesions must be confirmed on multiple radiographs as peristaltic waves lead to transient gastric wall thickening which may give rise to false-positive diagnoses.

9.8 Gastric luminal filling defects

Smaller foreign bodies may initially be hidden by large-volume positive gastrograms.
1. Retained food.
2. Foreign bodies.
3. Pedunculated masses.
4. Blood clots and mucus.

9.9 Abnormal gastric mucosal pattern

Mild ulcerative gastritis and shallow ulcers may be difficult to detect; consider using endoscopy instead. The mucosal pattern is normally of parallel bands of barium in the inter-rugal clefts, with rugae seen as parallel-sided, band-like filling defects. Rugae are sparse near the pylorus and are less obvious in cats than in dogs.

1. Normal variant – the presence of ingesta or mucus creates an irregular, patchy rugal fold pattern mimicking pathology
2. Gastritis – irregular, patchy rugal fold pattern (Figure 9.6); barium persists after the stomach has largely emptied as it adheres to inflamed or ulcerated areas.
3. Ulceration – crater-like in profile and circular seen *en face* (Figure 9.7). Barium persists in the ulcer crater long after stomach

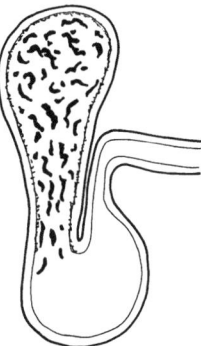

Figure 9.6 Severe gastritis on a barium or double-contrast gastrogram – poorly distensible stomach with an irregular mucosal surface and a broken-up rugal fold pattern.

SMALL ANIMAL RADIOLOGICAL DIFFERENTIAL DIAGNOSIS

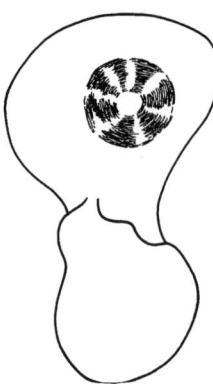

Figure 9.7 Gastric ulcer on a barium or double-contrast gastrogram – barium collects in the centre of the ulcer and rugal folds are "gathered" towards it.

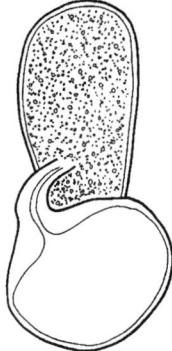

Figure 9.8 Pyloric stenosis on a barium gastrogram – the pyloric antrum is distended and little barium enters the duodenum. In the case of malignant neoplasia, the pylorus may be poorly distended and irregularly marginated (see also Figure 9.4).

has emptied (12–24-hour films are therefore useful)
   a. Neoplastic – the usual cause of gastric ulcers in dogs and cats
   b. Secondary to mast cell tumours elsewhere
   c. Due to the presence of abrasive foreign material
   d. Secondary to chronic renal disease.
4. Chronic hyperplastic gastropathy – giant rugal folds; may cause secondary pyloric stenosis.

9.10 Variations in stomach emptying time

If the stomach was empty prior to administration of the contrast medium, barium suspensions should begin to exit within 30 minutes (provided an adequate quantity was given) and the stomach should be completely empty by 4 hours. Hypertonic iodine solutions empty faster as they induce hyperperistalsis. Barium mixed with food (or food alone) empties more slowly, taking up to 12 hours to empty completely. When food and BIPS are fed together, half the BIPS should have left the stomach by 6 hours (+/– 3 hours) and three-quarters by 8.5 hours (+/– 2.75 hours).
1. Rapid gastric emptying
   a. Normal variant – barium suspension given on an empty stomach
   b. Gastroenteritis.
2. Delayed gastric emptying with decreased gastric motility (seen with fluoroscopy or serial radiographs)
   a. Sedation or general anaesthesia
   b. Nervous pylorospasm – highly strung animal
   c. Gastric or duodenal ulceration
   d. Gastritis
      • parvovirus
      • cats – panleucopenia
   e. Small intestinal obstruction
   f. Pancreatitis
   g. Peritonitis.
3. Delayed gastric emptying with normal or increased gastric motility
   a. Pyloric obstructions and stenoses (Figure 9.8)
      • foreign bodies
      • pyloric muscular or mucosal hypertrophy
      • neoplasia of the pylorus, duodenum, pancreas or gall bladder
      • pyloric or duodenal scar tissue
      • pyloric or duodenal ulceration
      • pyloric or duodenal granulomata
      • chronic hyperplastic gastropathy
   b. Pylorospasm
      • nervous pylorospasm – highly strung animal
      • small intestinal obstruction.

9.11 Ultrasonographic examination of the stomach

The patient should ideally be fasted for 12 hours before ultrasonographic examination of the stomach, but allowed free access to water. The presence of food and/or gas in the stomach will result in acoustic shadowing, and therefore prevent complete examination of the gastric lumen and wall.

The hair should be clipped from the cranial ventral abdomen, between the xiphisternum and the umbilicus, the skin cleaned with surgical spirit and liberal quantities of acoustic gel applied. The transducer should be placed just behind the xiphisternum and the sound beam angled craniodorsally to image the stomach. The entire stomach should be imaged, in both longitudinal and transverse planes relative to the luminal axis. It may be helpful to vary the position of the animal in order to allow fluid to drop into different regions of the stomach.

A sector or curvilinear transducer of as high a frequency as possible compatible with adequate tissue penetration should be used (7.5 MHz in cats or small/medium dogs; 5 MHz in large or obese dogs). Endoscopic ultrasonography is especially useful but is still not widely available in veterinary medicine.

9.12 Normal ultrasonographic appearance of the stomach

The gastric wall has a characteristic layered appearance when imaged with a high-resolution system. The ultrasonographic layers are generally considered to correspond to histological regions (Figure 9.9).

The gastric wall is arranged to form rugal folds, but should otherwise be smooth and of uniform thickness. The thickness of the normal gastric wall, measured between rugal folds, is between 3 and 5 mm in the dog. If the stomach is empty and contracted, the wall will appear thicker than if the stomach is distended. Peristaltic and segmental contractions are normally seen at a rate of 4–5 contractions per minute in the normal dog.

9.13 Variations in gastric contents on ultrasonography

1. Anechoic with hyperechoic specks – (indicates fluid contents with air bubbles/debris/mucus)
   a. Normal with recent ingestion of fluid
   b. Retained fluid secondary to gastric outflow obstruction or high small intestinal obstruction (peristalsis may be increased or diminished)
   c. Retained fluid secondary to functional ileus (peristalsis diminished or absent)
      • following abdominal surgery
      • peritonitis/pancreatitis
      • electrolyte disturbances
      • renal failure.
2. Solid material of variable echogenicity outlined by fluid
   a. Food remnants
   b. Foreign material
   c. Pedunculated gastric mass.
3. Heterogeneous material filling the stomach, with or without acoustic shadowing
   a. Recent ingestion of food
   b. Retained food secondary to gastric outflow obstruction
   c. Foreign material
   d. Blood clot.
4. Extensive acoustic shadowing preventing visualisation of contents
   a. Gastric gas
   b. Pneumoperitoneum.

9.14 Lack of visualisation of the normal gastric wall layered architecture on ultrasonography

1. Gas or food contents.
2. Use of a low frequency transducer (5 MHz or lower).
3. Generally poor image quality
   a. Poor skin preparation
   b. Poor skin–transducer contact
   c. Obese patient.
4. Gastric disease (see 9.15 and 9.16).

9.15 Focal thickening of the gastric wall on ultrasonography

1. Retention of the normal layered architecture
   a. Normal rugal folds
   b. Localised hyperplastic gastropathy
   c. Pyloric hypertrophy – circumferential thickening of the pylorus (in the dog, wall thickness ≥9 mm, with the muscular layer ≥4 mm).
   d. Chronic gastritis or a gastric ulcer

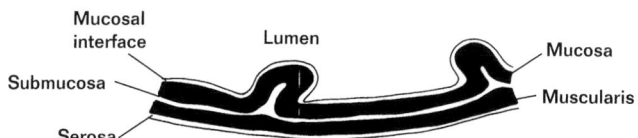

Figure 9.9 Gastric (or small intestinal) wall layers identified on ultrasonography.

SMALL ANIMAL RADIOLOGICAL DIFFERENTIAL DIAGNOSIS

   e. Neoplasia
      - polyp
      - leiomyoma/leiomyosarcoma.
2. Loss of the normal layered architecture
   a. Neoplasia
      - adenocarcinoma
      - leiomyoma/leiomyosarcoma
      - lymphosarcoma (typically symmetrical, hypoechoic thickening) – especially cats
   b. Gastric ulcer
   c. Necrotising gastritis
   d. Pyogranulomatous gastritis (e.g. gastrointestinal pythiosis*).

9.16 Diffuse thickening of the gastric wall on ultrasonography

1. Retention of the normal layered architecture
   a. Contracted, empty stomach
   b. Gastritis
   c. Chronic hyperplastic gastropathy.
2. Loss of the normal layered architecture
   a. Neoplasia
      - adenocarcinoma
      - leiomyoma/leiomyosarcoma
      - lymphosarcoma (typically symmetrical, hypoechoic thickening) – especially cats
   b. Necrotising gastritis
   c. Uraemic gastritis
   d. Pyogranulomatous gastritis (e.g. gastrointestinal pythiosis*).

SMALL INTESTINE

9.17 Normal radiographic appearance of the small intestine

The animal should ideally be fasted for 12 hours before the radiographic examination. When much faecal material is present in the colon, an enema may also be necessary and radiography repeated some hours later. Evaluation of the stomach contents should be made, as radio-opaque stomach contents and gas from aerophagia will also pass through to the small intestine.

The descending duodenum runs along the right abdominal wall and is slightly larger in diameter than the remaining small intestine. The jejunum and ileum cannot be differentiated except at the ileo-caeco-colic junction. The small intestine fills much of the abdominal cavity, lying caudal to the stomach and cranial to the urinary bladder. In obese animals, the small intestine lies more centrally.

9.18 Variations in the number of small intestinal loops visible

1. Increased number of small intestinal loops visible
   a. Normal – a false impression is given if the intestine is distended by gas, food or fluid; evaluate the stomach, which will contain similar material
   b. Mechanical obstruction (ileus)
   c. Functional obstruction (paralytic ileus).
2. Decreased number of small intestinal loops visible
   a. Normal, artefactual
      - small intestine empty and collapsed
      - obesity, making the intestine lie more centrally
      - poor abdominal detail in very thin or young animals
   b. Abnormal
      - abdominal effusion masking serosal detail
      - displacement through hernias or body wall ruptures
      - plication along a linear foreign body
      - intussusception
      - previous enterectomy.

9.19 Displacement of the small intestine

1. Small intestine displaced into the thoracic cavity
   a. Ruptured diaphragm
   b. Peritoneopericardial diaphragmatic hernia (PPDH)
   c. Congenital diaphragmatic hernia (incomplete formation of the diaphragm).
2. Cranial displacement of the small intestine
   a. Against the dorsal diaphragm, sometimes seen in normal deep-chested dogs when the stomach is empty
   b. Small liver
   c. Ruptured diaphragm, with displacement of the liver into the thorax allowing small intestines to lie more cranially

d. Distended urinary bladder
e. Uterine enlargement
- pregnancy
- pyometra
f. Ruptured attachment of abdominal muscles to ribs.
3. Caudal displacement of the small intestine
a. Liver enlargement
b. Stomach distension
c. Empty urinary bladder
d. Inguinal hernia
e. Large perineal hernia
f. Ruptured caudal abdominal muscles.
4. Displacement of the small intestine to the right or left
a. Previous prolonged lateral recumbency
b. Asymmetrical enlargement of liver
c. Enlargement of the spleen
d. Severe enlargement of a kidney
e. Rupture of right or left abdominal muscles.
5. Fixed location of distended small intestinal loops on serial radiographs
a. Prior surgery
b. Adhesions
c. Peritonitis.
6. Central bunching of the small intestine (see 9.20).

9.20 Bunching of small intestinal loops

1. Obesity causing intestines to lie centrally, especially in cats.
2. Plication along a linear foreign body – usually see teardrop-shaped gas bubbles (see 9.22.1 and 9.25.4 and Figures 9.11 and 9.13).
3. Adhesions.

9.21 Increased width of small intestinal loops

Sufficient abdominal fat is necessary to provide contrast to see the serosal surface of intestinal loops. On lateral radiographs, the small intestine usually has a diameter less than the height of lumbar vertebral bodies or two rib widths (in dogs) and less than 12 mm in cats. Generally, no loop should be more than twice the diameter of the other loops. Increased width of small intestinal loops may be due to dilation of the lumen, thickening of the wall or a combination of both processes. Fluid-filled dilation can only be differentiated from wall thickening using contrast studies or ultrasonography. Dilated loops of intestine tend to appear to stack up against one another and to curve abnormally (like a hairpin or paperclip) (Figure 9.10). The number of dilated loops should be assessed, as complete obstructions in the lower jejunum/ileum and generalised paralytic ileus will cause many loops to be dilated whilst higher obstructions and segmental paralytic ileus will affect fewer loops.

1. Single dilated or thickened small intestinal loop
a. Obstruction due to
- neoplasia: lymphosarcoma (especially cats), adenocarcinoma, leiomyoma/leiomyosarcoma
- foreign body (may be radiolucent)
- granuloma
- abscess
- intussusception – most common in young dogs or soon after surgery
b. Partial functional obstruction (paralytic ileus) – "sentinel loop" (e.g. due to localised peritonitis).
2. Few dilated small intestinal loops – localised dilation
a. Colon mistaken for small intestine
b. Normal peristalsis
c. High small intestinal obstruction
- foreign bodies
- neoplasia
- strangulation of a few loops in a hernia or mesenteric tear
d. Partial functional obstruction (paralytic ileus)
- severe gastroenteritis (e.g. parvovirus infection)
- recent abdominal surgery
- localised peritonitis
- pancreatitis
e. Adhesions.
3. Many dilated small intestinal loops – generalised dilation
a. Low acute small intestinal obstruction
- foreign bodies
- intussusception
- intestinal volvulus at the root of the mesentery (also partly functional obstruction)
- strangulation in a hernia or mesenteric tear
b. Low chronic partial obstruction (may finally become total) – "gravel sign" likely (see 9.4.2 and Fig. 9.3)
- foreign bodies
- intussusception
- neoplasia
- polyps
- adhesions/strictures
- granulomata
- caecal impaction (faecolithiasis)

SMALL ANIMAL RADIOLOGICAL DIFFERENTIAL DIAGNOSIS

c. Functional obstruction (paralytic ileus)
- GDV
- intestinal volvulus at the root of the mesentery (also partly mechanical obstruction)
- severe gastroenteritis (e.g. parvovirus infection)
- secondary to chronic mechanical obstruction
- recent abdominal surgery
- electrolyte imbalances
- dysautonomia
- peritonitis
- pancreatitis

d. Diffuse neoplasia – mainly lymphosarcoma.

9.22 Variations in small intestinal contents

In a fasted animal with an empty stomach, the small intestine should be of homogeneous fluid opacity with some gas-filled segments. Normally less gas is seen in the small intestine of the cat than the dog.

1. Gas-filled small intestine
   a. Normal diameter small intestine
      - normal
      - aerophagia (e.g. due to dyspnoea) – evaluate stomach contents
      - recent enema
      - enteritis
      - adhesions from previous surgery or peritonitis
      - incomplete obstruction
      - debilitated, recumbent animal
      - intussusception (crescentic gas shadow, lying between intussuscipiens and intussusceptum)
      - plication along a linear foreign body (gas bubbles small and triangular or teardrop-shaped, or forming a corkscrew pattern) (Figure 9.11)
   b. Small intestine of increased diameter
      - colon or caecum mistaken for small intestine
      - mechanical obstruction: foreign bodies, intussusception, neoplasia, polyps, adhesions, granulomata, intestinal volvulus at the root of the mesentery (also partly functional obstruction), strangulation in a hernia or mesenteric tear
      - functional obstruction (paralytic ileus): GDV, intestinal volvulus at the root of the mesentery (also partly mechanical obstruction), severe gastroenteritis (e.g. parvovirus infection), secondary to chronic mechanical obstruction, recent abdominal surgery, dysautonomia, peritonitis, pancreatitis
2. Fluid radio-opacity of the small intestine
   a. Normal-diameter small intestine
      - normal
      - intestinal disease without dilation of lumen or marked mural thickening
   b. Small intestine of increased diameter
      - colon mistaken for small intestine
      - uterine enlargement mistaken for small intestine
      - mechanical obstruction – see 9.22.1b for causes
      - functional obstruction (paralytic ileus) – see 9.22.1b for causes
      - severe gastroenteritis
      - diffuse neoplasia – mainly lymphosarcoma
      - other infiltrative bowel wall disease

When dilated intestine is filled with both gas and fluid, standing lateral abdominal radiographs made using a horizontal X-ray beam

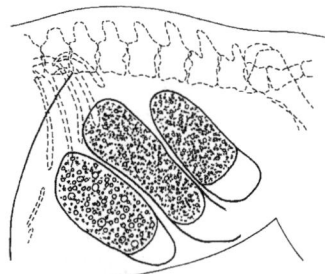

Figure 9.10 Dilated, gas- and fluid-filled small intestinal loops.

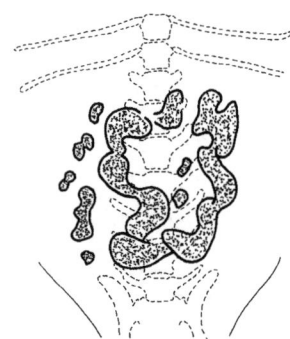

Figure 9.11 Linear foreign body seen on survey radiography; irregular accumulations of small intestinal gas, often in corkscrew or teardrop shapes (see also 9.25.4 and Figure 9.13).

can be useful. Mechanical obstructions tend to cause different levels between the gas-capped fluid lines in the same intestinal loop (look for inverted, U-shaped loops and compare the gas cap level on each vertical side). Functional obstructions (paralytic ileus) tend to have gas-capped fluid lines at the same level in a given U-shaped section of intestine.

3. Radio-opaque contents in the small intestine
   a. Small intestine of normal diameter
      - radio-opaque medications
      - barium or iodine contrast media
      - radio-opaque food
      - incidental foreign material
      evaluate stomach contents as well
      - faeces mistaken for small intestinal contents
      - incidental enterolith
   b. Small intestine of increased diameter
      - radio-opaque foreign bodies (fluid/gas dilated loops too) (Figure 9.12)
      - enterolith
      - food debris lodged proximal to an obstruction
      - focal accumulation of mineral debris ("gravel sign") – proximal to a chronic, partial obstruction
      - caecal impaction (faecolithiasis) mistaken for an area of small intestine.

9.23 Small intestinal contrast studies – technique and normal appearance

If rupture of the small intestine is suspected, iodinated contrast medium rather than barium should be used. If the procedure is elective, preparation should involve a fast of at least 12 hours and enemas to remove superimposed colonic faecal material followed by appropriate chemical restraint (usually mild sedation of a type which does not significantly affect transit time). Radiographs should be taken in lateral and dorsal recumbency at regular intervals to follow the passage of contrast medium along the gut (e.g. 15, 30, 60 minutes after dosing and then hourly until most of the contrast is in the colon). 30% w/v barium sulphate is given by stomach tube or oral syringing at a dose rate of 5–12 ml/kg depending on body weight (larger doses/kg for smaller breeds). An alternative technique is to use BIPS and to observe the passage of the radio-opaque spheres through the gastrointestinal tract. The small BIPS show transit rate of ingesta; the larger BIPS are used to demonstrate obstructions.

The normal appearance of the small intestine on a barium study is of a mass of sinuous tubes, with slight variations in radio-opacity as barium mixes with luminal gas. The diameter of the loops varies slightly due to peristalsis. A hazy, spiculated or brush-border appearance seen in some animals is normal, and is due to barium extending between clumps of intestinal villi, so-called *fimbriation*. Normal variants in the duodenum are pseudoulcers (dogs) and duodenal beading (cats) – see 9.25 and Fig. 9.13. With iodine studies, progressive dilution of the contrast medium as it passes along the gut creates a less radio-opaque and hazier appearance.

9.24 Technical errors with small intestinal contrast studies

1. Lack of survey (plain) radiographs
   a. Radio-opaque foreign bodies overlooked
   b. Incorrect exposure factors used for contrast study
   c. Animal not adequately fasted
   d. Much faecal material present – inadequate enema.
2. Inappropriate exposure factors – add 5–10 kVp to settings used to obtain survey radiographs.
3. Inadequate amount of contrast medium
   a. Underdosing
   b. Vomiting after administration.
4. Inadequate number of images (in absence of fluoroscopic evaluation) may preclude thorough evaluation; accurate diagnosis can be improved by taking sufficient radiographs and viewing them together for consistency of findings.

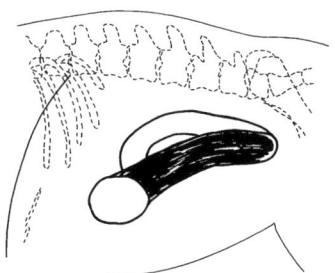

Figure 9.12 A radio-opaque small intestinal foreign body (stone) with dilated gas- and fluid-filled small intestine proximal to the obstruction.

SMALL ANIMAL RADIOLOGICAL DIFFERENTIAL DIAGNOSIS

5. Overdiagnosis based on single or few images because peristaltic waves may mimic lesions.

9.25 Variations in small intestinal luminal diameter

Normal intestinal diameter is approximately the same as the depth of a lumbar vertebra or twice the width of a rib in the dog and 12 mm in the cat. In dogs, a ratio of >1.6 between the diameter of the small intestine and the depth of the centrum of L5 at its narrowest point is highly suggestive of obstruction. The jejunum and ileum are similar in size; the duodenum is slightly wider.
1. Segmental narrowing of diameter
   a. Normal peristaltic waves – will be transient and symmetrical
   b. Cats – a bead-like "string of pearls" appearance to the duodenum is normal (duodenal segmentation – Figure 9.13a)
   c. Intestinal neoplasia
   d. Intestinal scarring following foreign body impaction or previous surgery.
2. Generalised narrowing of diameter
   a. Inadequate dose of contrast medium
   b. Contrast medium mixing with ingesta already present in the stomach and emptying at the slower rate of solid material
   c. Thickening of the intestinal wall (see 9.27).
3. Dilation of the small intestine (see 9.21).
4. Irregular luminal diameter
   a. Normal "pseudoulcers" in young dogs are outpouchings of the duodenal lumen along the antimesenteric border, due to mucosal thinning over submucosal lymphoid follicles (Figure 9.13b)
   b. Diffuse neoplasia (e.g. alimentary lymphosarcoma; Figure 9.13c)

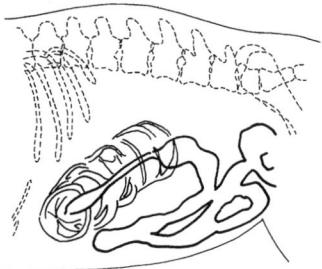

Figure 9.14 Intussusception at the ileo-caeco-colic junction. The intussusceptum is sometimes seen as a thin band of barium entering the intussusception, which produces a corrugated "watchspring" appearance due to barium passing back into the space between the two outer layers of intestinal wall.

   c. Linear foreign body – intestines bunched and plicated (Figure 9.13d)
   d. Ulceration.

9.26 Small intestinal luminal filling defects

1. Foreign bodies – variable in shape.
2. Worms – linear (transverse lines may be seen with tapeworms).
3. Intussusception (especially at ileo-caeco-colic junction) – luminal mass +/– "watchspring" appearance as the barium dissects between the intussusceptum and intussuscipiens (Figure 9.14).
4. Polyps.
5. Neoplasia.

9.27 Increased small intestinal wall thickness

Small intestinal wall thickness can be adequately assessed only using contrast studies or ultrasonography. On survey recumbent radiographs a linear gas bubble lying along the top of a partially filled intestinal loop will mimic intestinal wall thickening (Figure 9.15).
1. Severe chronic enteritis.
2. Ulcerative enteritis.
3. Severe inflammatory or infiltrative bowel wall disease.
4. Neoplasia
   a. Lymphosarcoma (especially in cats)
   b. Adenocarcinoma – focal thickening
   c. Leiomyoma/leiomyosarcoma – focal thickening.
5. Fungal infections*, especially phycomycosis.
6. Lymphangiectasia.

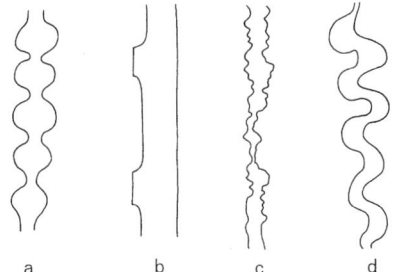

Figure 9.13 Variations in small intestinal luminal diameter: (a) "string of pearls" appearance in cat duodenum; (b) "pseudoulcers" in dog duodenum; (c) diffuse neoplasia; (d) linear foreign body.

9 GASTROINTESTINAL TRACT

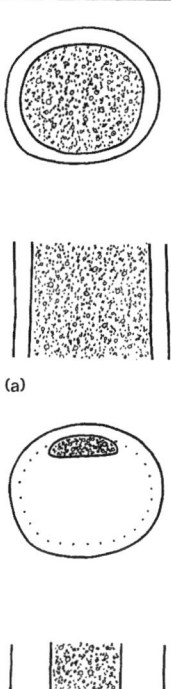

Figure 9.15 Formation of artefactual intestinal wall "thickening" on survey radiographs. (a) A gas-filled loop in which only the intestinal wall is of soft tissue radio-opacity; (b) a gas- and fluid-filled loop in which the soft tissue radio-opacity of the fluid lying beneath the gas summates with the intestinal wall, producing the false appearance of wall thickening.

9.28 Variations in small intestinal transit time

In dogs, barium sulphate should begin to reach the colon within 90–120 minutes; in cats the normal transit time is 30–60 minutes. Hypertonic iodinated media induce hyperperistalsis and reduce the transit time. Persistent accumulation of BIPS in a loop of small intestine is highly suggestive of physical obstruction. Scattered distribution of BIPS through the small intestine suggests increased transit time.
1. Reduced transit time (rapid transit)
   a. Hypermotility due to enteritis
   b. Prior surgical resection of significant lengths of intestine.
2. Increased small intestinal transit time (delayed transit)
   a. Sedation or general anaesthesia
   b. Partial obstruction

- foreign bodies
- neoplasia
- polyp
- intussusception
c. Inflammatory or infiltrative bowel wall disease
d. Pancreatitis
e. Hypomotility due to enteritis
   - parvovirus
   - cats – panleucopenia
f. Functional obstruction (paralytic ileus)
g. Peritonitis
h. Dysautonomia.

9.29 Ultrasonographic examination of the small intestine

In elective cases, the patient should be fasted for 12 hours, while allowing free access to water, and given an opportunity to defecate before carrying out the examination. Because barium sulphate interferes with image quality, the ultrasonographic examination should be performed before any barium contrast studies.

A ventral abdominal approach should be used, and a high-frequency (7.5 or 10 MHz) sector or curvilinear transducer chosen. The spleen may be used as an acoustic window to examine underlying intestinal loops. To avoid interference from intraluminal gas, the position of the patient may be varied so that fluid drops into, and gas rises away from the area of interest.

The descending loop of the duodenum may be identified in the right cranial abdomen as a superficially located, straight segment of small intestine. It is not usually possible to differentiate other specific intestinal regions, except perhaps the terminal ileum as it approaches the ileo-caeco-colic junction.

9.30 Normal ultrasonographic appearance of the small intestine

In good-quality images, layering of the small intestinal wall will be apparent as in the stomach (see 9.12 and Figure 9.9). In normal dogs, the thickness of the small intestinal wall varies between 2 and 5 mm, although the duodenal wall may be up to 6 mm thick. The normal proximal duodenum shows peristaltic waves at 4–5 contractions/minute. Small intestinal contractions in the mid-abdomen are generally seen 1–3 times per minute.

SMALL ANIMAL RADIOLOGICAL DIFFERENTIAL DIAGNOSIS

9.31 Variations in small intestinal contents on ultrasonography

1. Echogenic contents without acoustic shadowing
   a. Mucus
   b. Food material
   c. Foreign material.
2. Echogenic contents with significant acoustic shadowing
   a. Gas
   b. Bone fragments
   c. Foreign material.
3. Anechoic/hypoechoic contents
   a. Fluid.

9.32 Dilation of the small intestinal lumen on ultrasonography

Motility is generally decreased if the small intestine is dilated, but may be normal to increased in cases of acute mechanical obstruction.

1. Few dilated loops – localised dilation
   a. Normal peristalsis
   b. High obstruction
      - foreign bodies
      - neoplasia
      - strangulation of a few loops in a hernia or mesenteric tear
   c. Partial functional obstruction (paralytic ileus)
      - severe gastroenteritis (e.g. parvovirus infection)
      - recent abdominal surgery
      - localised peritonitis
      - pancreatitis
   d. Adhesions.
2. Many dilated loops – generalised dilation
   a. Low acute small intestinal obstruction
      - foreign bodies
      - intussusception
      - intestinal volvulus at the root of the mesentery (also partly functional obstruction)
      - strangulation in a hernia or mesenteric tear
   b. Low chronic partial obstruction (may become total)
      - foreign bodies
      - intussusception
      - neoplasia
      - polyps
      - adhesions
      - granulomata
   c. Functional obstruction (paralytic ileus)
      - GDV
      - intestinal volvulus at the root of the mesentery (also partly mechanical obstruction)
      - severe gastroenteritis (e.g. parvovirus infection)
      - secondary to chronic mechanical obstruction
      - recent abdominal surgery
      - electrolyte imbalances
      - dysautonomia
      - peritonitis
      - pancreatitis
   d. Diffuse neoplasia – mainly lymphosarcoma.

9.33 Lack of visualisation of the normal small intestinal wall layered architecture on ultrasonography

As for the stomach (see 9.14).

9.34 Abnormal arrangement of the small intestine on ultrasonography

1. Corrugated/plicated small intestine
   a. Secondary to peritonitis
   b. Linear foreign body.

9.35 Focal thickening of the small intestinal wall on ultrasonography

The small intestinal wall in the dog is generally considered to be abnormally thick if it is ≥5 mm (≥6 mm for the duodenum).

1. Retention of the normal layered architecture
   a. Enteritis/ulceration
   b. Duodenitis secondary to pancreatitis.
2. Loss of the normal layered architecture
   a. Neoplasia
      - adenocarcinoma (usually asymmetric thickening of wall)
      - lymphosarcoma (usually symmetric, hypoechoic thickening)
      - leiomyoma/leiomyosarcoma (leiomyosarcomas are described as exophytic, complex, cystic and solid masses)
   b. Severe duodenitis secondary to pancreatitis
   c. Fungal infections*, especially phycomycosis
   d. Ischaemic change.
3. Increased number of layers – intussusception (Figure 9.16).

9 GASTROINTESTINAL TRACT

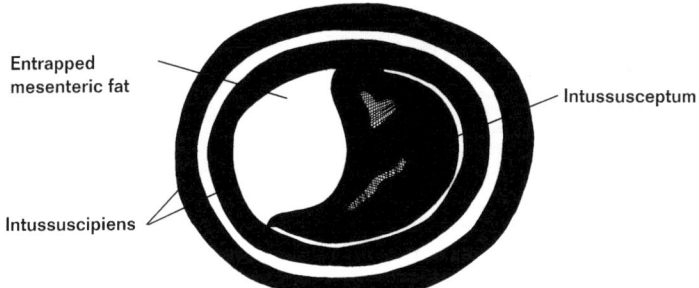

Figure 9.16 Intussusception on ultrasound examination – an increase in the number of concentric tissue layers visible.

9.36 Diffuse thickening of the small intestinal wall on ultrasonography

See 9.35 for normal measurements.
1. Retention of the normal layered architecture
   a. Enteritis
   b. Inflammatory bowel disease
   c. Lymphangiectasia
   d. Oedema secondary to portal hypertension.
2. Loss of normal layered architecture
   a. Severe, necrotising enteritis
   b. Lymphocytic/plasmacytic enteritis (decreased definition of layers has been described)
   c. Diffuse lymphosarcoma
   d. Fungal infections*, especially phycomycosis.

LARGE INTESTINE

9.37 Normal radiographic appearance of the large intestine

The caecum is located in the right side of the mid-abdomen at the level of L3 and is often gas-filled and corkscrew-shaped in dogs (Figure 9.17). In cats it is very small and usually not detectable. The ascending colon runs cranially and to the right of the spine adjacent to the duodenum and pancreas. The transverse colon crosses the cranial abdomen caudal to the stomach. The descending colon runs caudally to the left of the spine to the pelvic inlet. In large-breed dogs, the terminal descending colon may be observed to the right of the spine, especially if the dog lay in right lateral recumbency before the VD radiograph was obtained. Extra bends in the descending colon are termed "redundant colon" and occur more frequently in large breed dogs; this is normal unless there is simultaneous dilation. Through the pelvis the large intestine is called the rectum. The colon and rectum will be filled to a variable degree by gas and faeces; the radio-opacity of the faeces depends on diet and on faecal consistency.

9.38 Displacement of the large intestine

1. Displacement of the ascending colon
   a. Further to the right
      - enlarged right kidney
      - enlarged right colic lymph nodes
      - right adrenal masses
   b. Towards the midline
      - dilation of the duodenum
      - enlargement of the right limb of the pancreas
      - enlargement of the right side of the liver.
2. Displacement of the transverse colon
   a. Caudally
      - dilation of the stomach
      - enlarged liver
      - enlargement of the left limb of the pancreas
   b. Cranially
      - reduced liver size
      - ruptured diaphragm

SMALL ANIMAL RADIOLOGICAL DIFFERENTIAL DIAGNOSIS

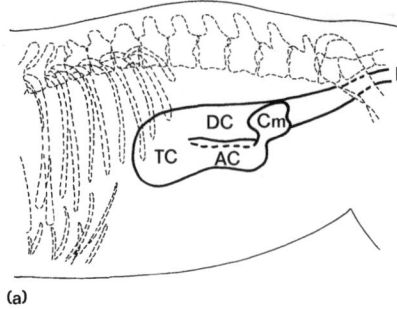

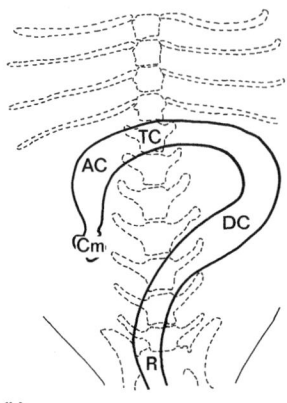

Figure 9.17 Normal large intestine in the dog. (a) Lateral view; (b) VD view. Cm = caecum; AC = ascending colon; TC = transverse colon; DC = descending colon; R = rectum. The appearance is similar in the cat, but the caecum is not usually visible.

- gross urinary retention
- uterine enlargement
- enlargement of the middle colic lymph nodes
- other mid-abdominal mass.
3. Displacement of the proximal descending colon
   a. Further to the left
      - enlarged left kidney
      - left adrenal masses
   b. Towards the midline or to the right side
      - enlargement of the left side of the liver
      - enlarged spleen
   c. Ventrally
      - enlarged left kidney.
4. Displacement of the distal descending colon
   a. Towards the midline
      - normal, especially in large-breed dogs and following previous right lateral recumbency
      - full bladder
      - enlarged prostate

b. Ventrally
   - enlarged medial iliac (sublumbar) lymph nodes
   - dorsal pelvic masses
   - severe spondylosis
   - retroperitoneal pathology (see 11.7)
c. Dorsally
   - full bladder
   - enlarged uterus
   - enlarged prostate.
5. Abnormally short colon
   a. Developmental anomaly which may predispose to soft, unformed faeces
   b. Severe colitis
   c. Previous surgical resection.
6. Displacement of the rectum
   a. Dorsally
      - enlarged prostate
      - intrapelvic paraprostatic cyst
      - retroflexed bladder (e.g. perineal hernia)
      - vaginal mass
      - urethral mass
      - pelvic bone mass
      - other intrapelvic masses (e.g. lipoma)
   b. Ventrally
      - dorsal intrapelvic soft tissue mass
      - sacral or caudal vertebral mass.

9.39 Large intestinal dilation

The colonic diameter should be less than 1.5 times the length of L7. A dilated colon is usually filled with faeces of increased radio-opacity.
1. Congenital conditions leading to large intestinal dilation
   a. Atresia ani or coli
   b. Myelodysplasia in Manx cats
   c. Spina bifida manifesta.
2. Acquired causes of large intestinal dilation (obstipation = mechanical obstruction to defecation; constipation = faecal retention without physical obstruction)
   a. Colonic or rectal stricture
   b. Pelvic canal deformity
      - traumatic fracture with malunion
      - folding fractures of the pelvis in puppies and kittens secondary to nutritional hyperparathyroidism
   c. Spinal cord/cauda equina pathology
   d. Lumbar nerve pathology
   e. Perineal hernia
   f. Colonic neuropathy – megacolon
   g. Psychogenic faecal retention in aged animals
   h. Pain on defecation

i. Neoplasia
   - colonic/rectal adenocarcinoma
   - pelvic canal neoplasia
j. Idiopathic.

9.40 Variations in large intestinal contents

Diarrhoea is often associated with a hypermotile colon which results in the colon being empty of faeces although it may be gas-filled to a variable degree. Colonic impaction can be diagnosed by observing a dilated colon filled with radio-opaque faecal material. Surprisingly, faecal impaction can also lead to diarrhoea.

1. Empty or gas-filled large intestine
   a. Normal – recent defecation
   b. Following enema
   c. Colitis
      - infectious
      - parasitic
      - abrasive dietary materials
      - ulcerative
      - lymphocytic/plasmacytic/ eosinophilic
   d. Diarrhoea
   e. Caecal inversion
   f. Intussusception
   g. Neoplasia
   h. Typhlitis (caecal inflammation).
2. Increased radio-opacity of the large intestine, normal diameter
   a. Bones in diet
   b. Constipation
      - lack of opportunity to defecate
      - psychogenic
      - old age
      - dietary
      - chronic abdominal pain or pain on defecation.
3. Increased radio-opacity of the large intestine, dilated
   a. Megacolon
   b. Obstipation
      - bony or soft tissue pelvic narrowing
      - colonic or rectal masses
   c. Caecal impaction (faecolithiasis) – focal area of soft tissue, faecal or mineralised radio-opacity.

9.41 Variations in large intestinal wall opacity

1. Reduced opacity – air (pneumatosis coli); leads to a linear, layered reduced radio-opacity of the colonic wall
   a. Ulcerative colitis
   b. Iatrogenic mucosal perforation.
2. Increased radio-opacity
   a. Artefactual due to adherent faeces
   b. Metastatic calcification
   c. Dystrophic calcification of colonic/rectal wall lesions.

9.42 Large intestinal contrast studies – technique and normal appearance

If colonic rupture is suspected, a contrast study should not be performed as it will encourage passage of faecal material into the peritoneal cavity, resulting in peritonitis. Colonic filling after oral contrast study is usually inadequate and misleading as the residual contrast medium is mixed with faeces. Thorough radiographic examination requires a large volume of contrast medium administered *per rectum*. The normal appearance of the large intestine is of a wide, gently curving tube with little variation in diameter and smooth, featureless walls and mucosal pattern.

Pneumocolon

A quick and useful study.

Pass a flexible catheter (e.g. Foley or urinary catheter) into the rectum and administer approximately 10 ml/kg room air to fill the colon.
- Differentiates colon from gas-filled small intestine
- Shows colonic/rectal strictures
- Shows colonic mass and ileo-caeco-colic intussusceptions
- Gives little or no information about the mucosal surface.

Barium enema

The animal should be fasted for 24 hours and the colon must be cleansed with warm water/saline enemas at least 6 hours before the study. The animal should be heavily sedated or anaesthetised. A balloon-tipped enema tube or Foley catheter is inserted into the rectum and 7–14 ml/kg of 10–20% w/v warmed barium sulphate suspension is run in under gravity. If the animal is anaesthetised and the anal sphincter relaxed, an anal purse-string suture may be required to prevent leakage. Radiographs are taken in lateral and dorsal recumbency.
- Differentiates colon from gas-filled small intestine
- Shows colonic/rectal strictures
- Shows large colonic/rectal masses and ileo-caeco-colic intussusceptions (small masses may be obscured)

- Gives more information about the mucosal surface than with pneumocolon.

Double-contrast enema
Following the above radiographs, barium is allowed to drain out of the anus (e.g. by placing the enema bag on the floor) and the large intestine is then distended with room air. Radiographs are repeated.
- Shows colonic/rectal masses and strictures
- Gives detailed visualisation of the mucosal surface.

9.43 Technical errors with large intestinal contrast studies

1. Lack of survey (plain) radiographs
   a. Incorrect exposure factors used for contrast study
   b. Animal not adequately cleansed of faeces, the retained faeces giving rise to filling defects in the contrast medium.
2. Inappropriate exposure factors – add 5–10 kVp to settings used to obtain survey radiographs for barium studies.
3. Small lesions masked by overlying barium – double-contrast studies overcome this problem.

9.44 Large intestinal luminal filling defects

1. Retained faeces.
2. Foreign bodies.
3. Masses
   a. Pedunculated (e.g. polyp, leiomyoma)
   b. Sessile (e.g. neoplasia of large intestinal wall; Figure 9.18) – often circumferential.
5. Intussusception.
6. Caecal inversion.

9.45 Increased large intestinal wall thickness

1. Diffuse thickening of the large intestinal wall
   a. Severe colitis
      - infectious
      - parasitic
      - abrasive dietary materials
      - ulcerative
      - lymphocytic/plasmacytic/eosinophilic
   b. Diffuse neoplasia.
2. Focal thickening of the large intestinal wall
   a. Neoplasia – usually asymmetric wall thickening, lumen narrowing +/– proximal obstipation
      - adenocarcinoma
      - lymphosarcoma
      - leiomyoma/leiomyosarcoma
   b. Focal colitis
      - histiocytic
      - granulomatous
      - fungal infections*, especially phycomycosis
   c. Scar tissue from a previous lesion or surgery (narrow lumen +/– wall thickening).

9.46 Abnormal large intestinal mucosal pattern

1. Artefactual – incomplete removal of faeces.
2. Colitis
   a. Mild colitis may not be detected – consider using proctoscopy/colonoscopy. Suggested by observing thickened mucosal folds and fine spiculation of the contrast/mucosal interface
   b. Severe, ulcerative colitis – deeper spiculation and ulceration at the contrast/mucosal interface; the colon may be rigid and shortened with a thickened wall and/or a corrugated mucosal pattern (Figure 9.19). Tends not to be focal, although may not involve the entire colon.

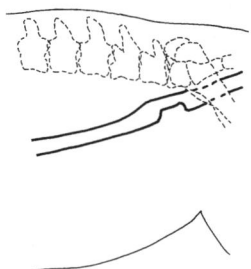

Figure 9.18 Large intestinal tumour shown on contrast enema – focal thickening of the colonic wall.

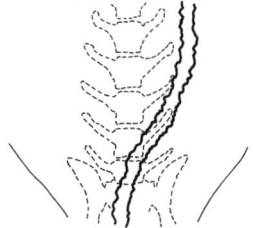

Figure 9.19 Severe colitis on a double-contrast enema – poor distension of the colon with a ragged and irregular mucosal pattern.

9.47 Ultrasonographic examination of the large intestine

As for the small intestine (see 9.29). A water enema may be used to aid imaging, but this may necessitate sedation or even general anaesthesia. Transrectal ultrasound can be used to image the wall of the rectum and descending colon.

9.48 Normal ultrasonographic appearance of the large intestine

The large intestine of the cat and dog does not have sacculations or bands as are seen in other species. Accordingly, the appearance of the large intestine is similar to that of the small intestine (see 9.30), although the diameter of the large intestine tends to be greater than that of the small intestine. The descending colon can be identified by its relationship to the bladder and often by the presence of hyperechoic gas shadows. The layers of the large intestinal wall are often not clearly visible due to the presence of gas and faecal material, causing acoustic shadowing and reverberation artefacts. Peristaltic contractions are not usually seen.

9.49 Ultrasonographic changes in large intestinal disease

Similar to those described for the small intestine (see 9.32–9.36).

FURTHER READING

General

Agut, A., Sanchez-Valverde, M.A., Lasaosa, J.M., Murciano, J. and Molina, F. (1993) Use of iohexol as a gastrointestinal contrast medium in the dog. *Veterinary Radiology and Ultrasound* **34** 171–177.

Borgarelli, M., Biller, D.S., Goggin, J.M. and Bussadori, C. (1996) Ultrasonographic examination of the gastrointestinal system: Part 1. Ultrasonographic anatomy and normal findings. Part 2. Ultrasonographic identification of gastrointestinal disease. *Veterinaria* **10** 37–47.

Dennis, R. (1992) Barium meal techniques in dogs and cats. *In Practice* **14** 237–248.

Gibbs, C. and Pearson, H. (1973) The radiological diagnosis of gastrointestinal obstruction in the dog. *Journal of Small Animal Practice* **14** 61–82.

Goggin, J.M., Biller, D.S., Debey, B.M., Pickar, J.G. and Mason, D. (2000) Ultrasonographic measurement of gastrointestinal wall thickness and the ultrasonographic appearance of the ileocolic region in healthy cats. *Journal of the American Animal Hospital Association* **36** 224–228.

Graham, J.P., Newell, S.M., Roberts, G.D. and Lester N.V. (2000) Ultrasonographic features of canine gastrointestinal pythiosis. *Veterinary Radiology and Ultrasound* **41** 273–277.

Grooters, A.M., Biller, D.S., Ward, H., Miyabayashi, T. and Couto, C. (1994) Ultrasonographic appearance of feline alimentary lymphoma. *Veterinary Radiology and Ultrasound* **35** 468–472.

Kleine, L.J. and Lamb, C.R. (1989) Comparative organ imaging: the gastrointestinal tract. *Veterinary Radiology* **30** 133–141.

Lamb, C.R. (1990) Abdominal ultrasonography in small animals: intestinal tract and mesentery, kidneys, adrenal glands, uterus and prostate (review). *Journal of Small Animal Practice* **31** 295–304.

Lamb, C.R. (1999) Recent developments in diagnostic imaging of the gastrointestinal tract of the dog and cat. *Veterinary Clinics of North America; Small Animal Practice* **29** 307–342.

Myers, N. and Penninck, D.G. (1994) Ultrasonographic diagnosis of gastrointestinal smooth muscle tumors in the dog. *Veterinary Radiology and Ultrasound* **35** 391–397.

Newell, S.M., Graham, J.P., Roberts, G.D., Ginn, P.E. and Harrison, J.M. (1999) Sonography of the normal feline gastrointestinal tract. *Veterinary Radiology and Ultrasound* **40** 40–43.

Penninck, D.G., Nyland, T.G., Fisher, P.E. and Kerr, L.Y. (1989) Ultrasonography of the normal canine gastrointestinal tract. *Veterinary Radiology* **30** 272–276.

Penninck, D.G., Nyland, T.G., Kerr, L.Y. and Fisher, P.E. (1990) Ultrasonographic evaluation of gastrointestinal diseases in small animals. *Veterinary Radiology and Ultrasound* **31** 134–141.

Penninck, D.G., Moore, A.S., Tidwell, A.S., Matz, M.E. and Freden, G.O. (1994) Ultrasonography of alimentary lymphosarcoma in the cat. *Veterinary Radiology and Ultrasound* **35** 299–304.

Penninck, D.G. (1998) Characterisation of gastrointestinal tumors. *Veterinary Clinics of North America; Small Animal Practice* **28** 777–798.

Robertson, I.D. and Burbidge, H.M. (2000) Pros and cons of barium-impregnated polyethylene spheres in gastrointestinal disease. *Veterinary Clinics of North America; Small Animal Practice* **30** 449–465.

Sparkes, A.H., Papasouliotis, K., Barr, F.J. and Gruffydd-Jones, T.J. (1997) Reference ranges for gastrointestinal transit of barium-impregnated polyethylene spheres in healthy cats. *Journal of Small Animal Practice* **38** 340–343.

Tidwell, A.S. and Penninck, D.G. (1992) Ultrasonography of gastrointestinal foreign bodies. *Veterinary Radiology and Ultrasound* **33** 160–169.

Stomach

Allan, F.J., Guilford, W.G., Robertson, I.D. and Jones, B.R. (1996) Gastric emptying time of solid radio-opaque markers in healthy dogs. *Veterinary Radiology and Ultrasound* **37** 336–344.

Barber, D.L. (1982) Radiographic aspects of gastric ulcers in dogs: a comparative review and report of 5 case histories. *Veterinary Radiology* **23** 109–116.

Biller, D.S., Partington, B.P., Miyabayashi, T. and Leveille, R. (1994) Ultrasonographic appearance of chronic hypertrophic pyloric gastropathy in the dog. *Veterinary Radiology and Ultrasound* **35** 30–33.

Evans, S.M. (1983) Double versus single contrast gastrography in the dog and cat. *Veterinary Radiology* **24** 6–10.

Evans, S.M. and Biery, D.N. (1983) Double contrast gastrography in the cat; technique and normal radiographic appearance. *Veterinary Radiology* **24** 3–5.

Funkquist, B. (1979) Gastric torsion in the dog. I. Radiological picture during nonsurgical treatment related to the pathological anatomy and to the further clinical course. *Journal of Small Animal Practice* **20** 73–91.

Grooters, A.M., Miyabayashi, T., Biller, D.S. and Merryman, J. (1994) Sonographic appearance of uremic gastropathy in four dogs. *Veterinary Radiology and Ultrasound* **35** 35–40.

Jakovljevic, S. and Gibbs, C. (1993) Radiographic assessment of gastric mucosal fold thickness in dogs. *American Journal of Veterinary Research* **54** 1827–1830.

Jakovljevic, S. (1988) Gastric radiology and gastroscopy in the dog. *Veterinary Annual* **28** 172–182.

Kaser-Hotz, B., Hauser, B. and Arnold, P. (1996) Ultrasonographic findings in canine gastric neoplasia in 13 patients. *Veterinary Radiology and Ultrasound* **37** 51–56.

Lamb, C.R. and Grierson, J. (1999) Ultrasonographic appearance of primary gastric neoplasia in 21 dogs. *Journal of Small Animal Practice* **40** 211–215.

Love, N.E. (1993) Radiology corner: The appearance of the canine pyloric region in right versus left lateral recumbent radiographs. *Veterinary Radiology and Ultrasound* **34** 169–170.

Penninck, D.G., Moore, A.S. and Gliatto, J. (1998) Ultrasonography of canine gastric epithelial neoplasia. *Veterinary Radiology and Ultrasound* **39** 342–348.

Stomach and small intestine

Baez, J.L., Hendrick, M.J., Walker, L.M. and Washabau, R.J. (1999) Radiographic, ultrasonographic, and endoscopic findings in cats with inflammatory bowel disease of the stomach and small intestine: 33 cases (1990–1997). *Journal of the American Veterinary Medical Association* **215** 349–354.

Miyabayashi, T. and Morgan, J.P. (1991) Upper gastrointestinal examinations: a radiographic study of clinically normal beagle puppies. *Journal of Small Animal Practice* **32** 83–88.

Small intestine

Gibbs, C. and Pearson, H. (1986) Localized tumours of the canine small intestine: a report of twenty cases. *Journal of Small Animal Practice* **27** 507–519.

Graham, J.P., Lord, P.F. and Harrison, J.M. (1998) Quantitative estimation of intestinal dilation as a predictor of obstruction in the dog. *Journal of Small Animal Practice* **39** 521–524.

Lamb, C.R. and Hansson, K. (1994) Radiology corner: Radiological identification of nonopaque intestinal foreign bodies. *Veterinary Radiology and Ultrasound* **35** 87–88.

Lamb, C.R. and Mantis, P. (1998) Ultrasonographic features of intestinal intussusception in 10 dogs. *Journal of Small Animal Practice* **39** 437–441.

Large intestine

Bruce, S.J., Guilford, W.G., Hedderley, D.L. and McCauley M. (1999) Development of reference intervals for the large intestinal transit of radio-opaque markers in dogs. *Veterinary Radiology and Ultrasound* **40** 472–476.

10

Urogenital tract

KIDNEYS

10.1 Non-visualisation of the kidneys
10.2 Variations in kidney size and shape
10.3 Variations in kidney radio-opacity
10.4 Upper urinary tract contrast studies – technique and normal appearance
10.5 Abnormal timing of the nephrogram
10.6 Absent nephrogram
10.7 Uneven radio-opacity of the nephrogram
10.8 Variations in the pyelogram
10.9 Ultrasonographic examination of the kidneys
10.10 Normal ultrasonographic appearance of the kidneys
10.11 Distension of the renal pelvis on ultrasonography
10.12 Focal parenchymal abnormalities of the kidney on ultrasonography
10.13 Diffuse parenchymal abnormalities of the kidney on ultrasonography
10.14 Perirenal fluid on ultrasonography

URETERS

10.15 Dilated ureter
10.16 Normal ultrasonographic appearance of the ureters
10.17 Dilation of the ureter on ultrasonography

URINARY BLADDER

10.18 Non-visualisation of the urinary bladder
10.19 Displacement of the urinary bladder
10.20 Variations in urinary bladder size
10.21 Variations in urinary bladder shape
10.22 Variations in urinary bladder radio-opacity
10.23 Urinary bladder contrast studies – technique and normal appearance
10.24 Reflux of contrast medium up a ureter following cystography
10.25 Abnormal bladder contents on cystography

10.26 Thickening of the urinary bladder wall on cystography
10.27 Ultrasonographic examination of the bladder
10.28 Normal ultrasonographic appearance of the bladder
10.29 Thickening of the bladder wall on ultrasonography
10.30 Cystic structures within or near the bladder wall on ultrasonography
10.31 Changes in urinary bladder contents on ultrasonography

URETHRA

10.32 Urethral contrast studies – technique and normal appearance
10.33 Irregularities on the urethrogram
10.34 Ultrasonography of the urethra

OVARIES

10.35 Ovarian enlargement
10.36 Ultrasonographic examination of the ovaries
10.37 Normal ultrasonographic appearance of the ovaries
10.38 Ovarian abnormalities on ultrasonography

UTERUS

10.39 Uterine enlargement
10.40 Variations in uterine radio-opacity
10.41 Radiographic signs of dystocia and foetal death
10.42 Ultrasonographic examination of the uterus
10.43 Normal ultrasonographic appearance of the uterus
10.44 Variations in uterine contents on ultrasonography
10.45 Thickening of the uterine wall on ultrasonography

PROSTATE

10.46 Variations in location of the prostate
10.47 Variations in prostatic size

SMALL ANIMAL RADIOLOGICAL DIFFERENTIAL DIAGNOSIS

10.48 Variations in prostatic shape and outline

10.49 Variations in prostatic radio-opacity

10.50 Ultrasonographic examination of the prostate

10.51 Normal ultrasonographic appearance of the prostate

10.52 Focal parenchymal abnormalities of the prostate on ultrasonography

10.53 Diffuse parenchymal changes of the prostate on ultrasonography

10.54 Paraprostatic lesions on ultrasonography

TESTES

10.55 Ultrasonographic examination of the testes

10.56 Normal ultrasonographic appearance of the testes

10.57 Testicular abnormalities on ultrasonography

10.58 Paratesticular abnormalities on ultrasonography

KIDNEYS

The kidneys lie in the retroperitoneal space and visualisation of the bean-shaped renal border depends on the presence of sufficient surrounding fat. In the dog the cranial pole of the right kidney lies in the renal fossa of the caudate lobe of the liver at the level of T13–L1 and may be difficult to discern, especially in thin or deep-chested dogs or if the gastrointestinal tract contains much ingesta. The left kidney usually lies approximately half a kidney length more caudally, and more ventrally. In cats the kidneys tend to be more easily visible as the right kidney is usually separated from the liver by fat. The kidneys appear smaller and more variable in location. On the lateral radiograph partial superimposition of the kidneys may mimic a smaller mass in both cats and dogs.

Kidney size should be assessed on the ventrodorsal radiograph (Figure 10.1). The canine kidney should be 2.5–3.5 times the length of L2; the normal feline kidney size range is 1.9–2.6 times the length of L2 in neutered cats and 2.1–3.2 in entire cats. The two kidneys should be the same size in a given patient.

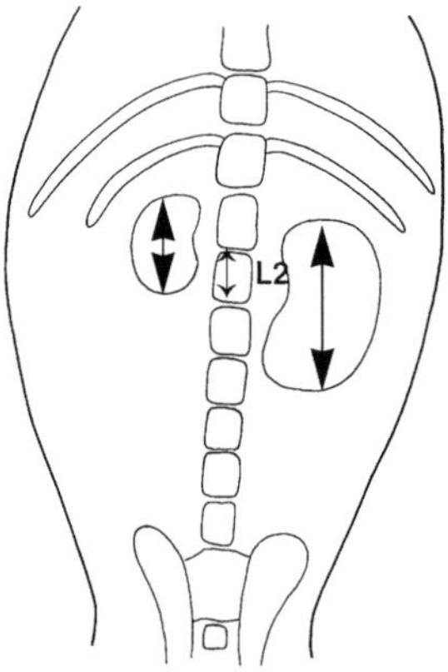

10.1 Non-visualisation of the kidneys

1. Normal variant (especially for the right kidney)
    a. Inappropriate exposure setting or processing (especially underexposure)
    b. Little abdominal fat
        * young animals
        * very thin animals
    c. Deep-chested conformation, kidneys lying more cranially
    d. Food, gas or faeces in the gastrointestinal tract obscuring a kidney.
2. Nephrectomy.
3. Very small kidney (see 10.2.5).
4. Unilateral renal agenesis.
5. Severe peritoneal effusion.
6. Retroperitoneal effusion
    a. Urine
    b. Haemorrhage.

10.2 Variations in kidney size and shape

1. Normal size kidney, smooth outline
    a. Normal
    b. Acute nephritis
    c. Acute renal toxicity
        * ethylene glycol (anti-freeze) poisoning
        * other toxins
        * certain drugs (e.g. gentamicin, cisplatin).
    d. Early stages of other disease processes.

Figure 10.1 Decreased and increased kidney size in the dog as assessed on the VD radiograph (normal size range 2.5–3.5 × L2).

2. Mildly enlarged kidney, smooth outline
   a. Nephrogram phase of intravenous urogram – bilateral
   b. Acute renal failure – bilateral
   c. Nephritis – often bilateral
   d. Acute pyelonephritis – often bilateral
   e. Hydronephrosis – unilateral or bilateral, depending on the cause
   f. Congenital portosystemic shunts – often bilateral kidney enlargement +/– urinary tract calculi and haematogenous osteomyelitis
   g. Amyloidosis – often bilateral
   h. Compensatory renal hypertrophy – unilateral – opposite kidney small or absent
   i. Renal neoplasia – usually unilateral; more often irregular than smooth (other than lymphosarcoma); in cats lymphosarcoma is the most common renal tumour and is usually bilateral
   j. Perirenal subcapsular abscess – unilateral.
3. Markedly enlarged kidney, smooth outline
   a. Hydronephrosis – uni- or bilateral, depending on the cause
   b. Renal tumour – usually unilateral – more often irregular than smooth
   c. Subcapsular haematoma or urine – uni- or bilateral depending on the cause
   d. Renal lymphosarcoma; common in cats; less so in dogs
   e. Cats – perirenal pseudocysts – usually elderly male cats
   f. Cats – feline infectious peritonitis (FIP), although the kidneys are more likely to be irregular in outline.
4. Enlarged kidney, irregular outline
   a. Primary renal neoplasia – usually unilateral but may be bilateral
      - renal cell carcinoma
      - transitional cell carcinoma
      - nephroblastoma
      - renal adenoma/haemangioma/papilloma
      - anaplastic sarcoma
      - hereditary cystadenocarcinoma – older German Shepherd dogs together with dermatofibrosis lesions
      - renal lymphosarcoma – especially cats, bilateral
   b. Metastatic neoplasia – uni- or bilateral
      - metastasis from a primary in the opposite kidney
      - many other primary tumours metastasise to the kidneys
   c. Renal abscess – usually unilateral
   d. Renal haematoma – usually unilateral
   e. Renal granuloma – uni- or bilateral
   f. Renal cyst(s)
   g. Polycystic kidney disease – heritable condition in long-haired cats, especially Persians and Persian crosses; usually bilateral.
5. Small kidney, smooth or irregular in outline
   a. Chronic renal disease
      - chronic glomerulonephritis
      - chronic pyelonephritis
      - chronic interstitial nephritis
   b. Parenchymal atrophy secondary to renal infarcts or chronic obstructive uropathy
   c. Developmental cortical hypoplasia/dysplasia – younger dogs, with a familial tendency in the Cocker Spaniel, Lhasa Apso, Shih Tzu, Norwegian Elkhound, Samoyed and Dobermann.

10.3 Variations in kidney radio-opacity

The radio-opacity of the kidneys is normally the same as for other soft tissue structures. On ventrodorsal radiographs, a slight radiolucency may be observed in the central medial area of each kidney due to fat within the pelvic region. Incidental adrenal gland mineralisation in older cats should not be mistaken for renal changes.

1. Focal increased radio-opacity of the kidney
   a. Artefactual due to superimposition of the other kidney (lateral view), nipple (ventrodorsal view) or ingesta (either view)
   b. Mineralised nephroliths in the renal pelvis – large ones can become "staghorn" in shape
   c. Mineralised nephroliths in the renal diverticula – often multiple (especially in cats)
   d. Dystrophic mineralisation
      - neoplasia
      - chronic haematoma, granuloma or abscess
   e. Parasitic granuloma (e.g. *Toxocara canis*)
   f. Osseous metaplasia.
2. Diffuse increased radio-opacity of the kidney – nephrocalcinosis
   a. Chronic renal disease
   b. Ethylene glycol poisoning
   c. Hyperparathyroidism
   d. Hyperadrenocorticism
   e. Hypercalcaemia syndromes
   f. Nephrotoxic drugs (e.g. gentamicin)

g. Hypervitaminosis D
h. Renal telangiectasia – Corgis.
3. Reduced radio-opacity of the renal pelvis
   a. Pelvic fat, especially in obese cats
   b. Reflux of air from pneumocystography of the urinary bladder under high pressure
      • overinflation of a normal bladder
      • inflation of a poorly distensible bladder
   c. Infection with gas-producing bacteria.

10.4 Upper urinary tract contrast studies – technique and normal appearance

Intravenous urography, or *IVU (excretion urography)*, is especially useful for evaluation of the renal pelvis and ureters. Lesions of the renal parenchyma are more difficult to diagnose and generally such diseases are more readily detected by ultrasound examination. Renal angiography is not often performed: contrast medium deposited near the renal artery via a femoral arterial catheter will outline the renal blood supply and demonstrate features of kidneys that are failing and therefore not likely to opacify well following an IVU.

During and immediately after the contrast medium injection the vascular supply to the kidney is outlined, forming the *angiogram* phase. This is quickly followed by a diffuse increase in radio-opacity of the kidney parenchyma, the *nephrogram* phase. Occasionally the cortex transiently appears more radio-opaque than the medulla. Within 1–2 minutes of the injection in normal kidneys the renal pelvis and ureters are outlined by contrast medium which is being concentrated in the urine; the *pyelogram* phase (Figure 10.2).

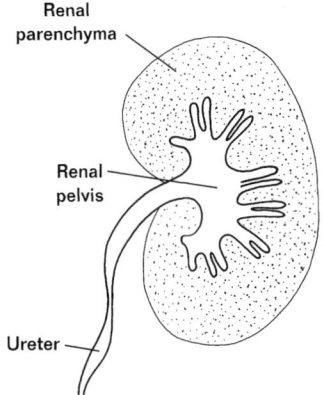

Figure 10.2 Nephrogram/pyelogram phase of IVU.

Preparation

• Blood tests: blood urea nitrogen level >17 mmol/l (>100 mg%) and/or blood creatinine levels >350 mmol/l (>4 mg%) indicate severe renal compromise, which is likely to preclude opacification of the upper urinary tract (if the urea and creatinine are only moderately increased consideration should be given to increasing the dose of iodine up to two-fold to improve visualisation of the urinary system).
• Assessment of circulation and hydration status: injection of hypertonic contrast medium should not be made in patients which are dehydrated or in hypotensive shock in case of induction of acute renal shut-down. Non-ionic (low osmolar) contrast media are safer for such patients, and for cats.
• Twelve-hour fast and colonic enema.
• Placement of an intravenous catheter: extravasation of contrast medium outside the vein is irritant.
• Sedation or anaesthesia of the patient, as appropriate.
• Lateral and VD survey radiographs.

Side effects

• Induction of dehydration.
• Acute renal failure, due to precipitation of proteins in renal tubules (more likely if the urine protein is elevated).
• Rare anaphylactic shock (severe reaction/death).

Bolus IVU [low volume, high concentration]

Inject approximately 850 mgI/kg bodyweight of 300–400 mgI/ml contrast medium rapidly with the patient in dorsal recumbency; take an immediate VD radiograph (kidneys not superimposed) followed by laterals and VDs as necessary. Identify the angiogram, nephrogram and pyelogram phases of opacification. Abdominal compression may be used to occlude the ureters and increase pelvic filling.

Infusion IVU [large volume, low concentration] – an alternative technique for the ureters

Inject approximately 1200 mgI/kg bodyweight of 150 mgI/ml contrast medium slowly as a drip infusion, creating more osmotic diuresis and better visualisation of the ureters. Rapid radiographic exposure is not necessary. The nephrogram and pyelogram phases only are seen.

Selective renal angiography

Catheterise the femoral artery and advance the catheter up the aorta until the tip is at the level of the renal arteries: inject a few ml of high-concentration contrast medium as a bolus and make an immediate VD radiograph. An angiogram phase is seen (unless the vascular supply is disrupted), and a nephrogram and pyelogram are subsequently seen in functioning kidneys. Fluoroscopy with image intensification and video recording may be helpful.

10.5 Abnormal timing of the nephrogram

Normal: uniformly increased kidney radio-opacity and improved visualisation of kidney outline should occur due to the presence of contrast medium in the renal vasculature and tubules. The opacity should be greatest initially, followed by a gradual decrease.
1. Poor initial kidney radio-opacity followed by gradual decrease
   a. Inadequate dose of contrast medium
   b. Polyuric renal failure.
2. Initial increase in kidney radio-opacity, which persists
   a. Systemic hypotension induced by the contrast medium
   b. Contrast medium-induced renal failure
   c. Acute tubular necrosis.
3. Kidney radio-opacity increases with time
   a. Contrast medium-induced renal failure
   b. Systemic hypotension induced by the contrast medium
   c. Renal ischaemia
   d. Slow opacification of abnormal and poorly vascularised tissue
      - neoplasia
      - abscess
      - granuloma
      - haematoma
      - cyst.

10.6 Absent nephrogram

1. Inadequate dose of contrast medium.
2. Severe renal disease with marked azotaemia.
3. Renal aplasia.
4. Prior nephrectomy.
5. Obstructed or avulsed renal artery.
6. Absence of functional renal tissue
   a. Extensive neoplasia
   b. Large abscess
   c. Extreme hydronephrosis.

10.7 Uneven radio-opacity of the nephrogram

1. Well-defined areas of non-opacification
   a. Renal cyst – solitary cysts are an occasional incidental finding
   b. Renal abscess
   c. Cats – polycystic kidney disease – heritable condition in long-haired cats especially Persians and Persian crosses; usually bilateral.
2. Poorly defined areas of non-opacification
   a. Renal neoplasia (may also see areas of increased opacity due to contrast medium extravasation and pooling)
      - renal cell carcinoma
      - transitional cell carcinoma
      - nephroblastoma
      - renal adenoma/haemangioma/papilloma
      - anaplastic sarcoma
      - hereditary cystadenocarcinoma – older German Shepherd dogs together with dermatofibrosis lesions
      - renal lymphosarcoma – especially cats, bilateral
   b. Renal infarcts: single or multiple – wedge-shaped areas with the apex directed towards the hilus
   c. Severe nephritis
   d. Cats – feline infectious peritonitis (FIP).
3. Peripheral rim of opacification only – severe hydronephrosis.
4. Peripheral rim of non-opacification – subcapsular fluid accumulation – e.g. perirenal pseudocysts (usually elderly male cats).

10.8 Variations in the pyelogram

The pyelogram (demonstrating renal diverticula, pelvis and ureters) should be visible approximately 1 minute after the injection and persist for up to several hours.
1. Dilation of the renal pelvis and diverticula
   a. Abdominal compression used
   b. Diuresis – bilaterally symmetrical and usually mild
   c. Hydronephrosis – pelvic dilation may become very gross, with only a thin rim of surrounding parenchymal tissue (Figure 10.3)
      - secondary to ureteric obstruction (see 10.15.3)
      - idiopathic
   d. Renal calculus (radio-opaque calculi may be obscured by the similar radio-opacity of the contrast medium)

SMALL ANIMAL RADIOLOGICAL DIFFERENTIAL DIAGNOSIS

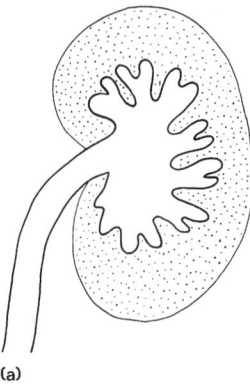

(a)

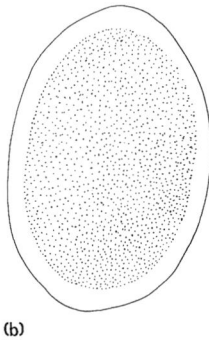

(b)

Figure 10.3 (a) Mild hydronephrosis on an IVU – slight distension and rounding of the renal pelvis and diverticula; dilation of the ureter.
(b) Severe hydronephrosis on IVU – only a thin rim of parenchyma remains. The ureter may not be visible if the kidney has become non-functional.

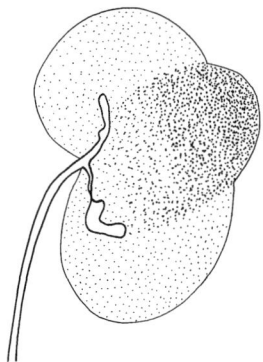

Figure 10.4 Renal tumour on IVU. The cranial and caudal poles of the kidney are normal but a central bulging and poorly opacifying area with distortion of the renal pelvis is visible.

  e. Chronic pyelonephritis – the pelvis may dilate with the diverticula remaining small
  f. Renal neoplasia
   • secondary dilation of the pelvis and proximal ureter is often seen
   • mechanical obstruction of the pelvis
  g. Ectopic ureter – due to stenosis of the ureter ending and/or ascending infection (see 10.15.1 and Fig. 10.8).
 2. Distortion of the renal pelvis
  a. Neoplasia (Figure 10.4)
  b. Other renal parenchymal mass lesions (cyst, abscess, granuloma)
  c. Large renal calculus
  d. Chronic pyelonephritis
  e. Blood clot
   • coagulopathy
   • bleeding neoplasm
   • trauma (or post biopsy)
   • idiopathic renal haemorrhage
  f. Cats – polycystic kidney disease – heritable condition in long-haired cats, especially Persians and Persian crosses; usually bilateral.
 3. Filling defects in the pyelogram
  a. Normal interlobar blood vessels – linear radiolucencies within the diverticula
  b. Air bubbles refluxed from over-distended pneumocystogram
  c. Calculi
  d. Debris due to pyelonephritis
  e. Blood clots
   • after renal biopsy
   • coagulopathy
   • bleeding neoplasm
   • idiopathic renal haemorrhage
   • trauma.

10.9 Ultrasonographic examination of the kidneys

The kidneys may be examined from either a ventral abdominal or flank approach. The advantages of the latter approach include the superficial location of the kidneys and the absence of intervening bowel. The main disadvantage is that the clipped areas of flank may be less acceptable to the owner.

Ideally, a high-frequency (7.5 MHz) sector or curvilinear transducer should be used. Each kidney should be imaged in transverse and either sagittal or dorsal (coronal) sections, ensuring that the entire renal volume is examined. Where possible, the renal artery and vein entering and leaving the hilus should be identified.

10.10 Normal ultrasonographic appearance of the kidneys

The normal kidney is smooth and bean-shaped. A thin echogenic capsule may be visible except at the poles, where the tissue interfaces are parallel to the ultrasound beam. The renal cortex is hypoechoic and finely granular in texture (Figure 10.5). It is usually isoechoic or hypoechoic relative to the liver if a 5 MHz transducer is used, but may appear mildly hyperechoic relative to the liver if a 7.5 MHz transducer is used. The renal cortex should normally be less echogenic than the spleen. The renal medulla is usually virtually anechoic, and divided into segments by the echogenic diverticula and interlobar vessels. A linear hyperechoic zone has been described, lying parallel to the corticomedullary junction in the medulla of some normal cats. Echogenic specks at the corticomedullary junction represent arcuate arteries. The renal sinus forms an intensely hyperechoic region at the hilus which may cast a faint acoustic shadow.

10.11 Distension of the renal pelvis on ultrasonography

The echoes of the renal pelvis become separated by an anechoic accumulation of fluid. As the severity of the dilation increases, there is progressive compression of the surrounding renal parenchyma. There may be associated ureteral dilation.
1. Diuresis – bilaterally symmetrical and usually mild.
2. Hydronephrosis – pelvic dilation may become very gross, with only a thin rim of surrounding parenchymal tissue (Figure 10.6)
   a. Idiopathic
   b. Secondary to ureteric obstruction (see 10.15.3).
3. Renal calculus – strongly reflective surface with distal acoustic shadowing also present.
4. Chronic pyelonephritis – the pelvis may dilate whilst the diverticula remain small.
5. Renal neoplasia
   a. Secondary dilation of the pelvis and proximal ureter is often seen
   b. Mechanical obstruction of the pelvis.
6. Ectopic ureter – due to stenosis of the ureter ending and/or ascending infection (see 10.15.1 and Figure 10.8).
7. Renal pelvic blood clot
   a. Following renal biopsy
   b. Coagulopathy
   c. Bleeding neoplasm
   d. Idiopathic renal haemorrhage
   e. Trauma.

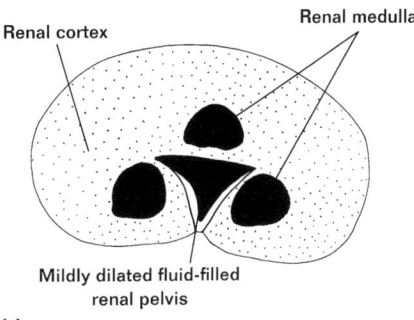

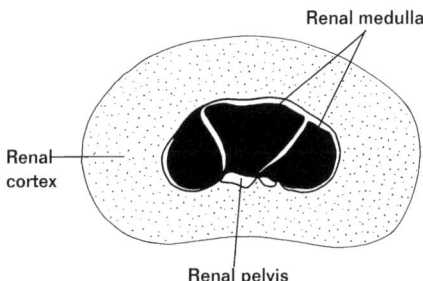

Figure 10.6 (a) Mild hydronephrosis on ultrasonography; anechoic fluid is visible in the renal pelvis (b) Severe hydronephrosis on ultrasonography; a thin rim of parenchyma surrounds a large collection of fluid.

Figure 10.5 Normal ultrasonographic appearance of the kidney in the dorsal plane: the medulla is almost anechoic, the cortex is hypoechoic and fat in the renal pelvis is hyperechoic.

10.12 Focal parenchymal abnormalities of the kidney on ultrasonography

1. Well circumscribed, anechoic parenchymal lesion
   a. Thin, smooth wall
      - cyst – single or multiple. Polycystic renal disease is heritable in Cairn terriers and long-haired cats, mainly Persians and Persian crosses. Cysts are also seen in familial nephropathy of Shih Tzus and Lhasa Apsos; solitary cysts may be seen in other breeds
   b. Thick/irregular wall
      - cyst
      - haematoma
      - abscess
      - neoplasia (e.g. cystadenocarcinoma, especially in the German Shepherd dog).
2. Hypoechoic parenchymal lesion
   a. Neoplasia
      - lymphosarcoma (nodular or wedge-shaped)
      - others (see 10.2.4).
3. Hyperechoic parenchymal lesion
   a. Neoplasia
      - primary (e.g. chondrosarcoma, haemangioma)
      - metastatic (e.g. haemangiosarcoma, thyroid adenocarcinoma)
   b. Chronic infarct (wedge-shaped)
   c. Parenchymal calcification/calculi
   d. Parenchymal gas
   e. A large number of very small cysts (polycystic disease) – especially Persian and Persian-cross cats
   f. Cats – feline infectious peritonitis (FIP).
4. Heterogeneous/complex parenchymal lesion
   a. Neoplasia
      - primary renal carcinoma
      - others (see 10.2.4)
   b. Abscess
   c. Haematoma
   d. Granuloma
   e. Acute infarct
   f. A large number of very small cysts (polycystic disease) – especially Persian and Persian-cross cats.
5. Medullary rim sign – an echogenic line in the outer zone of the renal medulla that parallels the corticomedullary junction.
   a. Cats – normal variant
   b. Nephrocalcinosis
   c. Ethylene glycol toxicity
   d. Chronic interstitial nephritis
   e. Cats – feline infectious peritonitis (FIP).
6. Acoustic shadowing
   a. Deep to pelvic fat
   b. Renal calculus – strongly reflective surface
   c. Nephrolithiasis – reflective surface.

10.13 Diffuse parenchymal abnormalities of the kidney on ultrasonography

1. Increased cortical echogenicity, with retained or enhanced corticomedullary definition
   a. Normal variant in cats (fat deposition)
   b. Inflammatory disease
      - glomerulonephritis
      - interstitial nephritis
      - cats – FIP
   c. Acute tubular necrosis/nephrosis due to toxins (e.g. ethylene glycol toxicity)
   d. Renal dysplasia
   e. Nephrocalcinosis
   f. Neoplasia
      - diffuse lymphosarcoma (especially cats)

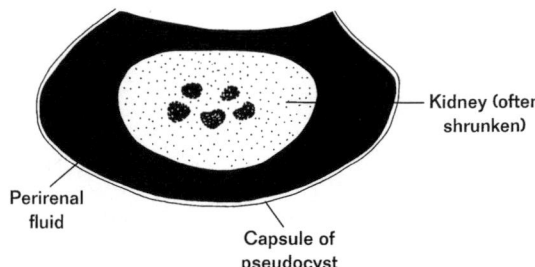

Figure 10.7 Perirenal fluid on ultrasonography – anechoic fluid outlines the kidney, which is often shrunken and hyperechoic.

- metastatic squamous cell carcinoma.
2. Reduced corticomedullary definition
   a. Chronic inflammatory and degenerative disease ("end-stage" kidneys)
   b. Multiple small cysts.

10.14 Perirenal fluid on ultrasonography

Encapsulated anechoic fluid surrounding the kidney, either subcapsular or extracapsular (Figure 10.7).

1. Perirenal pseudocyst (especially elderly male cats – unknown aetiology).
2. Smaller amounts of fluid (blood, urine, exudate, transudate)
   a. Trauma
   b. Neoplasia (e.g. lymphosarcoma)
   c. Ureteral obstruction/rupture
   d. Infection
   e. Toxicities (e.g. ethylene glycol).

URETERS

The ureters are not normally detected on survey radiographs unless they are obstructed and grossly dilated. Occasionally they may be seen as fine, radio-opaque lines in obese animals. An IVU is required for the assessment of ureteric location, diameter and patency. Normal ureters move urine to the bladder in peristaltic waves so only segments of each ureter may be visible on a single IVU radiograph. The normal termination of the ureter within the bladder wall is characteristically hook shaped, the right normally lying slightly more cranially than the left (see Figure 10.8).

Dislodged nephroliths may lead to ureteral obstruction and dilation but are easily confused with radio-opaque bowel contents on plain radiographs. They may be obscured by contrast medium on IVU (confirming their location) or seen as filling defects.

Traumatic rupture of a ureter will result in uroretroperitoneum and/or uroabdomen with loss of visualisation of retroperitoneal and/or abdominal detail. IVU shows contrast medium leakage.

10.15 Dilated ureter

Not seen on survey radiographs unless the dilation is gross, otherwise requires an IVU for demonstration.
1. Ectopic ureter – dilation due to stenosis at the ectopic ending and/or ascending infection (Figure 10.8). The ureter may open into the urethra, vagina or rectum; check location using concomitant pneumocystogram and/or retrograde (vagino)urethrogram. Unilateral or bilateral
   a. Congenital – animals usually show incontinence from a young age; females affected more often than males; dogs more often than cats (especially Golden Retriever)
   b. Acquired – accidental ligation of the ureters with the uterine stump at ovariohysterectomy.
2. Ascending infection (the ureters may also be narrow and/or lacking peristalsis) – pyelonephritis may also be present, causing pelvic dilation and filling defects.
3. Proximal to a ureteric obstruction (hydroureter)
   a. Calculus dislodged from kidney
   b. Ureteric stricture or obstruction
      • following calculus
      • following trauma
      • neoplasia of the ureter or surrounding tissues (bladder neck, urethra, prostate)
      • iatrogenic due to inadvertent ligation

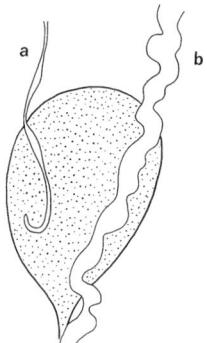

Figure 10.8 Normal and ectopic ureters shown by combined IVU and pneumocystogram. The normal ureter (a) is narrow and ends in a terminal "hook" in the trigone area of the bladder. The ectopic ureter (b) is dilated and tortuous and extends caudal to the bladder neck.

SMALL ANIMAL RADIOLOGICAL DIFFERENTIAL DIAGNOSIS

   c. Any abdominal mass causing extrinsic ureteric compression (e.g. uterine stump granuloma).
4. Ureterocoele – focal dilation of ureter at or near its entry into the bladder.
5. Ureteral diverticula – small sacculations protruding from the lumen secondary to chronic partial ureteral obstruction.

10.16 Normal ultrasonographic appearance of the ureters

The normal ureter is generally not visible ultrasonographically. Periodic flow of urine from the ureters into the bladder can be demonstrated using colour flow techniques (or occasionally without colour if the specific gravity of the urine entering from the ureters differs significantly from that in the bladder).

10.17 Dilation of the ureter on ultrasonography

This is most clearly seen proximally, as the ureter leaves the kidney, or distally as it passes dorsal to the bladder. For differential diagnoses see 10.15.

URINARY BLADDER

The urinary bladder is most easily seen on the lateral radiograph. The trigone (neck) of the bladder is located in the retroperitoneum and is more difficult to see than the more cranial portions of the bladder, especially if overlain by hindlimb musculature. In bitches, the trigone is located at or near the pelvic inlet; in entire male dogs the trigone is displaced cranially to a variable degree depending on the size of the prostate. In fat cats the bladder may lie far cranially with a long, thin bladder neck.

10.18 Non-visualisation of the urinary bladder

1. Technical factors
   a. Obscured by hindlimb musculature (lateral view) or faeces (VD view)
   b. Underexposure.
2. Empty bladder
   a. Normal – recent urination
   b. Severe cystitis
   c. Bilateral ectopic ureters.
3. Displacement through a hernia or rupture
   a. Perineal
   b. Inguinal
   c. Body wall.
4. Urinary bladder rupture – free abdominal fluid seen.

10.19 Displacement of the urinary bladder

1. Caudal displacement
   a. Perineal hernia (male dogs)
   b. Short urethra syndrome (bitches).
2. Ventral displacement
   a. Severe sublumbar lymphadenopathy

   b. Colonic distension
      • constipation/megacolon
      • colonic masses
   c. Uterine or uterine stump enlargement
   d. Prepubic tendon rupture
   e. Rupture of ventral abdominal wall muscles
   f. Inguinal hernia.
3. Cranial displacement
   a. Prostatomegaly
   b Ruptured/avulsed urethra
   c. Cats – obesity.

10.20 Variations in urinary bladder size

The bladder size is very variable as it depends on the rate of urine production, time elapsed since last urination and degree of dysuria. Housetrained animals may be reluctant to urinate in the confines of a veterinary hospital and so large bladders are often seen on radiographs.
1. Large urinary bladder
   a. Normal, lack of urination
   b. Non-obstructive urinary retention
      • psychogenic urinary retention
      • neurological dysfunction (e.g. cauda equina syndrome)
      • orthopaedic disease leading to reluctance or inability to adopt posture for urination
   c. Outflow obstruction
      • bladder neck tumour
      • urethral tumour
      • urethral calculus
      • large calculus lodged in the bladder neck

- urethral stricture
- mucosal slough
- prostatic disease (see 10.46–54)
- neurological dysfunction
- cats – penile urethral plug (males).
2. Small urinary bladder
   a. Recent urination
   b. Anuria
   c. Large tear in the bladder wall (free abdominal fluid present)
   d. Ureteric rupture (retroperitoneal and/or abdominal fluid present)
   e. Ectopic ureter(s)
   f. Non-distensible bladder
      - severe infectious or chemical cystitis
      - mechanical cystitis due to bladder calculi
      - traumatic cystitis
      - diffuse bladder wall neoplasia
   g. Bladder hypoplasia.

10.21 Variations in urinary bladder shape

1. Artefactual due to superimposition of a paraprostatic cyst, or cyst mistaken for bladder.
2. Extensive bladder neoplasia.
3. Bladder rupture.
4. Mucosal herniation through a muscular tear.
5. Congenital diverticula.
6. Patent urachus.

10.22 Variations in urinary bladder radio-opacity

Overlying objects – e.g. radio-opacities in the small and large intestine, nipples and dirt in the hair coat – can be mistaken for bladder calculi. Additional radiographs made after urination, other projections or simultaneous compression with a radiolucent paddle should help to differentiate opacities within the bladder from overlying structures.

1. Increased bladder radio-opacity
   a. Normal summating radio-opaque objects; see above
   b. Radio-opaque calculi
      - triple phosphate
      - calcium oxalate
      - ammonium urate
      - cystine
      - silica
   c. Dystrophic mineralisation in a tumour
   d. Dystrophic mineralisation secondary to severe cystitis

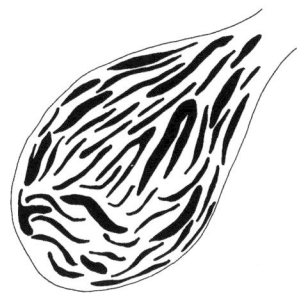

Figure 10.9 Emphysematous cystitis. Streaks of gas lucency are seen in the region of the bladder.

   e. Ballistics
   f. Cats – crystalline debris (standing lateral radiographs may help to show abnormal sediment).
2. Radiolucency associated with the bladder
   a. Iatrogenic from catheterisation or cystocentesis – most likely to be central in location on a recumbent lateral radiograph
   b. Emphysematous cystitis – infection with gas-producing bacteria, predisposed to by diabetes mellitus – streaks of gas lucency in the bladder wall and ligaments (Figure 10.9).

10.23 Urinary bladder contrast studies – technique and normal appearance

Cystography is used to demonstrate the location, integrity, wall thickness, lumenal filling defects and mucosal detail of the urinary bladder. Different techniques can be used depending on the requirement of the examination – e.g. pneumocystography is used for bladder location, positive cystography for small ruptures and double-contrast cystography for mucosal detail. Following administration of the contrast medium, additional oblique radiographs may be helpful to skyline other areas of bladder wall.

Bladder wall thickness is best assessed on a pneumocystogram or double-contrast study. The normal bladder wall is about 1–2 mm thick when the bladder is reasonably well distended. With a double-contrast study, the mucosal surface will be highlighted by a fine margin of contrast medium, residual contrast pooling centrally (in the dependent area) as a "contrast puddle".

SMALL ANIMAL RADIOLOGICAL DIFFERENTIAL DIAGNOSIS

Preparation
- Fasting to remove intestinal ingesta which may overlie the bladder.
- Enema.
- Sedation or anaesthesia of the patient, as appropriate.
- Lateral and VD survey films.
- Bladder catheterisation and urine drainage, noting the quantity removed (aids in establishing how much contrast can safely be instilled).

Pneumocystography
Good for location and shape of the bladder. Shows large luminal filling defects, mural masses and marked increase in wall thickness. Poor for mucosal detail, small filling defects and minor changes in wall thickness; small tears may be overlooked as escaping gas mimics intestinal gas.

The patient is laid in left lateral recumbency as this reduces the risk of significant air emboli in the lungs. Fatal air emboli have been reported when the bladder was overinflated with air, especially in cats. The bladder is inflated slowly with room air, until it feels turgid by abdominal palpation (cats 10–40 ml, dogs usually 50–300 ml depending on patient size and observation of the amount of urine removed). O_2, N_2O or CO_2 from cylinders can also be used. To avoid overexposure 30% less mAs should be used.

Positive contrast cystography
Good for location and shape of the bladder and for detecting small amounts of contrast leakage from the bladder or proximal urethra. Adequate for assessment of wall thickness and large filling defects. Poor for small filling defects, which may be "drowned" by contrast medium; poor for mucosal detail.

The bladder is inflated slowly, using iodinated positive contrast medium, best diluted to approximately 100–150 mgI/ml to avoid irritation of bladder wall due to high osmolarity. To avoid underexposure 30% higher mAs should be used.

Double contrast cystography
Good for all requirements; excellent for mucosal detail and for detection of small filling defects; free bodies will be seen within the central contrast puddle.

Positive contrast medium (5–20 ml) is instilled, the patient rolled or the bladder area massaged to encourage coating of the bladder wall, and the bladder inflated with air. Alternatively, a positive contrast study can be performed first, excess contrast drained and then the bladder inflated with air.

Cystogram following IVU
Undertaken if bladder catheterisation is impossible. Following an IVU, positive contrast will enter the bladder and mix with urine. There is no control over the degree of bladder distension.

10.24 Reflux of contrast medium up a ureter following cystography

1. Normal in immature animals and occasionally observed in normal adults.
2. Contrast medium under high pressure
   a. Overinflation of a normal bladder
   b. Inflation of a poorly distensible bladder.
3. Cystitis (likely to predispose to pyelonephritis).
4. Neoplasia of the trigone of the bladder.
5. Previous ureteral transplant surgery.
6. Accidental catheterisation of an ectopic ureter followed by injection of contrast medium.

10.25 Abnormal bladder contents on cystography

1. Opacities seen on pneumocystography
   a. Calculi – usually lie in the centre of the bladder shadow in lateral recumbency. Variable in opacity and may easily be overexposed (use a bright light)
   b. Blood clot – irregular in outline; any location (may be attached to the bladder wall); soft tissue opacity. DDx mural masses – try flushing bladder with saline and repeating the cystogram
   c. Bladder tumour – attached to the wall, usually near the bladder neck; soft tissue opacity
   d. Polyp – smooth, pedunculated, soft tissue opacity.
2. Filling defects seen on positive or double-contrast cystography (Figure 10.10)
   a. Artefactual from overlying gas-filled bowel or incomplete bladder distension
   b. Calculi – usually lie in the centre of the bladder shadow in lateral recumbency. Radiolucent compared with contrast medium; may be obscured by large amounts so better seen with a double-contrast cystogram
   c. Air bubbles – radiolucent "soap bubble" appearance, lying in the centre of

10 UROGENITAL TRACT

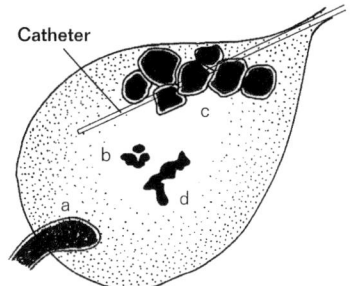

Figure 10.10 Various filling defects seen on double contrast cystography. (a) Overlying gas-filled bowel; (b) calculi – in the centre of the contrast puddle; (c) air bubbles – around the periphery of the contrast puddle; (d) blood clots – variable in location.

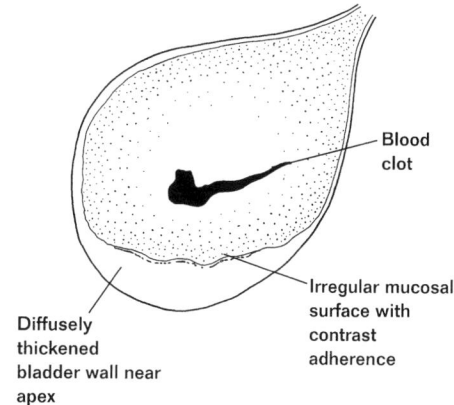

Figure 10.11 Chronic cystitis on double-contrast cystography.

the bladder shadow on a positive-contrast cystogram (rise to the highest point) and around the periphery of the contrast puddle on a double contrast cystogram
d. Blood clots
 • small, free clots simulate the appearance of calculi
 • large, free clots produce irregular filling defects
 • clots attached to the bladder wall mimic tumours; may be dislodged on bladder flushing
e. Fine, linear filling defects – mucosal slough
 • severe cystitis
 • iatrogenic from poor catheterisation technique.

10.26 Thickening of the urinary bladder wall on cystography

Best seen on a full double-contrast cystogram, when the bladder is distended to a normal capacity. However, chronic cystitis and neoplasia can result in a reduction in bladder capacity so proceed with caution when trying to distend the bladder, especially when only a small volume of urine has been obtained on catheterisation.
1. Diffuse bladder wall thickening with a smooth mucosal surface
   a. Normal, inadequately distended bladder
   b. Chronic cystitis (mainly cranioventral)
   c. Muscular hypertrophy due to chronic urinary outflow obstruction.
2. Diffuse bladder wall thickening with an irregular mucosal surface
   a. Chronic cystitis (mainly cranioventral) – Figure 10.11
   b. Diffuse neoplasia – unusual.
3. Diffuse bladder wall thickening with a nodular mucosal surface
   a. Ulcerative cystitis with adherent blood clots (cranioventral)
   b. Polypoid cystitis (cranioventral)
   c. Neoplasia (usually near the bladder neck).
4. Diffuse bladder wall thickening with contrast medium passing into or through the bladder wall
   a. Small bladder tear
   b. Congenital urachal diverticulum (cranioventral; may be associated with chronic cystitis)
   c. Severe, ulcerative cystitis.
5. Focal bladder wall thickening
   a. Neoplasia (usually near the bladder neck) – Figure 10.12
      • epithelial types are more common (transitional cell carcinoma, squamous cell carcinoma, adeno-

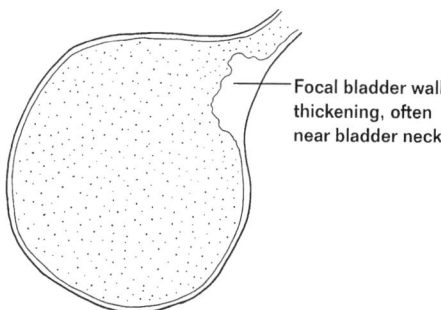

Figure 10.12 Bladder tumour on cystography.

SMALL ANIMAL RADIOLOGICAL DIFFERENTIAL DIAGNOSIS

carcinoma); often a roughened surface with contrast adherence
- mesenchymal types less common (leiomyoma, leiomyosarcoma, rhabdomyosarcoma, fibrosarcoma, metastatic tumours); usually a smoother mucosal surface

b. Polypoid cystitis
c. Ureterocoele – focal dilation of the ureter adjacent to or within the bladder wall.

10.27 Ultrasonographic examination of the bladder

Ideally urine should be present in the bladder, so avoid giving the patient the opportunity to urinate before carrying out ultrasonographic examination.

The bladder is imaged from the caudal ventral abdominal wall, adopting a parapreputial approach in the male dog. A high-frequency (7.5 MHz) sector or curvilinear transducer should be used and placed just cranial to the pubic brim, moving cranially until the bladder is identified. The bladder is imaged in both sagittal and transverse planes of section. If necessary, the position of the animal can be altered and/or imaging performed from the flank to ensure that all parts of the bladder wall and lumen are adequately evaluated.

10.28 Normal ultrasonographic appearance of the bladder

The bladder should be oval or ellipsoid in shape with thin, smooth walls. The normal wall thickness is 1–2 mm when fully distended, but may be up to 5 mm when empty. If a high-frequency transducer is used and the bladder is not full, three distinct wall layers may be seen – hyperechoic serosa, hypoechoic muscular layer and hyperechoic mucosa. However, these layers are not usually clear in the distended bladder.

10.29 Thickening of the bladder wall on ultrasonography

Thickening may be focal or diffuse, and smooth or irregular. See 10.26 for a list of differential diagnoses.

10.30 Cystic structures within or near the bladder wall on ultrasonography

1. Distinct from the bladder lumen
   a. Hydroureter (dorsal to bladder)
   b. Ureterocoele (in the region of the bladder trigone)
   c. Urachal cyst (cranial to the bladder)
   d. Prostatic or paraprostatic lesions (see 10.52–54 and Figure 10.19)
   e. Uterine or vaginal lesions (see 10.44 and Figure 10.16).
2. Extending from the bladder lumen
   a. Urachal diverticulum (cranioventral bladder)
   b. Traumatic diverticulum (any location).

10.31 Changes in urinary bladder contents on ultrasonography

1. Small, scattered echoes within the anechoic urine
   a. Slice thickness or reverberation artefact
   b. Sediment
      - blood/cellular debris
      - crystalline material
   c. Air bubbles (usually secondary to cystocentesis).
2. Hypo/hyperechoic masses, non-shadowing
   a. Blood clot (may be free in the lumen or adherent to the wall)
   b. Polyp/neoplasm (can usually be shown to be attached to wall).
4. Hyperechoic masses, shadowing
   a. Calculi (in the dependent part of the bladder)
   b. Full colon impinging on the bladder
   c. Calcified mural mass.

URETHRA

The male and female urethras are not visible on survey radiographs. Radio-opaque calculi may be seen in the region of the urethra. Mineralised structures in the distal urethral area may be due to a vestigial os penis in a hermaphrodite or pseudohermaphrodite animal. Large, intrapelvic masses associated with the urethra may be seen to displace the rectum, but further evaluation of the urethra requires examination with contrast medium. In male dogs the os penis is seen; its base may appear roughened or fragmented mimicking adjacent urethral calculi.

10.32 Urethral contrast studies – technique and normal appearance

Retrograde urethrography (males) and retrograde vaginourethrography (females) are used to examine the urethra, and with larger quantities of contrast medium the bladder will also be demonstrated *(retrograde urethrocystography)*.

In the male animal the urethra is seen as a smoothly bordered tube with occasional symmetrical narrowing due to peristalsis (Figure 10.13a). In male dogs the prostatic urethra is often of wider diameter. In the bitch, the urethra appears very narrow and the vestibule and vagina are spindle shaped, terminating in a spoon-shaped cervix (in both intact and neutered animals) (Figure 10.13b).

Preparation

- Enema to empty the rectum and distal colon of faeces.
- The urinary bladder should be reasonably full of urine or contrast medium to create a little backflow resistance and encourage urethral distension.

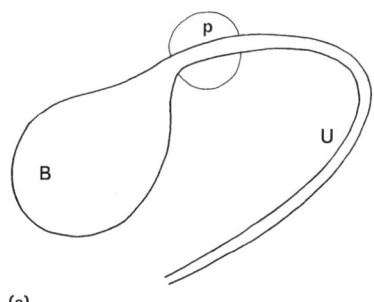

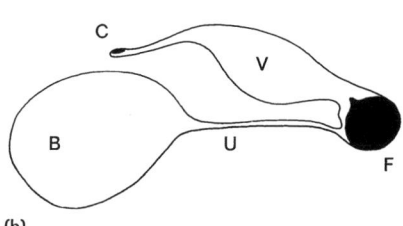

Figure 10.13 (a) Normal retrograde urethrogram – male dog (B = bladder; P = prostate; U = urethra). (b) Normal retrograde vaginourethrogram – bitch (B = bladder; U = urethra; V = vagina; C = cervix; F = bulb of Foley catheter).

- Sedate or anaesthetise the patient as appropriate.
- Take survey radiographs.
- Pre-fill the catheter with contrast medium to avoid introduction of air bubbles during the injection.

Retrograde urethrography (males)

The urethra is catheterised with the catheter tip lying distal to the area of interest. The external urethral orifice is occluded by a soft clamp during injection. Iodinated contrast medium (used alone, or mixed with an equal quantity of KY jelly) is injected at a dose rate of about 1 ml/kg body weight. Air should not be used as it can occasionally enter the corpus cavernosa of the penis. The exposure is made as soon as possible after injection, consistent with radiation safety of the operator.

In the male dog different positions, centring points and exposures may be needed to show different areas of the urethra in lateral recumbency. Oblique VD projections are used to avoid superimposition of the penile and prostatic urethra.

Retrograde vaginourethrography (females)

In bitches, a Foley catheter is inserted between the lips of the vulva and held in place with a soft clamp. The tip of the catheter distal to the bulb is cut off, to prevent it entering the vagina and occluding the urethra. The bulb is inflated. In cats, it may not be possible to use a Foley catheter. An alternative procedure is to inject contrast medium as the catheter is withdrawn from the bladder.

1 ml/kg bodyweight of iodinated contrast medium is injected carefully (vaginal rupture has been reported in Rough Collies and Shetland Sheepdogs). Lateral and oblique VD radiographs are obtained.

10.33 Irregularities on the urethrogram

1. Filling defects
   a. Air bubbles accidentally injected into the urethra (will not distend its lumen and will move freely up the urethra into the bladder)
   b. Calculi (may distend the urethra)
2. Strictures
   a. Simulated by a peristaltic wave – repeat the radiograph to see if it is consistent
   b. Previous calculus impaction
   c. Previous surgery

SMALL ANIMAL RADIOLOGICAL DIFFERENTIAL DIAGNOSIS

  d. Prostatic disease, especially neoplasia
  e. Urethral neoplasia
  f. Severe urethritis.
3. Irregular mucosal surface
  a. Severe urethritis
  b. Neoplasia of the urethra or prostate (Figure 10.14).
4. Displacement of the urethra
  a. Adjacent or encircling mass
  b. Perineal or inguinal hernia and bladder displacement
  c. Asymmetric prostatic disease (see 10.46–54)
    - prostatic cyst(s)
    - prostatic abscess(es)
    - prostatic neoplasia.
5. Contrast medium extravasation
  a. Normal – small amount of extravasation into prostatic ductules in male dogs
  b. Urethral rupture
    - trauma
    - iatrogenic from poor catheterisation technique
  c. Urethral fistula
  d. Urethrotomy/urethrostomy
  e. Prostatic disease (see 10.46–54)
    - cystic hyperplasia
    - prostatic neoplasia
    - prostatic abscess.

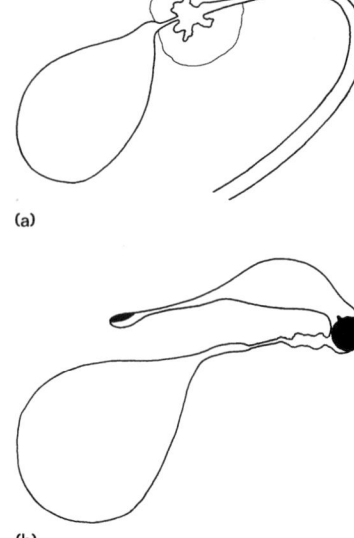

Figure 10.14 (a) Prostatic tumour seen on retrograde urethrography – extravasation of contrast medium, urethral stricture and irregular prostatic outline (cf. Figure 10.13a). (b) Urethral neoplasia seen on retrograde vagino-urethrography – narrow and irregular urethra (cf. Figure 10.13b).

10.34 Ultrasonography of the urethra

There is limited ultrasonographic visualisation of the urethra unless a high-frequency rectal or vaginal transducer is available. From a ventral abdominal approach, the prostatic urethra may be visible in the male dog.

OVARIES

Normal ovaries are not visible radiographically. Ovarian masses are usually located caudal to the ipsilateral kidney but may migrate ventrally if large.

10.35 Ovarian enlargement

For the radiographic appearance of ovarian masses, see 11.37.7.
1. Ovarian tumour
  a. Granulosa cell tumour
  b. Teratoma – may calcify.
2. Ovarian cyst(s) – may develop a calcified rim.
3. Mimicked by other mid-abdominal masses – use contrast techniques or ultrasonography to investigate further
  a. Composite shadow – rule out by taking the orthogonal view
  b. Enlarged kidney
  c. Enlarged lymph node
  d. Small intestinal mass.

10.36 Ultrasonographic examination of the ovaries

Ultrasonographic examination may be carried out with the animal in dorsal or lateral recumbency. A high-frequency (7.5 MHz) sector or curvilinear transducer is used, and each kidney identified. The region caudal and ventral to the caudal pole of each kidney is then searched. Normal ovaries may be particularly difficult to identify during anoestrus.

10.37 Normal ultrasonographic appearance of the ovaries

In anoestrus, the ovary is smoothly rounded and uniformly hypoechoic relative to the surrounding fat. Multiple follicles develop during pro-oestrus; these are thin walled and anechoic. During oestrus and dioestrus the follicles regress and corpora lutea develop, but immature corpora lutea and follicles have a very similar ultrasonographic appearance. Mature corpora lutea appear oval and hypoechoic.

10.38 Ovarian abnormalities on ultrasonography

1. Rounded foci, anechoic contents, thin walls – benign cysts. May be single or multiple, unilateral or bilateral
    a. Non-functional
    b. Functional.
2. Rounded foci, hypoechoic contents, thick irregular walls
    a. Neoplasia with a cystic component (granulosa cell tumour, adenocarcinoma, teratoma)
    b. Haemorrhagic cyst.
3. Hyperechoic foci (+/– shadowing)
    a. Teratoma containing fat, bone or tooth
    b. Dystrophic mineralisation (other tumours).
4. Solid mass, variable echogenicity
    a. Neoplasia
        - adenoma, adenocarcinoma (often bilateral)
        - granulosa cell tumour
        - teratoma
        - others.

UTERUS

A normal, non-gravid uterus is not seen radiographically except in very obese dogs, in which it may be outlined by fat. Mild uterine enlargement is best seen as a tubular soft tissue structure ventral to the descending colon and dorsal to the bladder neck; more cranially the uterine horns mimic fluid-filled small intestine. When enlargement of the uterine horns exceeds the diameter of small intestine they may be seen as convoluted soft tissue structures cranial to the bladder. On the VD view an enlarged uterus can give rise to kidney-shaped radio-opacities (the "extra kidney sign").

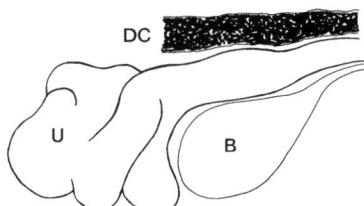

Figure 10.15 Uterine enlargement – the descending colon and bladder are separated by a soft tissue viscus, which continues cranial to the bladder (U = uterus; B = bladder; DC = descending colon).

10.39 Uterine enlargement

1. Generalised uterine enlargement (Figure 10.15)
    a. Normal, gravid uterus before detection of foetal mineralisation (cats <35 days gestation, dogs <41 days gestation). A lobular shape may be noted by mid-pregnancy
    b. Normal post-partum uterus – the involuting uterus will remain visible for at least a week after parturition.
    c. Pyometra – the most common cause of pathological generalised enlargement
    d. Mucometra
    e. Haemometra
    f. Hydrometra – secondary to uterine neoplasia.
2. Focal uterine enlargement
    a. Small litter size
    b. Mid pregnancy, before foetal ossification
    c. Pyometra localised to one uterine horn
    d. Stump pyometra or granuloma – mass lesion dorsal or craniodorsal to the bladder neck
    e. Uterine neoplasia.

10.40 Variations in uterine radio-opacity

Foetal mineralisation will be detected from 35 days gestation in the cat and 41 days in dogs. It is easier to detect on lateral radiographs because the spine is partly superimposed over the abdomen on the VD view. Increasing bone opacity develops during the last trimester – the skull, vertebrae and long bones being the most apparent. Just before parturition mineralisation of the bones of the paws will become apparent. Assessment of foetal numbers is best achieved by counting the number of skulls.

1. Increased uterine radio-opacity – mineralisation
   a. Mimicked by mineralisation in the stomach from an ingested bird, rodent, foetus or other foreign object
   b. Third trimester pregnancy
   c. Foetal mummification especially if ectopic – coiled and sclerotic foetal skeletal remnants.
2. Decreased uterine radio-opacity – gas
   a. Mimicked by overlying bowel gas
   b. Foetal death – gas in foetal heart cavities or cranium
   c. Physometra – gas in the uterus due to metritis and/or foetal death.

10.41 Radiographic signs of dystocia and foetal death

Radiographs are useful to evaluate the number of foetuses, their size relative to the pelvic diameter, their presentation to the pelvic canal and the size and shape of the pelvic canal. Live foetuses normally lie in a neutral or semi-flexed position. Ultrasonography is needed to check for foetal distress or recent death.

1. Foetal oversize – a pregnancy with single or few foetuses tends to result in larger foetuses which are more likely to lead to dystocia.
2. Foetal malpresentation (e.g. lying at the pelvic inlet but with head or limb back).
3. Maternal dystocia
   a. Uterine inertia – foetuses normal but none close to pelvic inlet
   b. Physical obstruction (e.g. pelvic fracture malunion).
4. Foetal death
   a. Foetal or uterine gas
   b. Abnormal position of the foetus (e.g. hyperextension)
   c. Disintegration of the foetus
   d. Overlapping of foetal cranial bones – "Spalding's sign"
   e. Demineralisation of foetal bones
   f. Mummification – dense, compacted foetuses.

10.42 Ultrasonographic examination of the uterus

The cervix and body of the uterus are located dorsal to the bladder and ventral to the descending colon. The uterine horns cranial to the bladder are not usually recognised unless distended; they are typically less than 1 cm in diameter, and are hidden amongst the small intestine and mesenteric fat.

10.43 Normal ultrasonographic appearance of the uterus

The normal non-gravid uterus is a hypoechoic tubular structure, with a focal thickening at the cervix. A central linear echo may be apparent during pro-oestrus, oestrus and dioestrus.

During pregnancy, the uterus begins to enlarge within days. This is, however, a non-specific effect due to hormonal changes. Pregnancy can be positively confirmed only when gestational sacs (comprising the foetus surrounded by foetal fluids and membranes) become visible – at around 20–25 days after the last mating (sometimes earlier). Foetal cardiac activity and generalised foetal movements indicate viability. As pregnancy progresses, the foetus grows and differentiation of foetal organs and mineralisation of the foetal skeleton become apparent.

10.44 Variation in uterine contents on ultrasonography

1. Anechoic uterine contents (fluid)
   a. Early pregnancy (10–20 days after mating, before the foetus is visible)
   b. Pyometra
   c. Haemometra
   d. Hydrometra
   e. Mucometra.
2. Hypoechoic uterine contents (fluid containing variable quantities of swirling echoes)

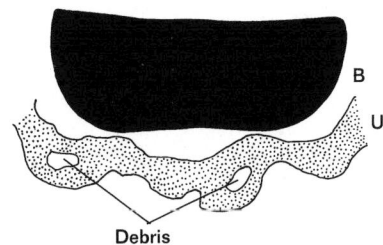

Figure 10.16 Pyometra on ultrasonography – a hypoechoic tubular structure deep to the anechoic bladder (B = bladder; U = uterus).

a. Pyometra (Figure 10.16)
b. Haemometra
c. Mucometra.
3. Mixed echogenicity uterine contents
   a. Normal pregnancy (defined foetal structures surrounded by fluid, foetal cardiac activity)
   b. Dead foetuses (foetal structure becomes progressively less well defined as decomposition or mummification occurs, no foetal cardiac activity)
   c. Pyometra (fluid with unstructured debris)
   d. Post-partum uterus (fluid with unstructured debris).

10.45 Thickening of the uterine wall on ultrasonography

1. Diffuse thickening of the uterine wall
   a. Early pregnancy
   b. Post-partum
   c. Endometritis/cystic endometrial hyperplasia (may be heterogeneous, may see multiple small cysts).
2. Focal thickening of the uterine wall – may be isoechoic with the surrounding uterine wall or of complex echogenicity. May have a cystic component
   a. Uterine neoplasia
   b. Uterine granuloma/abscess.

PROSTATE

Radiographic examination of the male reproductive organs is limited to the prostate gland in dogs. Prostatic disease is very rare in cats. The prostate lies in the caudal retroperitoneum caudal to the bladder neck and ventral to the descending colon. It is normally, smooth, rounded, bilobed and symmetrical about the urethra. As it enlarges, it will displace the bladder cranially and a larger proportion will be seen cranial to the pelvic brim. Prostate size is variable and related to age, breed, presence of disease and benign hyperplasia, which occurs from middle age. Radiography is insensitive for precise diagnosis of prostatic disease because different conditions can produce similar changes (e.g. increase in size). Prostatic disease can be investigated further using retrograde urethrography to assess the location, diameter and integrity of the prostatic urethra (see 10.32, 10.33 and Figs 10.13, 10.14). Ultrasonographic examination of the prostate often yields further information.

10.46 Variations in location of the prostate

1. Cranial displacement of the cranial margin of the prostate
   a. Full bladder
   b. Ventral abdominal wall weakness (e.g. hyperadrenocorticism)
   c. Prostatomegaly.
2. Caudal displacement of the prostate
   a. Small and caudally located in castrated dogs (not usually visible)
   b. Perineal hernia.

10.47 Variations in prostatic size

Prostatic size can be assessed on a lateral radiograph by comparing the craniocaudal prostate dimension to the pelvic inlet dimension (the distance between the ventral border of the sacrum and the cranial tip or promontory of the pubis). In normal intact males, the craniocaudal prostate dimension should not exceed 70% of the pelvic inlet dimension (Figure 10.17). Severe prostatomegaly may compress the descending colon, leading to obstipation, and may cause chronic dysuria and bladder dilation.

1. Normal size
   a. Normal
   b. Enlargement due to disease in a dog previously castrated

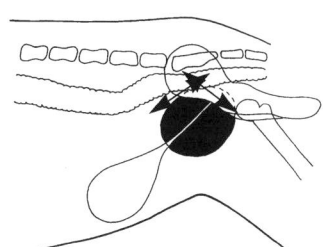

Figure 10.17 Measurement of prostatic size. The craniocaudal prostatic dimension should not exceed 70% of the pelvic inlet dimension. This figure shows prostatomegaly, with cranial displacement of the bladder and dorsal displacement of the colon.

SMALL ANIMAL RADIOLOGICAL DIFFERENTIAL DIAGNOSIS

   c. Neoplasia – may be present without obvious enlargement
   d. Chronic prostatitis.
2. Enlarged prostate
   a. Normal size but cranial displacement due to a full bladder or abdominal weakness
   b. Benign prostatic hyperplasia – smooth, symmetrical about the urethra, remains bilobed
   c. Prostatitis – irregular, ill-defined +/– caudal peritonitis
   d. Prostatic cyst(s) – may be asymmetric about the urethra
   e. Prostatic abscess(es) – may be asymmetric about the urethra
   f. Prostatic neoplasia – may be asymmetric about the urethra; may see periosteal new bone on caudal lumbar spine, sacrum, tail base and pelvis (see 5.4.3 and Figure 5.7)
   g. Androgen-producing testicular neoplasia.
3. Small or non-visible prostate
   a. Poor radiographic technique (e.g. hind legs not pulled far enough caudally)
   b. Normal
      • young dog – prostate small and intra-pelvic
      • castrated dog
   c. Caudal displacement
      • perineal hernia.

10.48 Variations in prostatic shape and outline

1. Asymmetry of the prostate about the urethra
   a. Prostatic abscess
   b. Intra-prostatic cyst
   c. Paraprostatic cyst – cystic vestiges of the Wolffian duct or uterus masculinus. Large paraprostatic cysts mimic "extra" bladder shadows (Figure 10.18)
   d. Prostatic neoplasia
2. Irregularity or loss of clarity of the prostatic margins
   a. Prostatitis
   b. Neoplasia.

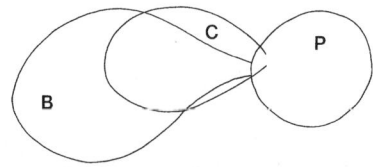

Figure 10.18 Paraprostatic cyst – "extra" bladder shadow.

10.49 Variations in prostatic radio-opacity

1. Increased prostatic radio-opacity – mineralisation
   a. Eggshell-like rim radio-opacity
      • paraprostatic cyst (may be intra-abdominal or intrapelvic)
      • resolving abscess
   b. Irregular patches or nodules of mineralisation
      • dystrophic mineralisation due to neoplasia
      • severe, chronic prostatitis
      • prostatic calculi – may be incidental.
2. Decreased prostatic radio-opacity – gas
   a. Normal – iatrogenic reflux of air into prostatic ductules during pneumocystography
   b. Prostatitis or abscessation.

10.50 Ultrasonographic examination of the prostate

No special patient preparation is required, although it can be useful to allow defecation before the examination. A high-frequency (7.5 MHz or, in large dogs, 5 MHz) sector or curvilinear transducer is placed on one side of the prepuce, cranial to the pubic brim, to locate the bladder. Having found the bladder neck, the transducer is moved caudally to identify the prostate. If the prostate is small or intrapelvic, it may be helpful to push it forwards gently using a gloved finger per rectum. The prostate is imaged in both the sagittal and transverse planes of section, ensuring that the entire volume of the gland is imaged.

A transrectal approach can be used to image the prostate if an appropriate transducer is available.

10.51 Normal ultrasonographic appearance of the prostate

The normal canine prostate is smooth in outline, and oval or bilobed in shape. The parenchyma is moderately echoic with an evenly granular texture. A central linear echo, the 'hilar echo', may be evident. The open prostatic urethra is usually only seen in sedated or anaesthetised animals.

For differential diagnoses related to changes in size of the prostate, see 10.47.

10 UROGENITAL TRACT

10.52 Focal parenchymal changes of the prostate on ultrasonography

1. Anechoic contents, smooth thin walls
   a. Intraprostatic cyst (<1 cm diameter considered normal)
   b. Haematocyst
   c. Abscess.
2. Anechoic/hypoechoic contents, thick irregular walls
   a. Abscess
   b. Neoplasm with necrotic centre or cystic component.
3. Hyperechoic
   a. Prostatic calculus
   b. Focal calcification (see 10.49).

10.53 Diffuse parenchymal changes of the prostate on ultrasonography

1. Normal echogenicity and echotexture
   a. Normal prostate
   b. Benign prostatic hyperplasia.
2. Increased echogenicity, uniform echotexture
   a. Benign prostatic hyperplasia.
3. Increased echogenicity, disturbed echotexture
   a. Chronic bacterial prostatitis
   b. Granulomatous prostatitis (blastomycosis*, cryptococcosis*)
   c. Neoplasia (may contain focal mineralisation, leading to acoustic shadowing).
4. Decreased echogenicity, disturbed echotexture
   a. Acute inflammation/abscessation
   b. Neoplasia (less common).

10.54 Paraprostatic lesions on ultrasonography

1. Paraprostatic cysts – vary in appearance from simple cysts to complex septated structures (Figure 10.19). May be benign or malignant.

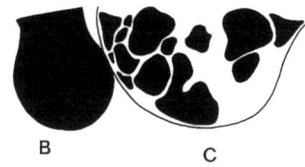

Figure 10.19 Paraprostatic cyst on ultrasonography. Internal septation is often seen, with variable amounts of solid tissue (B = bladder; C = paraprostatic cyst).

TESTES

10.55 Ultrasonographic examination of the testes

The testicles normally lie in the scrotum and so may be imaged by placing a high-frequency transducer directly on the scrotal skin. If a testicle is not fully descended, then a search may be made starting in the inguinal region and progressing to the abdominal cavity. Within the abdomen, the testicle most commonly lies near the bladder, but may lie anywhere between the kidneys and the bladder.

10.56 Normal ultrasonographic appearance of the testes

The normal canine testis is smoothly rounded and moderately echoic with an even, granular echotexture. A central linear echo may be seen, representing the mediastinum testis. The epididymis, found at the head and tail of the testis, is less echoic and more coarsely textured.

10.57 Testicular abnormalities on ultrasonography

1. Focal parenchymal abnormalities
   a. Neoplasia (interstitial cell, Sertoli cell, seminoma) – may be single or multiple, and of variable echogenicity. Very large lesions tend to have a complex appearance.
   b. Abscess – anechoic/hypoechoic contents, irregular wall
   c. Infarct – hyperechoic, wedge shaped.
2. Diffuse parenchymal abnormalities
   a. Orchitis – patchy hypoechoic appearance, often associated with epididymitis
   b. Torsion – diffusely hypoechoic, concurrent enlargement of epididymis
   c. Atrophy – hypoechoic/isoechoic
      • senile
      • neoplasm in contralateral testis.

10.58 Paratesticular abnormalities on ultrasonography

1. Enlargement of epididymis
   a. Epididymitis
   b. Torsion.
2. Abnormal scrotal contents
   a. Scrotal hernia (mixed echogenicity, often with shadowing or reverberation due to gas)
   b. Haemorrhage (usually anechoic)
      - trauma
      - extension from abdominal or retroperitoneal haemorrhage (see 11.4.1 and 11.7.2).

FURTHER READING

General

Johnston, G.R., Walter, P.S. and Feeney, D.A. (1986) Radiographic and ultrasonographic features of uroliths and other urinary tract fillings defects. *Veterinary Clinics of North America; Small Animal Practice* **16** 261–292.

Lamb, C.R. (1990) Abdominal ultrasonography in small animals: intestinal tract and mesentery, kidneys, adrenal glands, uterus and prostate (review). *Journal of Small Animal Practice* **31** 295–304.

Pugh, C.R., Rhodes, W.H. and Biery, D.N. (1993) Contrast studies of the urogenital system. *Veterinary Clinics of North America; Small Animal Practice* **23** 281–306.

Silverman, S. and Long, C.D. (2000) The diagnosis of urinary incontinence and abnormal urination in dogs and cats. *Veterinary Clinics of North America; Small Animal Practice* **30** 427–448.

Kidneys

Barr, F.J. (1990) Evaluation of ultrasound as a method of assessing renal size in the dog. *Journal of Small Animal Practice* **31** 174–179.

Barr, F.J., Holt, P.E. and Gibbs, C. (1990) Ultrasonographic measurement of normal renal parameters. *Journal of Small Animal Practice* **31** 180–184.

Biller, D.S., Schenkman, D.I. and Bortnoski, H. (1991) Ultrasonographic appearance of renal infarcts in a dog. *Journal of the American Animal Hospital Association* **27** 370–372.

Biller, D.S., Bradley, G.A. and Partington, B.P. (1992) Renal medullary rim sign: ultrasonographic evidence of renal disease. *Veterinary Radiology* **33** 286–290.

Felkai, C.S., Voros, K., Vrabely, T. and Karsai, F. (1992) Ultrasonographic determination of renal volume in the dog. *Veterinary Radiology and Ultrasound* **33** 292–296.

Forrest, L.J., O'Brien, R.T., Tremelling, M.S., Steinberg, H., Cooley, A.J. and Kerlin, R.L. (1998) Sonographic renal findings in 20 dogs with leptospirosis. *Veterinary Radiology and Ultrasound* **39** 337–340.

Grandage, J. (1975) Some effects of posture on the radiographic appearance of the kidneys of the dog. *Journal of the American Veterinary Medical Association* **166** 165–166.

Grooters, A.M., Cuypers, M.D., Partington, B.P., Williams, J. and Pechman, R.D. (1997) Renomegaly in dogs and cats. Part II. Diagnostic approach. *Compendium of Continuing Education for the Practicing Veterinarian (Small Animal)* **19** 1213–1229.

Konde, L.J., Wrigley, R.H., Park, R.D. and Lebel, J.L (1984) Ultrasonographic anatomy of the normal canine kidney. *Veterinary Radiology* **25** 173–178.

Moe, L. and Lium, B. (1997) Hereditary multifocal renal cystadenocarcinomas and nodular dermatofibrosis in 51 German shepherd dogs. *Journal of Small Animal Practice* **38** 498–505.

Nyland, T.G., Kantrowitz, B.M., Fisher, P., Olander, H.J. and Hornof, W.J. (1989) Ultrasonic determination of kidney volume in the dog. *Veterinary Radiology* **30** 174–180.

Ochoa, V.B., DiBartola, S.P., Chew, D.J., Westropp, J., Carothers, M. and Biller, D.S. (1999) Perinephric pseudocysts in the cat: a retrospective study and review of the literature. *Journal of Veterinary Internal Medicine* **13** 47–55.

Rivers, B.J. and Johnston, G.R. (1996) Diagnostic imaging strategies in small animal nephrology. *Veterinary Clinics of North America; Small Animal Practice* **26** 1505–1517.

Triolo, A.J., and Miles, K.G. (1995) Renal imaging techniques in dogs and cats. *Veterinary Medicine* **13** 959–966.

Ureters

Dean, P.W., Bojrab, M.J. and Constantinescu, G.M. (1988) Canine ectopic ureter. *Compendium of Continuing Education for the Practicing Veterinarian (Small Animal)* **10** 146–157.

Holt, P.E., Gibbs, C. and Pearson, H. (1982) Canine ectopic ureter – a review of twenty-nine cases. *Journal of Small Animal Practice* **23** 195–208.

Holt, P.E. and Gibbs, C. (1992) Congenital urinary incontinence in cats: a review of 19 cases. *Veterinary Radiology* **130** 437–442.

Lamb, C.R. and Gregory, S.P. (1994) Ultrasonography of the ureterovesicular junction in the dog: a preliminary report. *Veterinary Record* **134** 36–38.

Lamb, C.R. and Gregory, S.P. (1998) Ultrasonographic findings in 14 dogs with ectopic ureter. *Veterinary Radiology and Ultrasound* **39** 218–223.

Lamb, C.R. (1998) Ultrasonography of the ureters. *Veterinary Clinics of North America; Small Animal Practice* **28** 823–848.

Bladder

Atalan, G., Barr, F.J. and Holt, P.E. (1998) Estimation of bladder volume using ultrasonographic determination of cross-sectional areas and linear measurements. *Veterinary Radiology and Ultrasound* **39** 446–450.

Feeney, D.A., Weichselbaum, R.C., Jessen, C.R. and Osborne, C.A. (1999) Imaging canine urocystoliths. *Veterinary Clinics of North America; Small Animal Practice* **29** 59–72.

Geisse, A.L., Lowry, J.E., Schaeffer, D.J. and Smith, C.W. (1997) Sonographic evaluation of urinary bladder wall thickness in normal dogs. *Veterinary Radiology and Ultrasound* **38** 132–137.

Hanson, J.A. and Tidwell, A.S. (1996) Ultrasonographic appearance of urethral transitional cell carcinoma in ten dogs. *Veterinary Radiology and Ultrasound* **37** 293–299.

Johnston, G.R., Feeney, D.A., Rivers, W.J. and Weichselbaum, R. (1996) Diagnostic imaging of the feline lower urinary tract. *Veterinary Clinics of North America; Small Animal Practice* **26** 401–415.

Lamb, C.R., Trower, N.D. and Gregory, S.P. (1996) Ultrasound-guided catheter biopsy of the lower urinary tract: technique and results in 12 dogs. *Journal of Small Animal Practice* **37** 413–416.

Leveille, R., Biller, D.S., Partington, B.P. and Miyabayashi, T. (1992) Sonographic investigation of transitional cell carcinoma of the urinary bladder in small animals. *Veterinary Radiology and Ultrasound* **33** 103–107.

Leveille, R. (1998) Ultrasonography of urinary bladder disorders. *Veterinary Clinics of North America; Small Animal Practice* **28** 799–822.

Mahaffey, M.B., Barsanti, J.A., Crowell, W.A., Shotts, E. and Barber, D.L. (1989) Cystography: effect of technique on diagnosis of cystitis in dogs. *Veterinary Radiology and Ultrasound* **30** 261–267.

Scrivani, P.V., Chew, D.J., Buffington, C.A.T. and Kendall, M. (1998) Results of double-contrast cystography in cats with idiopathic cystitis: 45 cases (1993–1995) *Journal of the American Veterinary Medical Association* **212** 1907–1909.

Urethra

Holt, P.E., Gibbs, C. and Latham, J. (1984) An evaluation of positive contrast vaginourethrography as a diagnostic aid in the bitch. *Journal of Small Animal Practice* **25** 531–549.

Scrivani, P.V., Chew, D.J., Buffington, C.A.T., Kendall, M. and Leveille, D.M. (1997) Results of retrograde urethrography in cats with idiopathic non obstructive lower urinary tract disease and their association with pathogenesis in 53 cases (1993–1995). *Journal of the American Veterinary Medical Association* **211** 741–748.

Ticer, J.W., Spencer, C.P. and Ackerman, N. (1980) Positive contrast retrograde urethrography: a useful procedure for evaluating urethral disorders in the dog. *Veterinary Radiology* **21** 2–11.

Genital system – general

Kneller, S.K. (1986) Radiologic examination, in *Small Animal Reproduction and Infertility*, pp. 158–185, ed. Burke, T.J. Lea and Febiger.

Root, C.R. and Spaulding, K.A. (1994) Diagnostic imaging in companion animal theriogenology. *Seminars in Veterinary Medicine and Surgery (Small Animals)* **9** 7–27.

Female genital system

Diez-Bru, N., Garcia-Real, I, Martinez, E.M., Rollan, E., Mayenco, A. and Llorens, P. (1998) Ultrasonographic appearance of ovarian tumors in 10 dogs. *Veterinary Radiology and Ultrasound* **39** 226–233.

England, G.C.W. and Allen, W.E. (1989) Ultrasonographic and histological appearance of the canine ovary. *Veterinary Record* **125** 555–556.

England, G.C.W. and Yeager, A.E. (1993) Ultrasonographic appearance of the ovary and uterus of the bitch during oestrus, ovulation and early pregnancy. *Journal of Reproduction and Fertility Supplement* **47** 107–117.

England, G.C.W. (1998) Ultrasonographic assessment of abnormal pregnancy. *Veterinary Clinics of North America; Small Animal Practice* **28** 849–868.

Fayrer-Hosken, R.A., Mahaffey, M., Miller-Liebl, D. and Caudle, A.B. (1991) Early diagnosis of canine pyometra using ultrasonography. *Veterinary Radiology and Ultrasound* **32** 287–289.

Ferretti, L.M., Newell, S.M., Graham, J.P. and Roberts, G.D. (2000) Radiographic and ultrasonographic evaluation of the normal feline postpartum uterus. *Veterinary Radiology and Ultrasound* **41** 287–291.

Kydd, D.M. and Burnie, A.G. (1986) Vaginal neoplasia in the bitch: a review of forty clinical cases. *Journal of Small Animal Practice* **27** 255–263.

Miles, K. (1995) Imaging pregnant dogs and cats. *Compendium of Continuing Education for the Practicing Veterinarian (Small Animal)* **17** 1217–1226.

Pharr, J.W. and Post, K. (1992) Ultrasonography and radiography of the canine post partum uterus. *Veterinary Radiology and Ultrasound* **33** 35–40.

Male genital system

Atalan, G., Barr, F.J. and Holt, P.E. (1999) Comparison of ultrasonographic and radiographic measurements of canine prostatic dimensions. *Veterinary Radiology and Ultrasound* **40** 408–412.

Atalan, G., Holt, P.E. and Barr, F.J. (1999) Ultrasonographic estimation of prostate size in normal dogs, and relationship to bodyweight and age. *Journal of Small Animal Practice* **40** 119–122.

Dorfman, M. and Barsanti, J. (1995) Diseases of the canine prostate gland. *Compendium of Continuing Education for the Practicing Veterinarian (Small Animal)* **17** 791–810.

Feeney, D.A., Johnston, G.R., Klausner, J.S., Perman, V., Leininger, J.R. and Tomlinson, M.J. (1987) Canine prostatic disease – comparison of ultrasonographic appearance with morphologic and microbiologic findings: 30 cases (1981–1985). *Journal of the American Veterinary Medical Association* **190** 1027–1034.

Feeney, D.A., Johnston, G.R., Klausner, J.S. and Bell, F.W. (1989) Canine prostatic ultrasonography. *Seminars in Veterinary Medicine and Surgery (Small Animals)* **4** 44–57.

Johnston, G.R., Feeney, D.A., Johnston, S.D. and O'Brien, T.D. (1991) Ultrasonographic features of testicular neoplasia in dogs: 16 cases (1989–1988). *Journal of the American Veterinary Medical Association* **198** 1779–1784.

Pugh, C.R., Konde, L.J. and Park, R.D. (1990) Testicular ultrasound in the normal dog. *Veterinary Radiology* **31** 195–199.

Pugh, C.R. and Konde, L.J. (1991) Sonographic evaluation of canine testicular and scrotal abnormalities: a review of 26 case histories. *Veterinary Radiology* **32** 243–250.

Ruel, Y., Barthez, P.Y., Mailles, A. and Begon, D. (1998) Ultrasonographic evaluation of the prostate in healthy intact dogs. *Veterinary Radiology and Ultrasound* **39** 212–216.

Stowater, J.L. and Lamb, C.R. (1989) Ultrasonographic features of paraprostatic cysts in nine dogs. *Veterinary Radiology* **30** 232–239.

Williams, J. and Niles, J. (1999) Prostatic disease in the dog. *In Practice* **21** 558–575.

11

Other abdominal structures – abdominal wall, peritoneal and retroperitoneal cavities, parenchymal organs

ABDOMINAL WALL

11.1 Variations in shape of the abdominal wall
11.2 Variations in radio-opacity of the abdominal wall
11.3 Ultrasonographic examination of the abdominal wall

PERITONEAL CAVITY

11.4 Increased radio-opacity of the peritoneal cavity and/or loss of visualisation of abdominal organs
11.5 Decreased radio-opacity of the peritoneal cavity
11.6 Ultrasonographic examination of the peritoneal cavity

RETROPERITONEAL SPACE

11.7 Enlargement of the retroperitoneal space
11.8 Increased radio-opacity of the retroperitoneal space and/or loss of visualisation of the retroperitoneal structures
11.9 Decreased radio-opacity of the retroperitoneal space
11.10 Ultrasonographic examination of the retroperitoneal space
11.11 Ultrasonographic examination of the lymph nodes in the retroperitoneal space
11.12 Ultrasonographic examination of the abdominal aorta and caudal vena cava.

LIVER

11.13 Displacement of the liver
11.14 Variations in liver size
11.15 Variations in liver shape
11.16 Variations in liver radio-opacity
11.17 Hepatic contrast studies

11.18 Ultrasonographic examination of the liver
11.19 Normal ultrasonographic appearance of the liver
11.20 Hepatic parenchymal abnormalities on ultrasonography
11.21 Biliary tract abnormalities on ultrasonography
11.22 Hepatic vascular abnormalities on ultrasonography

SPLEEN

11.23 Absence of the splenic shadow
11.24 Variations in location of the tail of the spleen
11.25 Variations in splenic size and shape
11.26 Variations in splenic radio-opacity
11.27 Ultrasonographic examination of the spleen
11.28 Normal ultrasonographic appearance of the spleen
11.29 Ultrasonographic abnormalities of the spleen

PANCREAS

11.30 Pancreatic radiology
11.31 Ultrasonographic examination of the pancreas
11.32 Normal ultrasonographic appearance of the pancreas
11.33 Ultrasonographic abnormalities of the pancreas

ADRENAL GLANDS

11.34 Adrenal gland radiology
11.35 Ultrasonographic examination of the adrenal glands

ABDOMINAL MASSES

11.36 Cranial abdominal masses (largely within the costal arch)

SMALL ANIMAL RADIOLOGICAL DIFFERENTIAL DIAGNOSIS

11.37 Mid-abdominal masses
11.38 Caudal abdominal masses

MISCELLANEOUS

11.39 Calcification on abdominal radiographs

ABDOMINAL WALL

The abdominal wall is formed by the diaphragm and rib cage cranially, abdominal muscles ventrally and laterally, sublumbar muscles dorsally and peritoneum caudally.

11.1 Variations in shape of the abdominal wall

1. Generalised distension of the abdominal wall
   a. Obesity – abdominal viscera well outlined by fat; large falciform fat pad
   b. Loss of muscle tone, resulting in sagging of abdominal structures
      * old age
      * Cushing's syndrome (hyperadrenocorticism) – naturally occurring or iatrogenic
   c. Large abdominal mass, especially splenic
   d. Gastric distension by food or gas (see 9.3.4 and 5 and Figure 9.2)
   e. Small intestinal distension (see 9.21.3 and Figure 9.10) – e.g. low obstruction
   f. Severe faecal retention (see 9.39, 9.40.3)
   g. Uterine distension in female animals
      * mid- to late-term pregnancy
      * large pyometra
      * large hydrometra, mucometra or haemometra
   h. Severe peritoneal effusion
      * right heart failure
      * liver disease
      * nephrotic syndrome
      * other causes of hypoproteinaemia
      * obstruction of the caudal vena cava
      * ruptured urinary bladder
      * intra-abdominal haemorrhage
      * cats – feline infectious peritonitis (FIP)
   i. Severe pneumoperitoneum.
2. Focal distension of the abdominal wall
   a. Umbilical hernia
   b. Inguinal hernia (Figure 11.1)
   c. Traumatic rupture of abdominal or intercostal muscles
   d. Surgical wound breakdown.

   In a–d, viscera may be contained within the focal distension (contrast media or ultrasonography may be helpful if this is unclear on survey radiographs)

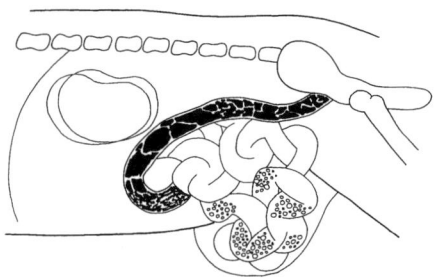

Figure 11.1 Inguinal hernia. The viscera extend beyond the normal abdominal boundary and the line of the abdominal wall is lost.

   e. Abdominal wall abscess
   f. Abdominal wall haematoma
   g. Abdominal wall seroma
   h. Abdominal wall neoplasia
   i. Lipoma – fat opacity.
3. Inward displacement of the abdominal wall
   a. Emaciation
   b. Diaphragmatic rupture with herniation of abdominal viscera into the thoracic cavity
   c. Severe inspiratory dyspnoea.

11.2 Variations in radio-opacity of the abdominal wall

In a well-nourished adult animal, fat interspersed between the fascial planes allows visualisation of the various muscle layers.
1. Increased soft tissue radio-opacity and loss of distinction of muscle layers of the abdominal wall
   a. Trauma with oedema or haemorrhage of the soft tissues
   b. Abdominal wall neoplasia
   c. Large volumes of fluid administered subcutaneously
   d. Cellulitis
   e. Healed laparotomy.
2. Mineralised radio-opacity of the abdominal wall
   a. Overlying wire skin sutures or staples
   b. Calcinosis cutis associated with Cushing's disease (hyperadrenocorticism)
   c. Foreign material e.g. bullets or dirt on the hair coat

11 OTHER ABDOMINAL STRUCTURES

   d. Overlying wet hair mimicking mineralised radio-opacity.
3. Decreased radio-opacity of the abdominal wall
   a. Fat – lipoma
   b. Gas
      - local skin lacerations
      - subcutaneous emphysema extending from a wound elsewhere
      - gas dissecting along fascial planes from a pneumomediastinum or pneumoretroperitoneum
      - recent surgical incision
      - gas within a hernia which contains small intestine.

11.3 Ultrasonographic examination of the abdominal wall

Interpretation is similar to that of ultrasonography of the soft tissues of the thoracic wall (see 8.24).

PERITONEAL CAVITY

The abdominal cavity is lined by peritoneum, and the areas between the major organs and the intestine are known as the peritoneal cavity. In the normal adult animal, serosal detail of abdominal viscera is demonstrated by intra-abdominal fat.

11.4 Increased radio-opacity of the peritoneal cavity and/or loss of visualisation of abdominal organs

All causes of increased intra-abdominal radio-opacity result in loss of serosal detail by obscuring intra-abdominal fat, which normally provides contrast with soft tissues. A diffuse and homogeneous increase in intra-abdominal opacity and loss of serosal detail is sometimes referred to as a "ground glass" appearance and is usually due to free abdominal fluid. Increase in opacity may also be patchy or mottled.

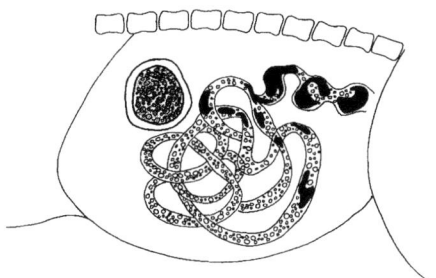

Figure 11.2 Ascites – loss of abdominal serosal detail and diffuse soft tissue (fluid) radio-opacity with only enteric gas, ingesta and faeces being visible. The abdomen is usually distended (cf. emaciation).

1. Generalised and homogeneous increase in radio-opacity of the peritoneal cavity
   a. Normal animal – suboptimal radiograph
      - underexposure
      - underdevelopment
      - kVp setting too high, leading to reduced contrast
      - scattered radiation if no grid has been used with a large abdomen
   b. Diffusely wet hair coat
   c. Normal puppy or kitten – lack of abdominal fat due to young age
   d. Emaciation and lack of abdominal fat – abdominal wall tucked inwards
   e. Peritoneal effusion – often abdominal distension too
      - ascites (hydroperitoneum) – Figure 11.2: right heart failure, liver disease, nephrotic syndrome, other causes of hypoproteinaemia, obstruction of the caudal vena cava (see 11.14.1), obstruction of lymphatics by neoplasia
      - haemoperitoneum: ruptured abdominal tumour, especially splenic haemangiosarcoma (especially German Shepherd dogs); coagulopathy – Warfarin poisoning, thrombocytopenia, disseminated intravascular coagulation, congenital bleeding disorders; trauma
      - uroabdomen – ruptured urinary bladder
      - bile peritonitis – ruptured gall bladder or bile duct
      - chylous effusion
      - cats – FIP
   f. After peritoneal dialysis or other intraperitoneal fluid administration.
2. Generalised but heterogeneous increase in radio-opacity of the peritoneal cavity

SMALL ANIMAL RADIOLOGICAL DIFFERENTIAL DIAGNOSIS

   a. Artefactual due to overlying wet or dirty hair coat
   b. Peritonitis
      - recent laparotomy
      - intestinal rupture – dilated intestinal loops and free gas in the peritoneal cavity are also likely; these findings warrant immediate surgical exploration
      - trauma (e.g. bite wounds, shot wounds, arrows)
      - pancreatitis
      - bile or urine peritonitis
      - small peritoneal effusion – see above for list of possible causes (ultrasonography is more sensitive than radiography for the detection of small effusions)
   c. Carcinomatosis
   d. Cats – steatitis – large amounts of intra-abdominal fat of increased opacity
      - vitamin E deficiency
      - fish diet.
3. Localised increase in radio-opacity of the peritoneal cavity – often heterogeneous
   a. Localised abdominal trauma
   b. Intestinal perforation walled off by mesentery
   c. Pancreatitis – right cranial quadrant of abdomen
   d. Peritoneal spread from adjacent neoplastic mass
   e. Walled-off abscess
   f. Mesenteric lymphadenopathy – the individual enlarged lymph nodes often blend together to create the appearance of an ill-defined opacity in the mid abdomen at the root of the mesentery
   g. Prostatitis
   h. Retained surgical swab.
4. Mineralised opacity in the peritoneal cavity
   a. Mineralised ingesta in the bowel
   b. Mineralised foreign bodies in the bowel
   c. Dystrophic or metastatic mineralisation of soft tissues (see 12.2.2)
      - neoplasia
      - chronic haematoma or abscess
      - hyperparathyroidism
   d. Barium or iodinated contrast medium leaking from perforated gut.

11.5 Decreased radio-opacity of the peritoneal cavity

1. Fat opacity – intra-abdominal lipoma; viscera will be displaced by the lipoma.
2. Gas opacity – a small volume of free gas is detected most accurately by taking a standing lateral radiograph or a left lateral recumbent VD projection with a horizontal beam. With both projections gas will rise to the highest part of the peritoneal cavity once the patient has maintained the position for a few minutes.
   a. Iatrogenic
      - post laparotomy
      - post peritoneal dialysis
      - post paracentesis (small amounts of gas)
   b. Perforated hollow viscus (trauma, neoplasia, ulceration) – increased radio-opacity may also be present due to peritonitis or free fluid
      - perforated stomach – large volume of gas causing abdominal distension and spontaneous pneumoperitoneogram effect
      - perforated small or large intestine
      - ruptured bladder with pneumocystogram performed
   c. Leakage of gas from emphysematous stomach, colon or uterus
   d. Entry of air through the abdominal wall
      - penetrating wound
      - around an abdominal drain or feeding tube
   e. Infection with gas-producing organisms; abdominal abscess
   f. Pneumothorax with a diaphragmatic rupture
   g. Leakage of gas through an intact, distended stomach wall.

11.6 Ultrasonographic examination of the peritoneal cavity

Use a sector or curvilinear transducer for optimal body contact. A frequency of 7.5 MHz may be used in cats and small to medium-sized dogs; 5 MHz may be required in larger dogs.

1. Peritoneal fluid: Fluid is generally anechoic, but may contain echoes depending on its cellular content or the presence of debris or small gas bubbles. Fluid surrounds and separates the abdominal organs, often enhancing visibility of these structures. In order to detect small quantities of fluid, search in dependent portions of the abdomen. In particular, look for small accumulations of fluid between the liver lobes, between the liver and the diaphragm, and around the urinary bladder (Figure 11.3). For differential diagnoses for the causes of peritoneal effusions, see 11.4.1.

11 OTHER ABDOMINAL STRUCTURES

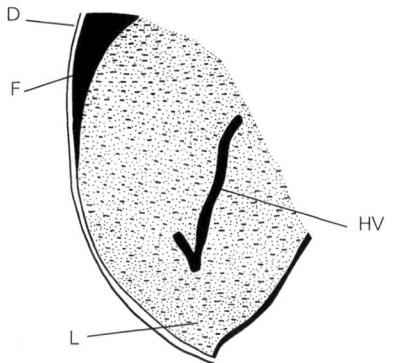

Figure 11.3 Mild ascites on ultrasonography – a small amount of anechoic fluid is seen between the liver and diaphragm. (D= diaphragm; F = free abdominal fluid trapped between the liver and the diaphragm; HV = hepatic vein; L = liver parenchyma.)

2. Free gas: This results in a poor-quality image and multiple artefacts (shadowing and reverberation). The effect of free gas on image quality can be reduced by altering the position of the patient and imaging from the dependent parts. Radiography is more sensitive than ultrasound for the detection of small quantities of free gas in the peritoneal cavity. For differential diagnoses for the causes of free gas, see 11.5.2.

RETROPERITONEAL SPACE

The retroperitoneal space (retroperitoneum) is the region of the abdomen ventral to the spine and dorsal to the intestines, lying outside the peritoneal cavity. The kidneys and prostate protrude into the peritoneal cavity from the retroperitoneal space and are covered by peritoneum. Retroperitoneal fat outlines the kidneys and ventral musculature of the spine. In fat animals, the deep circumflex arteries seen end-on ventral to the caudal lumbar vertebrae may simulate the appearance of mineral opacities such as ureteric calculi. The aorta, caudal vena cava and ureters are occasionally seen running through the retroperitoneal space in obese animals, but other retroperitoneal structures such as the adrenal glands and lymph nodes are not detectable when normal. The overall radiopacity of the retroperitoneal space should be similar to that of the peritoneal cavity.

11.7 Enlargement of the retroperitoneal space

1. Generalised retroperitoneal enlargement of fat opacity; normal visualisation of the kidneys and sublumbar musculature; ventral displacement of the intestines
   a. Normal, obese animal; the kidneys are clearly seen and occasionally blood vessels and ureters are visible.

2. Generalised retroperitoneal enlargement of soft tissue opacity; loss of visualisation of the kidneys and sublumbar musculature; ventral displacement of the intestines (Figure 11.4)
   a. Retroperitoneal haemorrhage
      • trauma to the kidneys
      • trauma to retroperitoneal blood vessels
      • coagulopathy
   b. Retroperitoneal urine
      • trauma to the ureters (rupture or avulsion from the kidneys or bladder); intravenous urography will demonstrate urine leakage

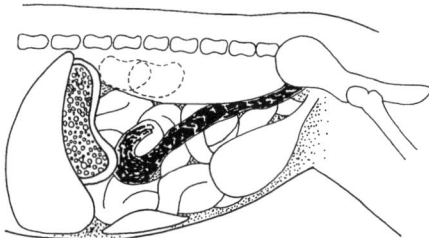

Figure 11.4 Generalised enlargement of the retroperitoneal space – loss of kidney outline (represented by dotted lines) and ventral displacement of intra-peritoneal viscera.

213

SMALL ANIMAL RADIOLOGICAL DIFFERENTIAL DIAGNOSIS

    c. Inflammation/abscessation
- migrating foreign body (e.g. grass awn); a periosteal reaction may be present along the ventral margins of lumbar vertebrae, especially L3 and L4 (DDx normal ill-defined ventral margins of these vertebrae where the diaphragmatic crura attach – see 5.4.4 and Figure 5.7)
- bite wounds

    d. Neoplasia of sublumbar muscle or lumbar vertebrae (the latter would also show bony changes).

3. Focal retroperitoneal enlargement of soft tissue opacity
   a. Renal mass (see 10.2.3, 10.2.4, 11.37.3 and Figure 11.16)
   b. Enlargement of the medial iliac (sublumbar) lymph nodes ventral to L6–7; ventral displacement +/– compression of the descending colon
      - lymphosarcoma
      - metastasis from malignant neoplasia in the hindquarters: prostate, urinary bladder, rectum and perianal region, pelvic canal, pelvic bones, hind legs, tail
   c. Abscess or focal inflammation
   d. Adrenal mass; mass medial or craniomedial to ipsilateral kidney; may show wispy mineralisation
      - adenocarcinoma
      - adenoma
      - phaeochromocytoma
   e. Mass or swelling of sublumbar muscle (see 11.7.2)
      - inflammation/abscessation
      - neoplasia of sublumbar muscle or lumbar vertebrae
   f. Soft tissue swelling associated with a vertebral lesion – look for bone changes too
      - spondylitis
      - spinal trauma
      - neoplasia.

11.8 Increased radio-opacity of the retroperitoneal space and/or loss of visualisation of the retroperitoneal structures

1. Soft tissue opacity of the retroperitoneal space with loss of visualisation of the kidneys and sublumbar musculature
   a. Overlying severe peritoneal effusion
   b. Retroperitoneal haemorrhage
      - trauma to the kidneys
      - trauma to retroperitoneal blood vessels
      - coagulopathy
   c. Retroperitoneal urine
      - trauma to the ureters (rupture or avulsion from the kidneys or bladder); intravenous urography will demonstrate urine leakage
   d. Inflammation/abscessation (see 11.7.2)
   e. Neoplasia of sublumbar muscle or lumbar vertebrae (see 11.7.2).

2. Focal mineralised opacity of the retroperitoneal space
   a. Artefactual due to blood vessels seen end-on
   b. Overlying intestinal contents
   c. Incidental mineralisation of adrenals in aged animals, more often in cats (bilateral, dumbbell-shaped)
   d. Ureteral calculus; intravenous urography needed to demonstrate its ureteral location, but the osmotic diuresis induced may flush the calculus into the bladder
   e. Mineralisation of a tumour (e.g. adrenal tumour); especially in dogs (unilateral, wispy or patchy mineralisation)
   f. Vertebral pathology with new bone extending into the sublumbar soft tissues.

11.9 Decreased radio-opacity of the retroperitoneal space

1. Fat opacity in the retroperitoneal space
   a. Excessive sublumbar fat in an obese animal
   b. Retroperitoneal lipoma.
2. Gas lucency in the retroperitoneal space (pneumoretroperitoneum)
   a. Extension of pneumomediastinum through the aortic or caval hiatus of the diaphragm
   b. Penetrating wound.

11.10 Ultrasonographic examination of the retroperitoneal space

The retroperitoneal space may be imaged from a ventral abdominal or flank approach. A high-frequency (7.5 MHz) sector or curvilinear transducer should be used.

11 OTHER ABDOMINAL STRUCTURES

1. Retroperitoneal fluid. Fluid is generally anechoic but may contain a variable number of echoes depending on the presence of cells, debris and/or gas bubbles. Fluid accumulations may be throughout the retroperitoneal space or localised. For differential diagnoses for the causes of retroperitoneal fluid accumulation, see 11.7.2.

A migrating foreign body may be seen as a hyperechoic structure, with or without acoustic shadowing, within an accumulation of fluid.

2. Retroperitoneal mass
   a. Tumour
   b. Granuloma
   c. Abscess
   d. Haematoma.

11.11 Ultrasonographic examination of the lymph nodes in the retroperitoneal space

The medial iliac lymph nodes lie close to the abdominal aorta and caudal vena cava at their caudal bifurcation. They may be visible in normal animals as well defined, elongated, hypoechoic structures. The lumbar lymph nodes extend along the paralumbar tissues, but are usually only recognised ultrasonographically when enlarged.

1. Enlargement of lymph nodes – tend to become more rounded as they enlarge, but they may also become irregular in shape and heterogeneous in echogenicity.
   a. "Reactive" enlargement, in response to an inflammatory lesion in the pelvis or hindquarters
   b. Metastasis from malignant neoplasia in the hindquarters (see 11.7.3 for list of differential diagnoses)
   c. Multicentric lymphosarcoma.

11.12 Ultrasonographic examination of the abdominal aorta and caudal vena cava

The aorta lies dorsal and to the left of the caudal vena cava in the retroperitoneal space. Pulsations of both vessels may be evident, due to referred aortic pulsation affecting the caudal vena cava. The caudal vena cava is more easily compressed by pressure from the transducer. Doppler ultrasound allows definitive differentiation between the two.

1. Vascular intraluminal mass
   a. Thrombus
   b. Neoplastic invasion from an adjacent mass.
2. Vascular narrowing
   a. Extrinsic compression by a mass.

LIVER

Radiographic examination of the liver is often unrewarding because the gall bladder, bile ducts and hepatic vessels are not detectable on plain radiographs and parenchymal changes can be suspected only when obvious focal or generalised hepatomegaly or reduction in liver size is present. Assessment of liver size is best made on a right lateral recumbent radiograph by noting the position of the stomach axis (see Chapter 9) and the thickness of the liver between the diaphragm and abdominal structures caudal to the liver. The ventral and caudal edges of the two medial liver lobes are well visualised on lateral radiographs, forming a sharp and acute angle (the hepatic angle) near the costal arch. In deep-chested dogs the hepatic angle lies cranial to the costal arch; in other breeds and in cats it protrudes a variable distance beyond the costal arch. In dogs with pendulous abdomens, or if there is caudal displacement of the liver due to thoracic expansion, the hepatic angle will be located more caudally.

Generalised hepatomegaly leads to an increase in the hepatic angle, with rounding of the liver margins and caudal displacement of the adjacent abdominal organs, especially the stomach. The position of the diaphragm, stomach and spleen allows evaluation of the size of the left side of the liver. Assessment of the right side is more difficult on the lateral radiograph although gross enlargement will displace the right kidney, pylorus and cranial duodenum caudally. Right-sided hepatomegaly is better seen on VD radiographs, displacing the stomach to the left.

SMALL ANIMAL RADIOLOGICAL DIFFERENTIAL DIAGNOSIS

11.13 Displacement of the liver

1. Cranial displacement of the liver
   a. Loss of integrity of the diaphragm
      - diaphragmatic hernia or rupture
      - peritoneopericardial hernia
   b. Enlargement of other abdominal organs, including advanced pregnancy
   c. Severe ascites.
2. Caudal displacement of the liver – expansion of the thorax
   a. Iatrogenic overinflation of lungs for thoracic radiography
   b. Pulmonary emphysema
   c. Large pleural effusion
   d. Large intrathoracic mass.
3. Displacement of a single liver lobe – lobar rupture or torsion.

11.14 Variations in liver size

Liver enlargement may be due to primary liver disease, or secondary to disease in another organ system. Enlargement usually has to be severe and/or extensive before changes can be detected on radiographs. Generalised changes in liver size may be inferred from the position of the stomach (see 9.2).

1. Generalised liver enlargement (usually causes left-caudal gastric displacement) (Figure 11.5)
   a. Venous congestion
      - right-sided heart failure (see 7.12 and Figure 7.7)
      - pericardial effusion or constrictive pericarditis reducing right atrial filling (cardiac tamponade) (see 7.6.2 and Figure 7.4)
      - post caval syndrome (caudal vena cava occlusion); in humans, hepatic vein or inferior vena cava occlusion leading to passive congestion of the liver is termed Budd–Chiari syndrome, a term sometimes used also in veterinary medicine. Caudal vena cava occlusion may be caused by compression by a diaphragmatic rupture or hernia, heartworms, compression by thoracic masses, caudal vena cava thrombosis, cardiac neoplasia, congenital cardiac anomalies, pericardial diseases, migrating foreign bodies and adhesions or kinking of the caudal vena cava cranial to the liver (e.g. following trauma)

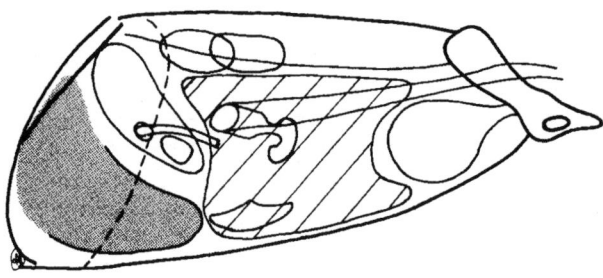
(a)

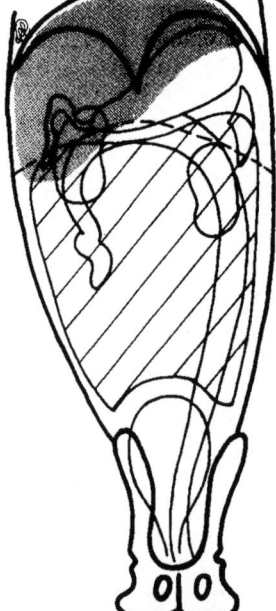
(b)

Figure 11.5 Generalised liver enlargement: (a) lateral view; (b) VD view. The body and pylorus of the stomach are displaced dorsally, caudally and to the left, and the ventral hepatic angle is rounded. In severe cases, other viscera may also be displaced caudally (reproduced with permission from *Textbook of Veterinary Diagnostic Radiology*, 3rd edition. Ed. D.E. Thrall, Philadelphia: W.B. Saunders).

11 OTHER ABDOMINAL STRUCTURES

    b. Cushing's disease (hyperadrenocorticism) – naturally occurring or iatrogenic
    c. Diabetes mellitus
    d. Neoplasia
- lymphosarcoma (usually with enlarged spleen +/– lymph nodes)
- haemangiosarcoma (may be also enlarged spleen +/– free fluid)
- other primary and metastatic tumours
- malignant histiocytosis – especially Bernese Mountain dogs, Golden and Flatcoated retrievers and Rottweilers

    e. Severe nodular hyperplasia
    f. Hepatitis
    g. Cirrhosis – in the early stages, hepatomegaly may be seen
    h. Cholestasis
    i. Storage diseases
    j. Amyloidosis
    k. Fungal infection*
    l. Cats – hepatic lipidosis
    m. Cats – FIP
    n. Cats – lymphocytic cholangitis.

2. Focal liver enlargement (see Figures 11.12 and 11.13)
    a. Focal neoplasia
- hepatoma – may be pedunculated and lie caudal to stomach
- various carcinomas (hepatocellular, cholangiocellular, adenocarcinoma)
- haemangiosarcoma
- lymphosarcoma – often with enlargement of the spleen, abdominal and thoracic lymph nodes and pulmonary changes too
- malignant histiocytosis – especially Bernese Mountain dogs, Golden and Flatcoated retrievers and Rottweilers; changes in other organs too, as with lymphosarcoma
- biliary cystadenoma
- metastatic neoplasia

    b. Intrahepatic abscess
    c. Biliary or parenchymal cyst
    d. Large area of hyperplastic/regenerative nodule formation
    e. Haematoma
    f. Granuloma
    g. Liver lobe torsion
    h. Biloma (biliary pseudocyst) – usually secondary to trauma or iatrogenic injury to the hepatic parenchyma
    i. Hepatic arteriovenous fistula.

3. Reduced liver size (Figure 11.6)
    a. Normal radiographic appearance, especially in deep-chested dogs

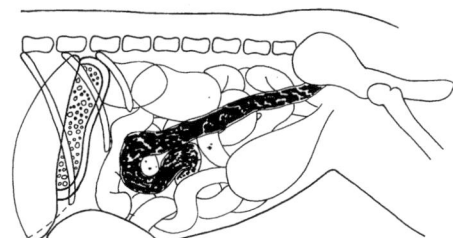

Figure 11.6 Reduced liver size. The gastric axis is displaced cranially and may slope cranioventrally. Other viscera also lie more cranially than normal, especially the spleen and small intestine.

    b. Diaphragmatic rupture or hernia with liver entering the thorax
    c. Portosystemic shunt – usually occurs in young animals due to anomalous development of vessels associated with the hepatic portal vein; less often acquired due to portal hypertension as a result of chronic liver disease (acquired shunts are rare in cats)
- intra-hepatic shunts: large breeds more often affected than small breeds, especially Irish Wolfhound and Golden Retriever; usually a persistent ductus venosus (left-sided) between the intrahepatic portions of the hepatic portal vein and the caudal vena cava; right-sided and central shunts are sometimes seen
- extrahepatic shunts: affect small dog breeds and cats more often than large breeds; between the extrahepatic portions of the hepatic portal vein and caudal vena cava
- porto-azygos shunts between the hepatic portal vein and the azygos vein
- multiple extrahepatic portosystemic shunts – opening of normally non-functional portocaval and porto-azygos connections – may develop secondary to congenital or acquired liver disease

    d. Cirrhosis in its later stages – concurrent ascites is common
    e. Idiopathic hepatic fibrosis – young dogs, especially German Shepherd dog; ascites common.

Portosystemic shunts may be associated with renomegaly, urinary tract calculi and haematogenous osteomyelitis. Ultrasonography may be used to diagnose shunts, especially those

SMALL ANIMAL RADIOLOGICAL DIFFERENTIAL DIAGNOSIS

located intrahepatically. Alternatively, radiographic contrast studies of the portal vein can be undertaken (*portal venography*, see 11.17).

11.15 Variations in liver shape

1. Rounding of the caudoventral liver margin (the hepatic angle)
   a. Any disease causing generalised liver enlargement (see 11.14.1 and Fig. 11.5).
2. Irregularity of the liver margins
   a. Any disease causing focal liver enlargement
   b. Any lesion near the liver surface
   c. Cirrhosis
   d. In normal cats, a full gall bladder may protrude ventral to the liver margin and be highlighted against falciform fat as a smooth, rounded structure.

11.16 Variations in liver radio-opacity

1. Branching mineralised radio-opacities in the liver
   a. Choledocholithiasis (biliary tree mineralisation)
   b. Incidental hepatic mineralisation mainly in older, obese dogs – especially the Yorkshire Terrier (possibly due to chronic hepatopathy).
2. Focal, unstructured or shell-like mineralised radio-opacities in the liver
   a. Cholelithiasis (gallstones) – right cranioventral liver shadow; those in the common bile duct are located near the pyloroduodenal junction
   b. Chronic cholecystitis, gall bladder neoplasia or cystic hyperplasia of the gall bladder wall
   c. Chronic hepatopathy
   d. Mineralised neoplasia (e.g. extraskeletal osteosarcoma)
   e. Chronic abscess, granuloma or haematoma
   f. Mineralised regenerative nodules
   g. Parasitic cysts.
3. Metallic radio-opacities in the liver – swallowed needles and wires may perforate the gastric wall and become embedded in the liver; usually incidental findings.
4. Fat radio opacity in the liver
   a. Lipoma forming between liver lobes or around gall bladder.
5. Branching or linear gas lucencies in the liver
   a. Gas in the biliary tree (pneumobilia)
      - previous surgery
      - reflux of gas from the duodenum due to an incompetent sphincter of Oddi
      - chronic bile duct obstruction with erosion into the duodenum
      - emphysematous cholecystitis/cholangitis – especially patients with diabetes mellitus
   b. Gas in the hepatic portal venous system (warrants a grave prognosis)
      - gastric torsion
      - necrotising gastroenteritis
      - clostridial infections
      - secondary to functional ileus
      - secondary to air embolisation during pneumocystography or pneumoperitoneography.
6. Focal, patchy or streaky gas lucencies in the liver
   a. Hepatic abscess
      - penetrating injury
      - haematogenous infection
   b. Infection with gas-producing organisms
      - emphysematous cholecystitis in association with diabetes mellitus or clostridial infections
      - haematogenous infection
      - spread from an adjacent organ
   c. Vascular compromise due to liver lobe entrapment.

11.17 Hepatic contrast studies

Contrast studies for the liver have largely been replaced by ultrasonography, and screening for portosystemic shunts can also be performed using scintigraphy. Portal venography for the diagnosis of shunts remains the most widely performed hepatic contrast technique (Figure 11.7).

Portal venography (operative portography)

This technique is used for the detection of portosystemic shunts and may be performed using equipment readily available in general practice. After laparotomy, a sterile intravenous catheter is placed into the splenic vein or a large mesenteric vein and directed towards the liver. A lateral abdominal radiograph is exposed at the end of a rapid injection of iodinated contrast medium at a dose of 1 ml/kg body weight. Shunting vessels are usually well outlined, with sparse or absent opacification of normal hepatic vessels. An additional injection for a ventrodorsal radi-

11 OTHER ABDOMINAL STRUCTURES

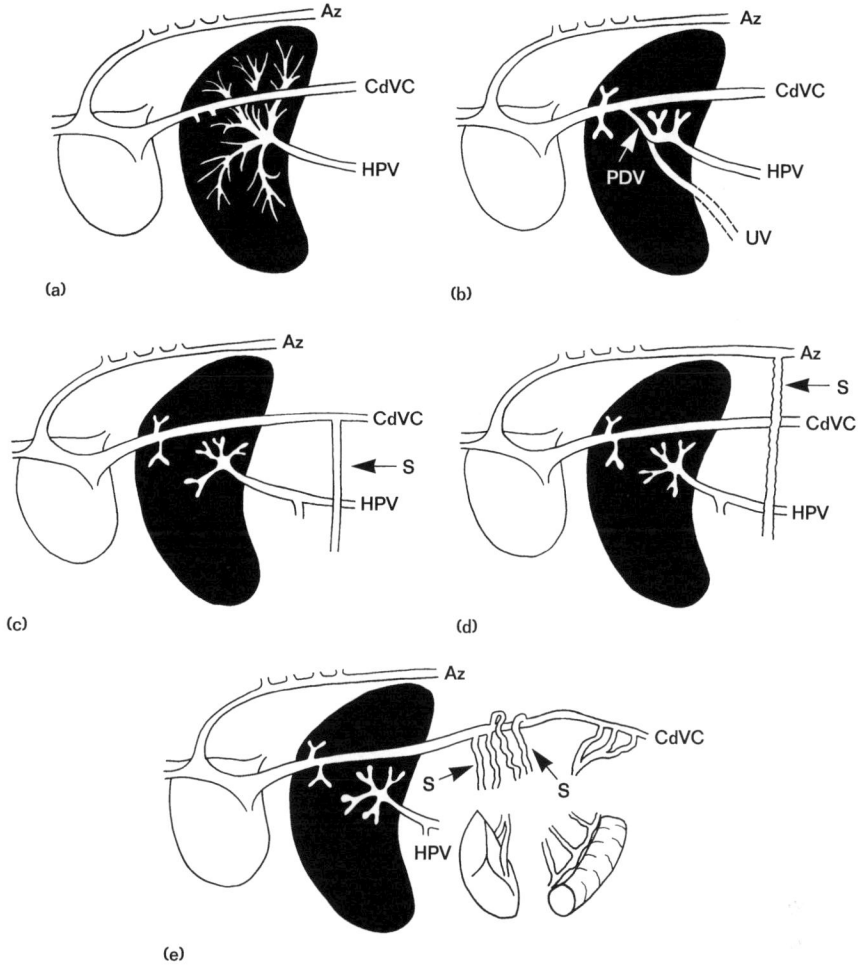

Figure 11.7 (a) Normal portal venogram – the hepatic portal vein enters the liver and branches extensively within the parenchyma. (b) Intrahepatic portosystemic shunt – patent ductus venosus. Most of the blood entering the liver in the hepatic portal vein passes directly to the caudal vena cava through the shunting vessel. The position of the foetal umbilical vein which gave rise to the ductus venosus is indicated. (c) Extrahepatic portosystemic shunt – an anomalous vessel carries blood from the viscera directly into the caudal vena cava, bypassing the hepatic portal vein and liver. Greatly reduced amounts of blood enter the liver. (d) Portoazygos shunt – similar to (c) but the anomalous vessel enters the azygos vein and not the caudal vena cava. (e) Multiple acquired extrahepatic portosystemic shunts – liver disease results in portal hypertension, reducing the amount of blood entering the liver via the hepatic portal vein and encouraging the opening up of collateral blood vessels in the mesentery. (Az = azygos vein; CdVC = caudal vena cava; HPV = hepatic portal vein; PDV = patent ductus venosus; S = shunting vessel; UV = foetal umbilical vein, which atrophies after birth.)

ograph enables more accurate localisation of the shunt. Shunts whose caudal limit lies cranial to T13 are usually intrahepatic; those whose caudal limits extend to T13 or beyond are likely to be extrahepatic. Surgical partial ligation of a single extrahepatic shunt can easily be performed; surgical correction of intrahepatic shunts is much more difficult. Cirrhosis and diffuse hepatic vascular diseases result in attenuation of intrahepatic portal circulation and the formation of numerous tortuous mesenteric collateral vessels.

Splenoportography

Also for the detection of portosystemic shunts. Contrast medium is injected directly into the splenic parenchyma either via laparotomy or percutaneously; however, this technique is associated with greater patient morbidity than portal venography.

Cholecystography
Cholecystography allows visualisation of the gall bladder and common bile duct, and assessment of patency of the latter. Contrast medium may be administered orally, intravenously or percutaneously using ultrasound guidance. Rarely performed nowadays.

Coeliography (peritoneography)
The main indications of this technique are for assessment of the liver when abdominal detail is poor, and for the integrity of the diaphragm. Coeliography uses negative or positive contrast medium with conventional radiographic positioning and erect, horizontal beam radiography. Administration of a large volume of air is contraindicated if the diaphragm is not intact.

Coeliac or cranial mesenteric arteriography
Mainly for investigation of arteriovenous malformations.

11.18 Ultrasonographic examination of the liver

The patient should be fasted before ultrasonographic examination of the liver, although free access to water may be given. The liver is usually imaged from a ventral abdominal approach; the transducer is placed just caudal to the xiphisternum and angled craniodorsally to image the liver. Sweeps of the sound beam are made throughout the organ in at least two planes of section. If the liver is very small, it may be preferable to examine it from a lateral intercostal approach, although it is then more difficult to ensure that the entire organ is inspected. A right intercostal approach can be particularly useful for evaluation of the caudate liver lobe, the caudal vena cava and portal vein, and for the detection of any anomalous shunting vessels.

11.19 Normal ultrasonographic appearance of the liver

The normal liver is moderately echoic with an even, granular texture (Figure 11.8). The lobes should be smooth in outline and sharply pointed. The gall bladder appears rounded or pear-shaped, depending on the plane of section, and lies just to the right of the midline.

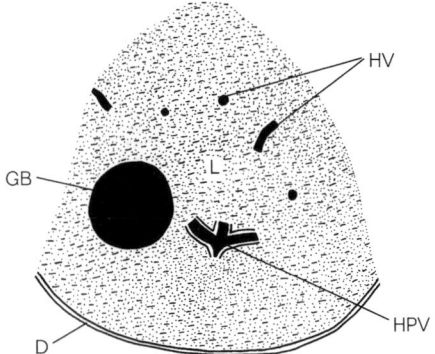

Figure 11.8 Normal liver ultrasonogram (see text for description). (D = diaphragm; GB = gall bladder; HV = hepatic veins; HPV = hepatic portal veins at the orta hepatis – echogenic walls; L = normal liver parenchyma (hypoechoic, coarsely granular).)

The walls of the gall bladder should be thin and smooth, and the contents are usually anechoic. The cystic duct may occasionally be seen leading from the gall bladder, especially in cats. The common bile duct runs caudally, ventral to the portal vein, but is not usually visible in normal animals. Intrahepatic bile ducts are not seen in the normal animal.

The portal vein enters the liver at the *porta hepatis*, where it branches. Intrahepatic veins are seen as anechoic tubes; the portal veins have echogenic borders, while the hepatic veins for the most part do not. The larger hepatic veins may be followed to their junction with the caudal vena cava. Intrahepatic arteries are not usually seen in the normal animal.

11.20 Hepatic parenchymal abnormalities on ultrasonography

1. Irregular hepatic margins on ultrasonography
   a. Neoplasia
   b. Fibrosis (irrespective of primary cause)
   c. Nodular hyperplasia
   d. Abscess
   e. Granuloma
   f. Cyst
   g. Haematoma.
2. Focal hepatic lesions on ultrasonography (single or multiple). There is wide variation in the ultrasonographic appearance of focal liver lesions, and the sonographic features are not usually specific for a particular disease process. The lists below therefore give the most probable differentials for a given ultrasonographic appearance.

11 OTHER ABDOMINAL STRUCTURES

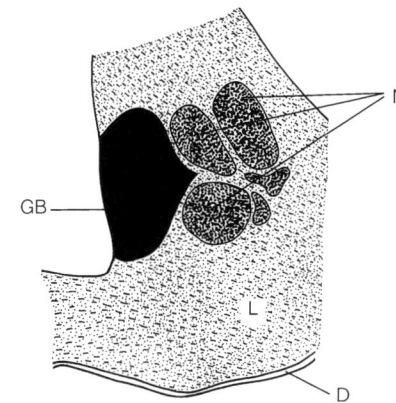

Figure 11.9 Focal hypoechoic liver nodules on ultrasonography. (D = diaphragm; GB = gall bladder deformed by adjacent nodules; L = normal liver parenchyma; N = hypoechoic liver nodules.)

  a. Anechoic
     - biliary cyst or pseudocyst
     - parenchymal cyst (may be associated with polycystic kidney disease in cats)
     - peliosis hepatis
  b. Hypoechoic (Figure 11.9)
     - primary hepatic or metastatic neoplasia
     - lymphosarcoma
     - nodular hyperplasia
     - abscess
     - granuloma
     - necrosis/acute infarction
     - hepatocutaneous syndrome
  c. Isoechoic/hyperechoic
     - primary hepatic or metastatic neoplasia
     - nodular hyperplasia
     - abscess
     - granuloma
     - organised infarct
     - acute parenchymal haemorrhage
  d. Complex
     - haemorrhagic or infected cyst
     - primary hepatic or metastatic neoplasia
     - abscess
     - organising haematoma.
     - telangiectasis
3. Diffuse hepatic changes on ultrasonography. In order to appreciate diffuse changes in echogenicity, the echogenicity of the liver should be compared with that of the renal cortex and the spleen at the same tissue depth and with the same machine settings. The normal liver is of the same echogenicity or slightly more echoic than the normal renal cortex, and slightly less echoic than the normal spleen.
  a. Increased echogenicity, normal architecture (portal vein margins tend to become obscured, sound attenuation may be increased)
     - chronic hepatitis
     - fatty infiltration
     - steroid hepatopathy
     - fibrosis (irrespective of primary cause)
     - lymphosarcoma
  b. Decreased echogenicity, normal architecture (portal vein margins tend to be enhanced)
     - acute hepatitis
     - diffuse infiltrative disease (e.g. lymphosarcoma)
     - passive congestion (usually see distended hepatic veins)
  c. Normal echogenicity, normal architecture
     - normal
     - acute hepatitis
     - toxic hepatopathy
     - diffuse infiltrative disease
  d. Disordered architecture
     - primary hepatic or widespread metastatic neoplasia
     - fibrosis with regenerative nodules
     - hepatocutaneous syndrome.

11.21 Biliary tract abnormalities on ultrasonography

1. Thickened gall bladder wall on ultrasonography
   a. Smooth
      - contracted gall bladder
      - oedema
      - cholecystitis
   b. Irregular
      - mucosal hyperplasia (incidental in middle-aged or older dogs)
      - neoplasia.
2. Echoes within the lumen of the gall bladder on ultrasonography
   a. Slice thickness artefact
   b. Sludge (in the dependent part of the gall bladder)
      - often seen in normal dogs
      - fasting
      - cholestasis
      - cholecystitis
   c. Choleliths (in the dependent part of the gall bladder; variable acoustic shadowing depending on mineral content)

SMALL ANIMAL RADIOLOGICAL DIFFERENTIAL DIAGNOSIS

   d. Mucosal hyperplasia
   e. Mucocoele
   f. Neoplasia.
3. Dilation of the biliary tract on ultrasonography
   a. Gall bladder alone
      - fasted/anorectic
      - early extrahepatic biliary obstruction
      - mucocoele
   b. Gall bladder and other parts of the biliary tract
      - extrahepatic biliary obstruction – e.g. due to pancreatitis, pancreatic neoplasia, choleliths, sclerosing cholangitis, lymphadenopathy (the first sign of obstruction is dilation of the gall bladder and cystic duct; then the common bile duct dilates; then the extra- and intrahepatic ducts dilate. The common bile duct may remain distended even after an obstruction is removed).

11.22 Hepatic vascular abnormalities on ultrasonography

1. Distension of hepatic veins and caudal vena cava on ultrasonography (often with ascites)
   a. Congestive heart failure
   b. Obstruction of caudal vena cava between the heart and the liver
      - thrombus
      - neoplasm
      - adhesions.
2. Distension of the hepatic portal vein on ultrasonography
   a. Portal hypertension secondary to liver disease (may see secondary shunting vessels, ascites)
   b. Obstruction of the portal vein near the *porta hepatis*
      - thrombus
      - neoplasm
      - adhesions
   c. Hepatic arteriovenous fistula.
3. Anomalous blood vessel(s) on ultrasonography
   a. Within the liver parenchyma
      - congenital intrahepatic portosystemic shunt
      - hepatic arteriovenous fistula
   b. Outside the liver parenchyma
      - congenital extrahepatic portosystemic shunt
      - acquired portosystemic shunts (usually multiple vessels)
      - arteriovenous fistula.

SPLEEN

The spleen in dogs is a proportionately larger organ than in cats. The spleen is triangular in cross-section and the head of the spleen lies in the left cranial abdomen between the fundus of the stomach cranially and the left kidney caudally (if the liver is small and the stomach is empty it may abut the diaphragm). It is visible on a VD radiograph in both dogs and cats as a triangular structure adjacent to the left body wall. The body and tail of the spleen are more variable in location, and in dogs are usually seen in the ventral abdomen on the lateral radiograph, lying caudal to the liver, especially on a right lateral recumbent radiograph. The body and tail of the spleen are rarely seen in cats, unless enlarged. The borders of the spleen should be smooth and sharply defined. Splenic size is very variable radiographically and so evaluation of size is very subjective. Splenic size increases with barbiturate anaesthesia.

11.23 Absence of the splenic shadow

1. Normal variation – the spleen is not usually seen on the lateral view in cats, and is less likely to be seen in a left lateral recumbent radiograph in dogs than in a right lateral. It is reliably seen on VD views in both dogs and cats
2. Previous splenectomy.
3. Displacement through a diaphragmatic or body wall rupture or hernia.

11.24 Variations in location of the tail of the spleen

The head of the spleen is attached to the stomach by the gastrosplenic ligament and will not be displaced unless rupture of the ligament or gastric displacement have occurred. The tail of the spleen is not usually seen in cats on the lateral radiograph.

11 OTHER ABDOMINAL STRUCTURES

1. Cranial displacement of the tail of the spleen
   a. Normal cranial location in deep-chested breeds of dog
   b. Displacement by caudal abdominal organomegaly
   c. Small liver, allowing spleen to slide cranially
   d. Diaphragmatic rupture or hernia
   e. Pericardioperitoneal diaphragmatic hernia.
2. Caudal displacement of the tail of the spleen
   a. Gastric distension (see 9.3.4 and 5)
   b. Enlarged liver
   c. Gastric mass.
3. Ventral displacement of the spleen
   a. Ventral body wall rupture
   b. Gastric dilation/volvulus.

11.25 Variations in splenic size and shape

Due to the normal wide variation in splenic size, substantial change must be present before it may be considered abnormal. An occasional variant is the development of ectopic splenic tissue giving a segmented appearance to the splenic shadow.
1. Generalised splenic enlargement with a normal shape and smooth outline
   a. Normal variant; especially in the German Shepherd dog and Greyhound
   b. Passive splenic congestion (spleen may be obscured by ascites)
      - right heart failure
      - portal hypertension
      - sedative, tranquillising and anaesthetic agents, especially barbiturates and phenothiazines
      - gastric dilation/volvulus involving the spleen (spleen in an abnormal location)
      - splenic thrombosis
      - splenic torsion (spleen C-shaped or in abnormal location)
   c. Neoplasia
      - lymphosarcoma (liver +/- lymph nodes also usually enlarged)
      - malignant histiocytosis; especially Bernese Mountain dog, Golden and Flatcoated retrievers and Rottweilers; concurrent pulmonary and hepatic masses and lymphadenopathy too
      - acute and chronic leukaemias
      - systemic mastocytosis
      - multiple myeloma
      - haemangioma/haemangiosarcoma/metastatic neoplasia more often results in an irregular liver outline
   d. Inflammatory splenomegaly – many causes, including
      - penetrating wounds
      - migrating foreign bodies
      - septicaemia and bacteraemia
      - toxoplasmosis*
      - salmonellosis
      - mycobacteriosis
      - brucellosis
      - leishmaniasis *
      - fungal infections*
      - ehrlichiosis*
      - babesiosis*
      - haemobartonellosis
      - infectious canine hepatitis
      - cats – FIP
   e. Chronic anaemia – splenic hyperplasia
   f. Chronic infection – splenic hyperplasia
   g. Severe nodular lymphoid hyperplasia (liver margins may be smooth or irregular)
   h. Extramedullary haemopoiesis
   i. Toxaemia
   j. Amyloidosis
   k. Systemic lupus erythematosus (SLE)
   l. Cats – hypereosinophilic syndrome.
2. Diffusely enlarged, C-shaped spleen
   a. Splenic torsion – ascites may obscure the spleen.
3. Focal or irregular splenic enlargement; splenic mass (see 11.37.2 and Figure 11.15)
   a. Neoplasia
      - haemangiosarcoma (especially German Shepherd dog); spleen may be obscured by abdominal fluid from splenic haemorrhage
      - haemangioma – as above
      - malignant histiocytosis; especially Bernese Mountain dog, Golden and Flatcoated retrievers and Rottweilers; concurrent pulmonary and hepatic masses and lymphadenopathy too
      - leiomyosarcoma
      - fibrosarcoma
      - other primary and metastatic tumours
   b. Nodular lymphoid hyperplasia
   c. Splenic haematoma
      - spontaneous
      - traumatic
      - secondary to splenic neoplasia
   d. Splenic abscess.

SMALL ANIMAL RADIOLOGICAL DIFFERENTIAL DIAGNOSIS

4. Reduction in splenic size
   a. Severe dehydration
   b. Severe shock.

11.26 Variations in splenic radio-opacity

Variations in splenic opacity are rare.
1. Mineralisation of the spleen
   a. Mineralisation of chronic haematoma or abscess – may be shell-like marginal mineralisation
   b. Histoplasmosis*
   c. Extra-skeletal osteosarcoma.
2. Gas lucency in the spleen – emphysema due to gas-forming organisms, secondary to splenic torsion.

11.27 Ultrasonographic examination of the spleen

The spleen lies superficially within the abdomen, so a high frequency transducer (7.5 MHz) may be used. The head of the spleen lies close to the gastric fundus in the left cranial abdomen. The body and tail of the spleen can be followed along the left flank or running obliquely across the floor of the abdomen.

11.28 Normal ultrasonographic appearance of the spleen

The spleen should be smooth in outline with a dense, even echotexture. The echogenicity of the spleen is usually greater that that of the liver at the same depth and machine settings. Splenic veins may be seen leaving the spleen at the hilus.

11.29 Ultrasonographic abnormalities of the spleen

1. Focal splenic parenchymal lesions on ultrasonography (Figure 11.10). Focal lesions may be single or multiple, and often distort the normal smooth outline of the spleen. They have a very variable ultrasonographic appearance, which is rarely specific for a particular disease process. The lists given below therefore give only the most probable differential diagnoses
   a. Anechoic/hypoechoic/isoechoic focal lesions

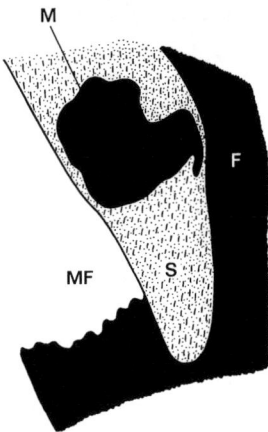

Figure 11.10 Splenic mass on ultrasonography. The splenic outline would be obscured radiographically by the abdominal effusion, but this enhances the ultrasonographic examination. (F = free abdominal fluid; M = focal splenic mass, deforming the outline of the spleen slightly; MF = mesenteric fat; S = tail of spleen.)

   - primary splenic neoplasia
   - metastatic neoplasia
   - lymphosarcoma
   - nodular lymphoid hyperplasia
   - small splenic haematoma
   - necrosis/acute infarct
   - splenic abscess
   - granuloma (e.g. histoplasmosis*)
   - splenic cyst (uncommon)

   b. Hyperechoic focal lesions
   - primary splenic neoplasia
   - metastatic neoplasia
   - myelolipomata
   - splenic abscess (with gas)
   - granuloma (with calcification)
   - organised infarct
   - acute intraparenchymal haemorrhage

   c. Complex lesions
   - primary splenic neoplasia
   - metastatic neoplasia
   - lymphosarcoma (less common)
   - splenic haematoma
   - splenic abscess
   - telangiectasia.

2. Diffuse splenic parenchymal changes on ultrasonography
   a. Reduced/normal echogenicity, normal architecture
   - passive splenic congestion (for differential diagnoses see 11.25.1)
   - acute systemic inflammatory diseases

11 OTHER ABDOMINAL STRUCTURES

- diffuse neoplastic infiltration
- arterial thrombosis
  b. Increased echogenicity, normal architecture
  - chronic congestion
  - chronic inflammatory diseases
  - chronic granulomatous diseases (e.g. histoplasmosis*)

  c. Disturbed architecture – hypoechoic
  - lymphosarcoma ("Swiss cheese" appearance)
  - splenic torsion ("starry sky" appearance)
  - arterial thrombosis.

PANCREAS

11.30 Pancreatic radiology

The normal pancreas is not visible radiographically due to its small size, although it can be imaged using ultrasound by experienced ultrasonographers.

Inflammatory or neoplastic pancreatic disease produces the radiographic appearance of focal peritonitis with or without a mild mass effect, in the right cranial quadrant of the abdomen. The adjacent descending duodenum may be displaced laterally and show focal, gas-dilated ileus, often assuming a C-shaped course with thickened and corrugated walls (barium may help in assessment of the duodenum) (Figure 11.11). Pancreatic mineralisation is rare, but may be caused by chronic pancreatitis, neoplasia or fat necrosis.

11.31 Ultrasonographic examination of the pancreas

The patient should ideally be fasted overnight to ensure that the stomach is empty, but may be allowed access to water. Acute cases are usually vomiting, so the stomach is often already empty. Ultrasonography of the pancreas should be scheduled before barium contrast studies, as barium will interfere with passage of the sound beam.

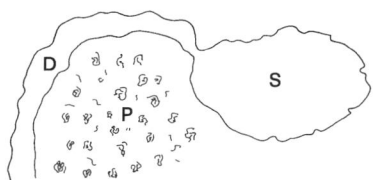

Figure 11.11 Pancreatic disease (detail) – VD view of barium study. The duodenum is dilated and spastic and follows a curved, "C-shaped" course. There is a mottled radio-opacity suggestive of peritonitis in the region of the pancreas (D = duodenum; P = pancreas, S = stomach)

In order to image the pancreas, a high-frequency (7.5 MHz or higher) transducer is essential. The animal may be placed on its right side to encourage gas to rise away from the area of interest in the right cranial abdomen; some operators prefer to perform the examination with the dog in dorsal recumbency. The stomach, descending duodenum and right kidney should be located as landmarks. The right limb of the pancreas lies dorsomedial to the descending duodenum and ventral to the right kidney, while the left limb of the pancreas lies caudal to the stomach and cranial to the transverse colon.

11.32 Normal ultrasonographic appearance of the pancreas

The pancreas is an ill-defined organ which may not be recognised if imaging conditions are not optimal. It is moderately echoic, usually intermediate in echogenicity between the liver and spleen, and of even echotexture. The pancreaticoduodenal vein running through the length of the right limb of the pancreas may aid in identification.

11.33 Ultrasonographic abnormalities of the pancreas

1. Pancreas not seen on ultrasonography
   a. Low-resolution imaging system
   b. Operator inexperience
   c. Patient factors such as obesity, gastrointestinal gas, panting, abdominal rigidity/pain
   d. Pancreatic atrophy.
2. Focal pancreatic lesions on ultrasonography
   a. Inflammatory pseudocysts
   b. Pancreatic abscess
   c. Small neoplasm (e.g. insulinoma)
   c. Nodular changes secondary to chronic pancreatitis
   e. Congenital cysts/retention cysts

225

SMALL ANIMAL RADIOLOGICAL DIFFERENTIAL DIAGNOSIS

3. Diffuse pancreatic disturbance on ultrasonography. Usually includes enlargement of the pancreas, of a heterogeneous, hypoechoic echogenicity and texture. There may be associated abdominal fluid, thickening and reduced motility of adjacent stomach and descending duodenum, and/or evidence of biliary obstruction. Inflammatory and neoplastic disease cannot be differentiated on ultrasonographic criteria alone
   a. Pancreatitis
   b. Pancreatic neoplasia
   c. Pancreatic oedema.

ADRENAL GLANDS

11.34 Adrenal gland radiology

The adrenal glands lie in the retroperitoneal space medial or craniomedial to the ipsilateral kidney. The normal adrenal gland is too small to be visible radiographically. Large adrenal masses be sometimes be recognised and may displace the adjacent kidney caudally or laterally (see 11.36.4 and Figure 11.14). Adrenal tumours often show wispy mineralisation.

11.35 Ultrasonographic examination of the adrenal glands

If the adrenal glands are to be identified ultrasonographically, it is essential that a high-frequency transducer is used (7.5 MHz) and that the operator has a clear understanding of the vascular anatomy of the retroperitoneal space. A ventral abdominal or flank approach may be used.

In the dog, the left adrenal gland is a bilobed or elongated oval shape, lying ventrolateral to the aorta, between the origins of the cranial mesenteric artery and the left renal artery. The right adrenal gland often has a triangular shape, and lies dorsolateral to the caudal vena cava, near the hilus of the right kidney. In the cat, both adrenal glands are a flattened oval shape. The adrenal glands are usually hypoechoic, but occasionally a hypoechoic cortex and a slightly more echoic medulla may be seen. The size of the adrenal glands in normal dogs and cats has been found to be variable and not proportional to bodyweight, although it has been reported that an adrenal gland greater than 2.4 cm long or 1 cm thick in a medium-sized dog may be considered enlarged. It is useful to compare the width to the length of the left adrenal. Hyperplasia and masses result in the width exceeding one third of the length.

1. Adrenal glands not seen on ultrasonography
   a. Low-resolution imaging system
   b. Poor image quality (e.g. bowel gas, obesity, panting)
   c. Inexperienced operator
   d. Adrenal atrophy (e.g. functional contralateral adrenal tumour)
   e. Previous adrenalectomy.
2. Adrenal glands enlarged on ultrasonography. Primary adrenal tumours may be uni- or bilateral, and of varying echogenicity. It is important to check ultrasonographically for invasion of adjacent blood vessels.
   a. Retention of normal basic shape
      - adrenal hyperplasia secondary to pituitary disease
      - small adrenal tumours
   b. Loss of normal basic shape
      - severe adrenal hyperplasia secondary to pituitary disease
      - adrenal tumour (adenoma, adenocarcinoma, phaeochromocytoma, metastasis).
3. Hyperechoic specks +/− acoustic shadowing
   a. Incidental, particularly in the cat
   b. Mineralisation of an adrenal tumour.

ABDOMINAL MASSES

Radiographic identification of the organ of origin of an abdominal mass is based upon location of the mass, displacement or compression of adjacent organs and absence of identification of normal organs. Further information may be obtained using other radiographic views, including horizontal beam projections, abdominal compression, radiographic and contrast techniques as well as ultrasonography. Ultrasonographic diagnosis is easiest if some normal organ tissue remains attached to the mass; if the entire organ is abnormal then diagnosis may be based on failure to identify a given organ.

11 OTHER ABDOMINAL STRUCTURES

The stomach, bladder and uterus are capable of considerable physiological enlargement, which should be differentiated from disease processes. The following sections are intended as a guide to the likely organ of origin of masses in various parts of the abdomen; having identified the likely organ(s) the relevant section of Chapters 9, 10 or 11 should be consulted for possible causes.

11.36 Cranial abdominal masses (largely within the costal arch)

1. Liver – the most cranial abdominal organ, lying immediately caudal to the diaphragm. The administration of barium may be helpful in showing the precise location of the stomach and by inference the caudal margin of the liver.
   a. Generalised liver enlargement (see 11.14.1 and Figure 11.5)
      Lateral view:
      - caudodorsal displacement of the pylorus: tilting of the gastric axis nearer to the horizontal plane
      - caudodorsal displacement of the cranial duodenal flexure
      - caudal displacement of small intestine

      VD view:
      - caudal and medial (left) displacement of the pylorus
      - caudal displacement of small intestine
   b. Right lateral or middle lobe enlargement (Figure 11.2)
      Lateral view:
      - caudodorsal displacement of the pylorus, small intestine and ascending colon
      - if large and pedunculated, the mass may lie caudal to the stomach mimicking a splenic mass

      VD view:
      - caudal and medial (left) displacement of the pylorus, small intestine and ascending colon
      - +/– caudal displacement of the right kidney
   c. Left lateral or middle lobe enlargement (Figure 11.3)
      Lateral view:
      - dorsal displacement of the fundus of the stomach
      - caudodorsal displacement of small intestine
      - may appear very similar to right-sided enlargement on this view, but differs on the VD view

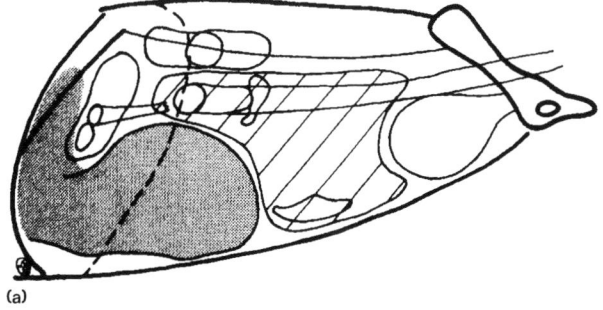

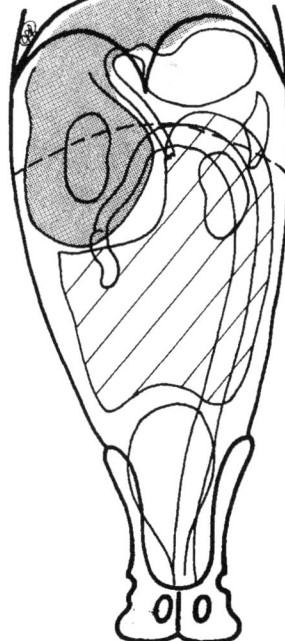

Figure 11.12 Right-sided liver enlargement: (a) lateral view; (b) VD view (reproduced with permission from *Textbook of Veterinary Diagnostic Radiology*, 3rd edition. Ed. D.E. Thrall, Philadelphia: W.B. Saunders).

SMALL ANIMAL RADIOLOGICAL DIFFERENTIAL DIAGNOSIS

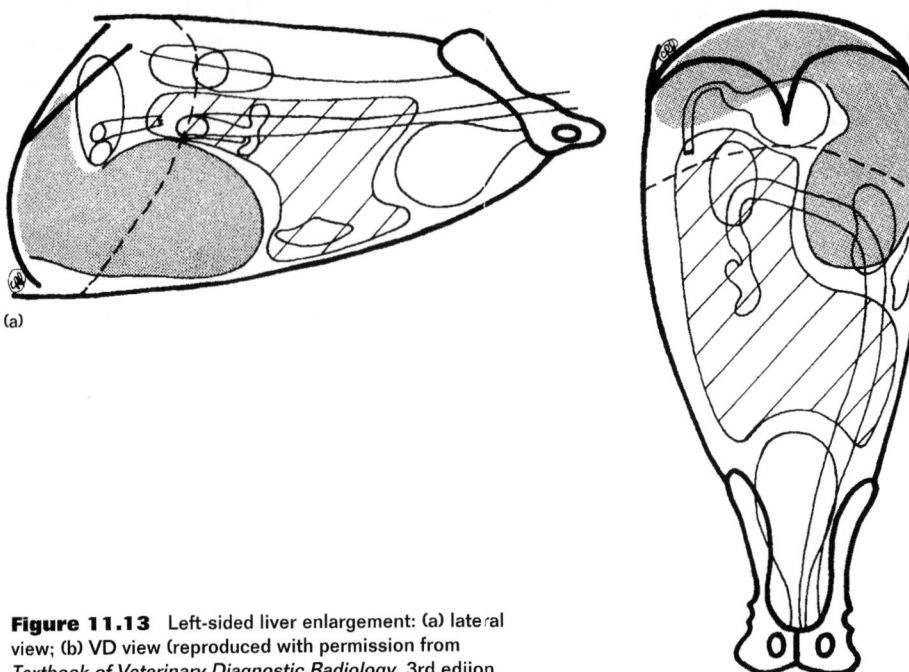

Figure 11.13 Left-sided liver enlargement: (a) lateral view; (b) VD view (reproduced with permission from *Textbook of Veterinary Diagnostic Radiology*, 3rd ediion. Ed. D.E. Thrall, Philadelphia: W.B. Saunders).

     VD view:
- caudal and medial (right) displacement of the fundus and small intestine
- caudal displacement of the head of the spleen
- +/− caudal displacement of the left kidney

  d. Central lobe enlargement
     Lateral view:
- caudodorsal displacement and indentation of the body of the stomach

     VD view:
- caudal displacement and indentation of the body of the stomach.

2. Stomach – lies immediately caudal to the liver
     Lateral view:
- caudal displacement of the small intestine, transverse colon and tail of spleen
- if the stomach is torsed, the spleen may also be displaced in other directions

     VD view:
- caudal displacement of the small intestine and transverse colon
- if the stomach is torsed, the spleen may also be displaced in other directions.

3. Pancreas – pancreatic masses are rarely seen as discrete soft tissue structures, but enlargement of the pancreas may be inferred by displacement of adjacent organs and localised loss of abdominal detail (see Fig 11.11)

  a. Right limb of pancreas
     Lateral view:
- ventral displacement of the duodenum

     VD view:
- lateral (right) displacement of the duodenum
- cranial and medial (left) displacement of the pylorus
- the pylorus and duodenum may form a wide, fixed "C" shape

  b. Left limb of pancreas
     Lateral view:
- ventral displacement of the duodenum
- caudal displacement of the transverse colon

     VD view:
- indentation of the caudal stomach wall
- caudal displacement of the small intestine and transverse colon.

4. Adrenal glands – lie in the retroperitoneal space craniomedial to the ipsilateral

11 OTHER ABDOMINAL STRUCTURES

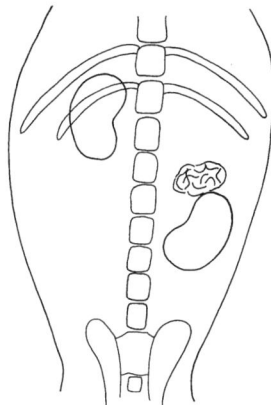

Figure 11.14 Left adrenal mass on the VD view – the ipsilateral kidney is displaced caudally and its cranial pole is often rotated outwards.

kidney. Adrenal masses which are visible radiographically are likely to be neoplastic, and are often mineralised
   Lateral view:
   • caudal displacement of the ipsilateral kidney, with ventral displacement of its cranial pole
   • ventral displacement of the small and large intestines
   VD view:
   • caudolateral displacement of the cranial pole of the ipsilateral kidney, so that the right kidney appears rotated anticlockwise and
   • the left kidney appears rotated clockwise, depending on which adrenal is enlarged (Figure 11.14).

11.37 Mid-abdominal masses

1. Liver – focal liver masses may occasionally extend into the mid-ventral abdomen, displacing the stomach cranially and mimicking other mid abdominal masses such as splenic lesions.
2. Spleen
   a. Head of spleen (proximal) – relatively immobile due to the gastrosplenic ligament
   Lateral view:
   • cranial displacement of the fundus of the stomach
   • caudal displacement of the left kidney
   • depending on the exact location of the mass within the spleen, small intestine may be displaced ventrally or dorsally

   VD view:
   • cranial displacement of the fundus of the stomach
   • caudal displacement of the left kidney
   • caudal and medial (right) displacement of the small intestine and adjacent parts of transverse and descending colon
   b. Body and tail (distal) – these portions of the spleen are highly mobile and masses can be seen in a variety of mid-abdominal locations (Figure 11.15)
   Lateral view:
   • dorsal and cranial and/or caudal displacement of small intestines, which may appear "draped" over a ventral abdominal mass
   • dorsal displacement of the large intestine
   • cranial displacement of the stomach, if the mass is large
   VD view:
   • small intestine most likely to be displaced to the right by a left-sided mass, but it may also be displaced to the left, cranially, caudally or peripherally
   • cranial displacement of the stomach, if the mass is large.
3. Kidneys – the kidneys lie in the retroperitoneal space, and so remain dorsally located in the abdomen, even when markedly enlarged
   a. Right kidney
   Lateral view:
   • ventral displacement of the small intestine and ascending and transverse colon
   VD view:
   • medial (left) displacement of the small intestine and ascending and transverse colon
   b. Left kidney (Figure 11.16 and 10.1)
   Lateral view:
   • ventral displacement of the small intestine and descending colon
   VD view:
   • medial (right) displacement of the small intestine and descending colon.
4. Small intestine – small intestinal masses are usually also associated with radiographic signs of intestinal obstruction (e.g. dilated loops and gravel signs)
   Lateral view:
   • displacement of other structures depending on size and location of mass

SMALL ANIMAL RADIOLOGICAL DIFFERENTIAL DIAGNOSIS

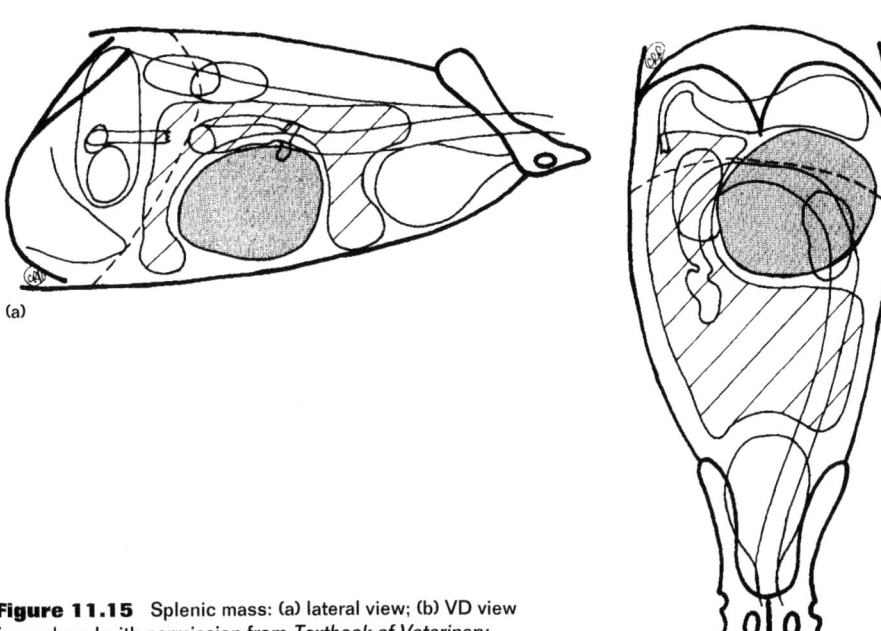

Figure 11.15 Splenic mass: (a) lateral view; (b) VD view (reproduced with permission from *Textbook of Veterinary Diagnostic Radiology*, 3rd edition. Ed. D.E. Thrall, Philadelphia: W.B. Saunders).

VD view:
- as for the lateral view.
5. Large intestine (including caecum) – the wide normal diameter of the large intestine means that without contrast studies, smaller masses may be overlooked
    Lateral view:
    - ventral displacement of small intestine
    VD view:
    - left, right or caudal displacement of small intestine, depending on the part of the large intestine affected.
6. Omentum and mesentery – variable effects, depending on the location of the mass
    a. Root of mesentery

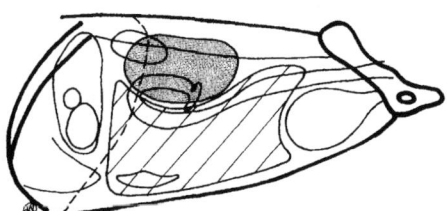

Figure 11.16 Left renal mass on the lateral view (see Figure 10.1 for VD view) (reproduced with permission from *Textbook of Veterinary Diagnostic Radiology*, 3rd edition. Ed. D.E. Thrall, Philadelphia: W.B. Saunders).

Lateral view:
- ventral mass with dorsal and cranial/caudal displacement of small intestine as for a splenic tail mass
VD view:
- mid-abdominal mass, displacing small intestines peripherally, which is unusual for a splenic mass
    b. Mesenteric lymph nodes
    Lateral view:
    - peripheral displacement of small intestines
    VD view:
    - as for the lateral view
    c. Colic lymph nodes
    Lateral view:
    - ventral displacement of the ascending colon, especially on the left lateral recumbent view
    VD view:
    - lateral (right) displacement of the ascending colon.
7. Ovaries – ovaries are intraperitoneal, therefore unlike the kidneys they may lie more ventrally in the abdomen when markedly enlarged. They arise caudal to the ipsilateral kidney
    a. Right ovary
    Lateral view:
    - variable ventral displacement of small intestine

11 OTHER ABDOMINAL STRUCTURES

- if large, cranial displacement of the right kidney +/− ventral deviation of its caudal pole
  VD view:
  - medial (left) displacement of the small intestine and ascending colon
  b. Left ovary
  Lateral view:
  - variable ventral displacement of small intestine
  - if large, cranial displacement of the left kidney +/− ventral deviation of its caudal pole
  VD view:
  - medial (right) displacement of the small intestine and descending colon.
8. Retained testicle − variable location between the caudal pole of the ipsilateral kidney and the inguinal region; displacement of other structures accordingly.
9. Retroperitoneal masses
  Lateral view:
  - ventral displacement of the kidneys and small intestine
  VD view:
  - less helpful, but there may be lateral (right or left) displacement of the kidneys or small intestine if the mass is lateralised.

11.38 Caudal abdominal masses

1. Urinary bladder − bladder masses are rarely visible on plain radiographs and require cystography for demonstration. The mass effect caused by distension of the bladder is described below; such distension may be physiological, or pathological due to inability to urinate
  Lateral view:
  - cranial displacement of small intestine
  - dorsal displacement of the descending colon
  VD view:
  - cranial displacement of small intestine
  - lateral (left or right) displacement of the descending colon.
2. Uterus − mild uterine enlargement may not be detected since uterine horns mimic the appearance of small intestinal loops. Most types of uterine enlargement affect the whole organ and are described below; focal masses will create effects depending on their location (see 10.39.1 and Figure 10.15)
  Lateral view:
  - cranial or craniodorsal displacement of small intestine

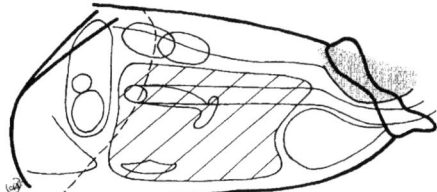

Figure 11.17 Sublumbar mass − lateral view (reproduced with permission from *Textbook of Veterinary Diagnostic Radiology*, 3rd edition. Ed. D.E. Thrall, Philadelphia: W.B. Saunders).

- dorsal displacement of the descending colon
- +/− separation of the descending colon and bladder by a soft tissue structure
VD view:
- cranial +/− medial displacement of small intestine.
3. Prostate − the location of the prostate gland varies depending on the degree of filling of the bladder; it lies more cranially when the bladder is full (see 10.47 and Figure 10.17)
  Lateral view:
  - cranial displacement of the bladder
  - asymmetric prostatic diseases (e.g. paraprostatic cysts) may also cause dorsal or ventral displacement of bladder; they may even lie cranial to the bladder and contrast studies or ultrasonography are required to locate the bladder (see 10.48.1 and Figure 10.18)
  - dorsal displacement +/− compression of the distal descending colon and rectum
  VD view:
  - cranial displacement of the bladder
  - asymmetric prostatic diseases may also cause displacement of the bladder to the right or left
  - lateral (left) displacement of the distal descending colon and rectum.
4. Large intestine − distal descending colon
  Lateral view:
  - ventral displacement of the bladder +/− prostate
  VD view:
  - little value; possible lateral displacement of the bladder.
5. Sublumbar area (Figure 11.17)
  Lateral view:
  - ventral displacement +/− compression of the distal descending colon
  - ventral displacement of the bladder if the mass is large

VD view:
- little value; possible further lateral (left) displacement of the distal descending colon.

11.39 Calcification on abdominal radiographs

The following list of causes of calcification seen on abdominal radiographs has been taken from the review paper Diagnosis of calcification on abdominal radiographs (Lamb et al., 1991 *Veterinary Radiology and Ultrasound* **32** 211–220, with permission), to which the reader is directed.

Intestinal tract:
    ingesta, e.g. bones (accumulation may indicate partial obstruction)
    foreign bodies (e.g. stones)
    medication (e.g. kaolin)
    enterolith
    uraemic gastritis.

Liver:
    cholelithiasis
    chronic cholecystitis
    chronic hepatopathy
    cyst (developmental or parasitic)
    hepatic nodular hyperplasia
    neoplasms (e.g. osteosarcoma)
    long-standing haematoma, abscess or granuloma.

Spleen:
    histoplasmosis*
    long-standing haematoma or abscess.

Pancreas:
    chronic pancreatitis (including pseudocyst)
    fat necrosis
    neoplasm (e.g. adenocarcinoma).

Kidney:
    nephrolithiasis
    nephrocalcinosis
        nephrotoxic drugs (e.g. gentamicin)
        hypervitaminosis D
        chronic nephritis (e.g. pyelonephritis)
        chronic renal insufficiency
        hyperparathyroidism
        hyperadrenocorticism
        renal telangiectasia of Corgis
    long-standing haematoma or abscess
    parasitic granuloma (e.g. *Toxocara canis*).

Ureter:
    calculus.

Urinary bladder:
    calculus
    chronic cystitis
    transitional cell carcinoma.

Adrenal:
    adrenocortical neoplasm (e.g. adenoma, carcinoma)
    idiopathic.

Ovary:
    neoplasm (e.g. teratoma)
    cyst.

Uterus:
    normal foetus (skeletal calcification is normally visible 38 days after mating in the cat, and approximately 46 days after mating in the dog).

Prostate:
    calculus
    chronic prostatitis
    neoplasm (e.g. adenocarcinoma)
    cyst (including paraprostatic cyst).

Vascular:
    chronic renal insufficiency
    hypervitaminosis D
    idiopathic.

Lymph node:
    chronic inflammation (e.g. fungal* infection)
    metastatic neoplasm (e.g. osteosarcoma, prostatic adenocarcinoma).

Peritoneum:
    chronic peritonitis
    previous barium extravasation may mimic peritoneal calcification.

Abdominal fat:
    idiopathic
    pansteatitis in cats.

Retained intra-abdominal testicle.

Penetrating foreign body.

Urethra:
    calculus
    chronic urethritis
    separate centres of ossification of the os penis.

Muscle:
    myositis ossificans (e.g. affecting the gluteal muscles)

Skin:
    calcinosis cutis associated with hyperadrenocorticism
    calcifying surgical scar
    chronic hygroma.

Rib:
    neoplasm (e.g. chondrosarcoma)
    fracture callus.

Mammary gland:
    neoplasm (e.g. mixed mammary tumour).

11 OTHER ABDOMINAL STRUCTURES

FURTHER READING

General

Blackwood, L., Sullivan, M. and Lawson, H. (1997) Radiographic abnormalities in canine multicentric lymphoma: a review of 84 cases. *Journal of Small Animal Practice* **38** 62–69.

Lamb, C.R. (1990) Abdominal ultrasonography in small animals: examination of the liver, spleen and pancreas (review). *Journal of Small Animal Practice* **31** 6–15.

Lamb, C.R. (1990) Abdominal ultrasonography in small animals: intestinal tract and mesentery, kidneys, adrenal glands, uterus and prostate (review). *Journal of Small Animal Practice* **31** 295–304.

Lamb, C.R., Kleine, L.J. and McMillan, M.C. (1991) Diagnosis of calcification on abdominal radiographs. *Veterinary Radiology and Ultrasound* **32** 211–220.

Lamb, C.R., Hartzband, L.E., Tidwell, A.S. and Pearson, S.H. (1991) Ultrasonographic findings in hepatic and splenic lymphosarcoma in dogs and cats. *Veterinary Radiology* **32** 117–120.

Lee, R. and Leowijuk, C. (1982) Normal parameters in abdominal radiology of the dog and cat. *Journal of Small Animal Practice* **23** 251–269.

Melian, C., Stefanacci, J., Petersen, M.E. and Kintzer, P.P. (1999) Radiographic findings in dogs with naturally occurring primary hypoadrenocorticism. *Journal of the American Animal Hospital Association* **35** 208–212.

Merlo, M. and Lamb, C.R. (2000) Radiographic and ultrasonographic features of retained surgical sponge in eight dogs. *Veterinary Radiology and Ultrasound* **41** 279–283.

Miles, K. (1997) Imaging abdominal masses. *Veterinary Clinics of North America; Small Animal Practice* **27** 1403–1431.

Root, C.R. and Lord, P.F. (1971) Peritoneal carcinomatosis in the dog and cat: its radiographic appearance. *Veterinary Radiology* **12** 54–59.

Root, C.R. (1998) Abdominal masses, in *Textbook of Diagnostic Radiology*, 3rd ed., pp. 417–439, ed. Thrall, D.E. Philadelphia: W.B. Saunders.

Saunders, H.M., Pugh, C.R. and Rhodes, W.H. (1992) Expanding applications of abdominal ultrasonography. *Journal of the American Animal Hospital Association* **28** 369–374.

Saunders, H.M. (1998) Ultrasonography of abdominal cavitary parenchymal lesions. *Veterinary Clinics of North America; Small Animal Practice* **28** 755–776.

Spaulding, K.A. (1993) Ultrasound corner: Sonographic evaluation of peritoneal effusion in small animals. *Veterinary Radiology and Ultrasound* **34** 427–431.

Shaiken, L.C., Evans, S.M. and Goldschmidt, M.H. (1991) Radiographic findings in canine malignant histiocytosis. *Veterinary Radiology* **32** 237–242.

Thrall, D.E. (1992) Radiology corner: Intraperitoneal vs. extraperitoneal fluid. *Veterinary Radiology and Ultrasound* **33** 138–140.

Liver

Barr, F.J. (1992) Ultrasonographic assessment of liver size in the dog. *Journal of Small Animal Practice* **33** 359–364.

Barr, F.J. (1992) Normal hepatic measurements in mature dogs. *Journal of Small Animal Practice* **33** 367–370.

Biller, D.S., Kantrowitz, B. and Miyabayashi, T. (1992) Ultrasonography of diffuse liver disease: a review. *Journal of Veterinary Internal Medicine* **6** 71–76.

Birchard, S.J., Biller, D.S. and Johnson, S.E. (1989) Differentiation of intrahepatic versus extrahepatic portosystemic shunts using positive contrast portography. *Journal of the American Animal Hospital Association* **25** 13–17.

Blaxter, A.C., Holt, P.E., Pearson, G.R., Gibbs, C. and Gruffydd-Jones, T.J. (1988) Congenital portosystemic shunts in the cat: a report of nine cases. *Journal of Small Animal Practice* **29** 631–645.

Broemel, C., Barthez, P.Y., Leveille, R. and Scrivani, P. (1998) Prevalence of gallbladder sludge in dogs as assessed by ultrasonography. *Veterinary Radiology and Ultrasound* **39** 206–210.

Evans, S.M. (1987) The radiographic appearance of primary liver neoplasia in dogs. *Veterinary Radiology* **28** 192–196.

Holt, D.E., Schelling, C.G., Saunders, H.M. and Orsher, R.J. (1995) Correlation of ultrasonographic findings with surgical, portographic, and necropsy findings in dogs and cats with portosystemic shunts: 63 cases (1987–1993). *Journal of the American Veterinary Medical Association* **207** 1190–1193.

Jacobson, L.S., Kirberger, R.M. and Nesbit, J.W. (1995) Hepatic ultrasonography and pathological findings in dogs with hepatocutaneous syndrome: new concepts. *Journal of Veterinary Internal Medicine* **9** 399–404.

Lamb, C.R. (1996) Ultrasonographic diagnosis of congenital portosystemic shunts in dogs: results of a prospective study. *Veterinary Radiology and Ultrasound* **37** 281–288.

Lamb, C.R., Forster-van Hyfte, M.A., White, R.N., McEvoy, F.J. and Rutgers, H.C. (1996) Ultrasonographic diagnosis of congenital portosystemic shunts in 14 cats. *Journal of Small Animal Practice* **37** 205–209.

Lamb, C.R., Wrigley, R.H., Simpson, K.W., Forster-van Hyfte, M., Garden, O.A., Smyth, B.A. et al. (1996) Ultrasonographic diagnosis of portal vein thrombosis in 4 dogs. *Veterinary Radiology and Ultrasound* **37** 121–129.

Lamb, C.R. (1998) Ultrasonography of portosystemic shunts in dogs and cats. *Veterinary Clinics of North America; Small Animal Practice* **28** 725–754.

Leveille, R., Biller, D.S. and Shiroma, J.T. (1996) Sonographic evaluation of the common bile duct in cats. *Journal of Veterinary Internal Medicine* **10** 296–299.

Newell, S.M., Selcer, B.A., Girard, E., Roberts, G.D., Thompson, J.P. and Harrison, J.M. (1998) Correlations between ultrasonographic findings and specific hepatic diseases in cats: 72 cases (1985–1997). *Journal of the American Veterinary Medical Association* **213** 94–98.

Nyland, T.G., Barthez, P.Y., Ortega, T.M. and Davis, C.R. (1996) Hepatic ultrasonographic and pathologic findings in dogs with canine superficial necrolytic dermatitis. *Veterinary Radiology and Ultrasound* **37** 200–205.

Nyland, T.G., Koblik, P.D. and Tellyer, S.E. (1999) Ultrasonographic features of splenic lymphosarcoma in dogs – 12 cases. *Journal of the American Veterinary Medical Association* **12** 1565–1568.

Partington, B.P. and Biller, D.S. (1995) Hepatic imaging with radiology and ultrasound. *Veterinary Clinics of North America; Small Animal Practice* **25** 305–335.

Reed, A.L. (1995) Ultrasonographic findings of diseases of the gallbladder and biliary tract. *Veterinary Medicine* October 1995 950–957.

Schwarz, L.A., Penninck, D.G. and Leveille-Webster, C. (1998) Hepatic abscesses in 13 dogs: a review of the ultrasonographic findings, clinical data and therapeutic options. *Veterinary Radiology and Ultrasound* **39** 357–365

Smith, S.A., Biller, D.S., Goggin, J.M., Kraft, S.L. and Hoskinson, J.J. (1998) Diagnostic imaging of biliary obstruction. *Compendium of Continuing Education for the Practicing Veterinarian (Small Animal)* **20** 1225–1234.

Suter, P.F. (1982) Radiographic diagnosis of liver disease in dogs and cats. *Veterinary Clinics of North America; Small Animal Practice* **12** 153–173.

Wrigley, R.H., Konde, L.J., Park, R.D. and Lebel, J.L. (1987) Ultrasonographic diagnosis of portacaval shunts in young dogs. *Journal of the American Veterinary Medical Association* **191** 421–424.

Spleen

Konde, L.J., Wrigley, R.H., Lebel, J.L., Park, R.D., Pugh, C. and Finn, S. (1989) Sonographic and radiographic changes associated with splenic torsion in the dog. *Veterinary Radiology* **30** 41–45.

Neath, P.J., Brockman, D.J. and Saunders, H.M. (1997) Retrospective analysis of 19 cases of isolated torsion of the splenic pedicle in dogs. *Journal of Small Animal Practice* **38** 387–392.

Saunders, H.M., Neath, P.J. and Brockman, D.J. (1998) B-mode and Doppler ultrasound imaging of the spleen with canine splenic torsion: a retrospective evaluation. *Veterinary Radiology and Ultrasound* **39** 349–353.

Stickle, R.L. (1989) Radiographic signs of isolated splenic torsion in dogs: eight cases (1980–1987). *Journal of the American Veterinary Medical Association* **194** 103–106.

Wrigley, R.H., Park, R.D., Konde, L.J. and Lebel, J.L. (1988) Ultrasonographic features of splenic haemangiosarcoma in dogs: 18 cases. *Journal of the American Veterinary Medical Association* **192** 1113–1117.

Wrigley, R.H., Konde, L.J., Park, R.D. and Lebel, J.L. (1988) Ultrasonographic features of splenic lymphosarcoma in dogs – 12 cases. *Journal of the American Veterinary Medical Association* **192** 1565–1568.

Pancreas

Hess, R.S., Saunders, H.M., Van Winkle, T.J., Shofer, F.S. and Washabau, R.J. (1998) Clinical, clinicopathologic, radiographic, and ultrasonographic abnormalities in dogs with fatal acute pancreatitis: 70 cases (1986–1995). *Journal of the American Veterinary Medical Association* **213** 665–670.

Lamb, C.R., Simpson, K.W., Boswood, A. and Matthewman, L.A. (1995) Ultrasonography of pancreatic neoplasia in the dog: a retrospective review of 16 cases. *Veterinary Record* **137** 65–68.

Adrenal glands

Barthez, P.Y., Nyland, T.G. and Feldman, E.C. (1995) Ultrasonographic evaluation of the adrenal glands in the dog. *Journal of the American Veterinary Medical Association* **207** 1180–1183.

Besso, J.G., Penninck, D.G. and Gliatto, J.M. (1997) Retrospective ultrasonographic evaluation of adrenal gland lesions in 26 dogs. *Veterinary Radiology and Ultrasound* **38** 448–455.

Douglass, J.P., Berry, C.R. and James, S. (1997) Ultrasonographic adrenal gland measurements in dogs without evidence of adrenal gland disease. *Veterinary Radiology and Ultrasound* **38** 124–130.

Grooters, A.M., Biller, D.S., Miyabayashi, T. and Leveille, R. (1994) Evaluation of routine abdominal ultrasonography as a technique for imaging the canine adrenal glands. *Journal of the American Animal Hospital Association* **30** 457–462.

Grooters, A.M., Biller, D.S. and Merryman, J. (1995) Ultrasonographic parameters of normal canine adrenal glands: comparison to necropsy findings. *Veterinary Radiology and Ultrasound* **36** 126–130.

Grooters, A.M., Biller, D.S., Theisen, S.K. and Miyabayashi, T. (1996) Ultrasonographic characteristics of adrenal glands in dogs with pituitary-dependent hyperadrenocorticism: comparison with normal dogs. *Journal of Veterinary Internal Medicine* **10** 110–115.

Schelling, C.G. (1991) Ultrasonography of the adrenal gland. *Problems in Veterinary Medicine* **3** 604–617.

Tidwell, A.S., Penninck, D.G. and Besso, J.G. (1997) Imaging of adrenal gland disorders. *Veterinary Clinics of North America; Small Animal Practice* **27** 237–254.

Abdominal blood vessels

Finn-Bodner, S.T. and Hudson, J.A. (1998) Abdominal vascular sonography. *Veterinary Clinics of North America; Small Animal Practice* **28** 887–942.

Spaulding, K.A. (1992) Ultrasound corner: Helpful hints in identifying the caudal abdominal aorta and caudal vena cava. *Veterinary Radiology and Ultrasound* **33** 90–92.

Spaulding, K.A. (1997) A review of sonographic identification of abdominal vessels and juxtavascular organs. *Veterinary Radiology and Ultrasound* **38** 4–23.

Abdominal lymph nodes

Pugh, C.R. (1994) Ultrasonographic examination of abdominal lymph nodes in the dog. *Veterinary Radiology and Ultrasound* **35** 110–115.

12

Soft tissues

12.1 Variations in thickness of soft tissues
12.2 Variations in radio-opacity of soft tissues
12.3 Contrast studies of sinus tracts and fistulae
12.4 Contrast studies of the lymphatic system (lymphography, lymphangiography)
12.5 Contrast studies of peripheral arteries and veins (angiography, arteriography, venography)
12.6 Ultrasonography of soft tissues
12.7 Ultrasonography of muscles and tendons

Soft tissues and fluid have a similar radio-opacity, which is less than that of bone and other mineralised material, and greater than that of gas. Fat is unusual in that it is slightly less radio-opaque than fluid and other soft tissues.

It is not usually possible, therefore, to distinguish different components of fluid or soft tissue structures within a region unless they are outlined by fat, gas or mineralised material, or unless contrast techniques are used.

12.1 Variations in thickness of soft tissues

1. Diffuse increase in thickness of soft tissue
   a. Fat deposition – obesity; distinguished by fat radio-opacity which is less than that of other soft tissues
   b. Muscular hypertrophy
      - in response to activity
      - cats – feline hypertrophic muscular dystrophy; uncommon, leads to progressive muscular hypertrophy
   c. Oedema
      - obstruction to venous drainage
      - congestive heart failure
      - hypoproteinaemia (secondary to renal, hepatic or intestinal disease)
   d. Lymphoedema
      - developmental anomaly of lymphatic drainage
      - acquired obstruction to lymphatic drainage
   e. Cellulitis
   f. Diffuse or extensive neoplasia
   g. Subcutaneous administration of fluids
   h. Emphysema (gas bubbles and streaks visible).
2. Focal increase in thickness of soft tissues
   a. Neoplasia
   b. Cellulitis or abscess
   c. Haematoma
   d. Granuloma
   e. Cyst
   f. Seroma (following surgery)
   g. Subcutaneous administration of fluids
   h. Skin folds – especially certain breeds, such as the English Bulldog and the Shar Pei.
3. Decrease in thickness of soft tissues
   a. Emaciation – loss of fat layer primarily
   b. Muscular atrophy
      - disuse (e.g. chronic lameness)
      - neurogenic
      - as a consequence of myositis.

12.2 Variations in radio-opacity of soft tissues

1. Increased radio-opacity – but still soft tissue opacity
   a. Increased thickness of soft tissues (e.g. given the same exposure, the soft tissues of the thigh will appear more radio-opaque than those of the distal limb, due to their increased bulk)
   b. Superimposition of skin or subcutaneous masses
   c. Superimposition of nipples
   d. Superimposition of engorged ticks
   e. Skin folds
   f. Positioning aids (e.g. foam wedges)
   g. Wet hair or fur – usually gives a streaky appearance.
2. Increased radio-opacity – unstructured mineral opacity due to deposition of calcium salts or other minerals
   a. Artefactual, due to dirty intensifying screens or cassettes

12 SOFT TISSUES

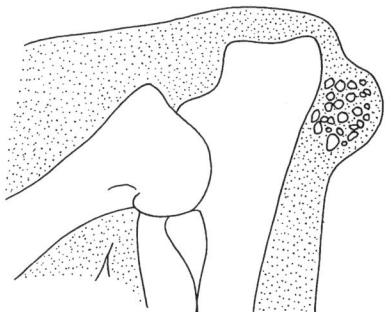

Figure 12.1 Calcinosis circumscripta near the elbow of a dog: a cluster of amorphous mineral opacities within an area of focal soft tissue swelling

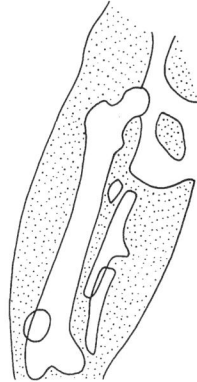

Figure 12.2 Myositis ossificans in the hindlimb of a cat – well-organised deposits of bone in the soft tissues of the medial thigh.

  b. Surface application of some lotions or ointments
  c. Secondary to injection of corticosteroids
  d. Dystrophic calcification. i.e. deposition of calcium salts in damaged or diseased tissue
     • secondary to trauma (e.g. calcifying tendinopathy)
     • within a haematoma
     • within a chronic abscess or granuloma
     • within a neoplasm
     • within the wall of a cyst
  e. Calcinosis circumscripta (tumoral calcinosis) (Figure 12.1) – young, large-breed dogs, especially German Shepherd dogs; amorphous calcium deposits within soft tissues. Commonly recognised sites include the extremities or prominences of the limbs, the neck and the tongue
  f. Calcinosis cutis – granular deposits of calcium in the skin and/or linear streaks of calcium in fascial planes; usually secondary to hyperadrenocorticism (Cushing's disease), but may also be seen secondary to hyperparathyroidism
  g. Metastatic calcification – calcification of soft tissues secondary to derangements of calcium metabolism (e.g. major blood vessels, gut wall)
  h. Chondrocalcinosis (pseudogout, calcium pyrophosphate deposition disease CPDD) – rare; unknown aetiology and mainly older animals; articular or peri-articular deposition of calcium pyrophosphate crystals
  i. Cats – hypervitaminosis A; there may be extensive periarticular mineralisation as well as periarticular and vertebral osteophytes
  j. Hypervitaminosis D
  k. Foreign material (e.g. dirt, glass).
3. Increased radio-opacity – structured mineral opacity with trabecular detail suggestive of bone formation
   a. Normal anatomical structures or variants (e.g. sesamoids, clavicle, hyoid apparatus, separate centres of ossification)
   b. Fragments of bone displaced from their normal position due to avulsion or other fractures
   c. Myositis ossificans (Figure 12.2) – formation of non-neoplastic bone within striated muscle; termed 'heterotopic' because it is in an abnormal position
      • idiopathic
      • secondary to trauma or chronic disease
   d. Cats – fibrodysplasia ossificans; rare, progressive disorder; differs from myositis ossificans in that the bone may displace muscle, but does not involve it. Typically multiple, symmetrical lesions unrelated to trauma
   e. Neoplasia
      • extraskeletal osteosarcoma
      • others.
4. Increased radio-opacity – metallic opacity
   a. Artefactual due to dirty intensifying screens or cassettes
   b. Surface application of lotions or ointments containing metallic salts
   c. Surface contamination with contrast medium
   d. Contrast medium within a sinus tract or fistula

SMALL ANIMAL RADIOLOGICAL DIFFERENTIAL DIAGNOSIS

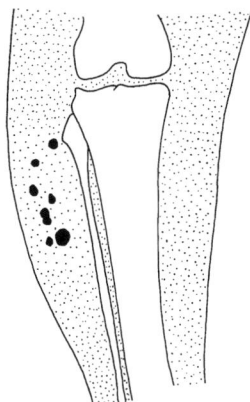

Figure 12.3 Subcutaneous emphysema secondary to a cat bite – multiple, small gas bubbles seen within the soft tissues lateral to the fibula.

   e. Foreign material (e.g. bullets, air-gun pellets, needles)
   f. Migration of metallic implants originally in skeletal structures
   g. Surgical staples or wire sutures
   h. Microchip.
5. Decreased radio-opacity of soft tissues
   a. Decreased thickness of soft tissues
   b. Presence of fat
      - normal/obese; linear fat deposits in a subcutaneous site and along fascial planes
      - localised fatty mass (lipoma, liposarcoma)
   c. Presence of gas (Figure 12.3)
      - puncture, laceration or incision of skin
      - secondary to subcutaneous or intramuscular injection
      - penetration of the pharynx, oesophagus or trachea
      - extension of pneumomediastinum
      - within intestinal loops within a hernia or rupture
      - infection with gas forming organisms (uncommon).

12.3 Contrast studies of sinus tracts and fistulae

A sinus tract is defined as a tract leading from a focus of infection to the lumen of a hollow organ, or to the body surface. A fistula runs from the lumen of a hollow organ or body cavity to another hollow organ or body cavity, or to the body surface.

Contrast studies may be used in either case to determine the route of the tract. In the case of a sinus tract, contrast material may, in addition, outline a foreign body at the site of the focus of infection. However, care must be taken with interpretation as the contrast medium does not always fill the tract(s) completely, and so may give a false impression of the extent of the lesion. In addition, it may be difficult to discriminate between foreign material and filling defects due to gas bubbles, purulent debris and fibrous tissue.

In order to perform a contrast study, a catheter is placed into the end of the tract opening at the body surface. The catheter is secured in place, either by a purse-string suture or by a balloon catheter. A water-soluble iodinated contrast medium is then injected slowly and a radiograph of the region taken towards the end of, or after completion of, the injection. The quantity of contrast medium used will depend on the suspected extent of the lesion.

12.4 Contrast studies of the lymphatic system (lymphography, lymphangiography)

This contrast technique is rarely used in veterinary medicine, but may be used to investigate causes of lymphoedema. A subcutaneous injection of methylene blue is given distal to the site of interest; this is taken up by the lymphatic vessels, which can then be identified, surgically exposed and cannulated. A water-soluble, iodinated contrast medium may then be injected, and radiographs of the region taken after completion of the injection.

An alternative method is to inject low-osmolar, water-soluble contrast medium intradermally distal to the site of the expected lesion. This may demonstrate lymphatics and lymph nodes.

12.5 Contrast studies of peripheral arteries and veins (angiography, arteriography, venography)

Contrast studies of peripheral blood vessels may be indicated when it is important to define the arterial supply or the venous drainage of a mass or extremity. If information regarding the arterial supply is required, then it is usually necessary to surgically expose and cannulate the feeder artery to the region. If information only about venous drainage is required, then it is sufficient to inject the con-

trast medium into a peripheral vein distal to the region of interest. Water-soluble iodinated contrast medium should be used in either case, and radiographs of the region taken towards the end of injection, or immediately upon completion of injection.
1. Failure of vessel(s) to fill completely with contrast
   a. Insufficient contrast medium used
   b. Leakage of contrast around the catheter
   c. Time delay between the completion of injection and the radiographic exposure too great
   d. Vessel occluded
      • by a mass within or outside it
      • by a ligature
      • by a thrombus
   e. Vessel disrupted.
2. Additional abnormal vessels seen
   a. Developmental anomaly of arterial supply and/or venous drainage
   b. Acquired anomaly of arterial supply and/or venous drainage
      • development of collateral circulation in response to disruption or occlusion of normal vessels
      • development of abnormal vessels supplying and draining a neoplasm
   c. Arteriovenous malformation
      • developmental
      • acquired (e.g. secondary to trauma, biopsy, surgery, neoplasia).

12.6 Ultrasonography of soft tissues

Changes in thickness of soft tissues (see 12.1) may be appreciated ultrasonographically and, in addition, it may be possible to determine which soft tissue component is responsible for the change in thickness. Changes in echogenicity may give added information.
1. Increased echogenicity of soft tissues, +/– acoustic shadowing
   a. Diffuse
      • inappropriate control settings
      • obesity
      • subcutaneous emphysema
   b. Localised
      • foreign material
      • localised subcutaneous emphysema
      • gas within herniated intestinal loops
      • localised calcification or ossification (see 12.2)
      • localised fibrosis
      • neoplasm
      • granuloma
      • abscess.
2. Decreased echogenicity of soft tissues
   a. Diffuse
      • inappropriate control settings
      • oedema
      • lymphoedema
      • obesity
   b. Localised
      • recently injected fluids
      • seroma post surgery
      • cyst
      • haematoma
      • abscess
      • neoplasm
      • granuloma.
3. Mixed echogenicity of soft tissues
   a. Abscess +/– foreign body (Figure 12.4)
   b. Haematoma
   c. Neoplasm.

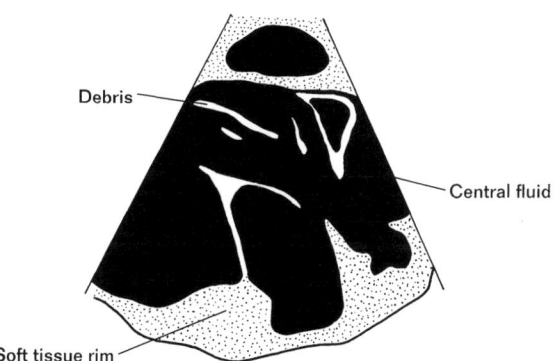

Figure 12.4 Ultrasound image of an abscess showing a soft tissue rim and central fluid containing some debris.

12.7 Ultrasonography of muscles and tendons

Ultrasonography of peripheral muscles is straightforward. Once the scanning site has been prepared by clipping and cleaning, a high-frequency (7.5 MHz) transducer is placed directly over the muscle of interest. Normal muscle appears hypoechoic, with a characteristic striated appearance in longitudinal section and a stippled appearance in transverse section. The hyperechoic striations and stipples represent fibrous tissue around muscle fibre bundles. The boundaries between different muscle bellies are hyperechoic. The tendons are relatively hyperechoic, with densely packed, parallel fibres apparent in longitudinal section. A little fluid around a tendon, within the tendon sheath, may be normal.

1. Hypoechoic focus within muscle, with disruption of fibre pattern
   a. Haematoma
      - trauma
      - coagulopathy
   b. Abscess
      - puncture wound
      - haematogenous infection
   c. Neoplasm
      - primary muscle tumour (rhabdomyoma, rhabdomyosarcoma)
      - metastatic tumour.

2. Hyperechoic focus within muscle, with disruption of fibre pattern: acoustic shadowing may or may not be present
   a. Fibrosis
   b. Calcification or ossification (see 12.2.2 and 12.2.3)
   c. Fracture fragments
   d. Metallic surgical implants
   e. Gas (see 12.2.5)
   f. Foreign body
   g. Neoplasm
      - primary muscle tumour (rhabdomyoma, rhabdomyosarcoma)
      - metastatic tumour.

3. Mixed echogenicity within muscle, with disruption of the fibre pattern
   a. Haematoma +/− muscle tearing
   b. Abscess
   c. Neoplasm.

4. Change in echogenicity of tendons (Figure 12.5) – damage to tendons is indicated by disruption of the normal tightly packed, hyperechoic fibres. Anechoic or hypoechoic lesions within the substance of the tendon represent haemorrhage or inflammatory exudate, progressing to granulation tissue. The lesions become more hyperechoic as fibrous tissue replaces granulation tissue, but the fibre alignment remains disrupted until the later stages of healing.

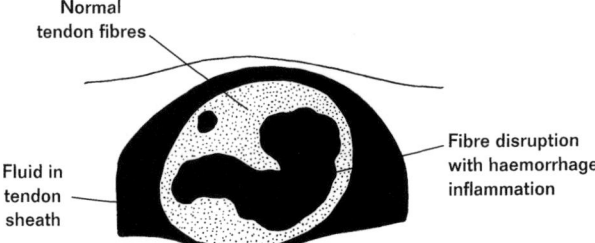

Figure 12.5 Ultrasonographic appearance of a damaged Achilles tendon (transverse section). The normal stippled pattern of the tendon fibres is replaced by a hypoechoic region representing fibre disruption and haemorrhage or inflammation. Fluid may be seen in the tendon sheath.

FURTHER READING

Boswood, A., Lamb, C.R. and White, R.N. (2000) Aortic and iliac thrombosis in six dogs. *Journal of Small Animal Practice* **41** 109–114.

de Bulnes, A.G., Fernandez, P.G., Aguirre, A.M.M. and de la Muela, M.S. (1998) Ultrasonographic imaging of canine mammary tumours. *Veterinary Record* **143** 687–689.

Fan, T.M., Simpson, K.W., Trasti, S., Birnbaum, N., Center, S.A. and Yeager, A. (1998) Calcipotriol toxicity in a dog. *Journal of Small Animal Practice* **39** 581–586.

Hay, C.W., Roberts, R. and Latimer, K. (1994) Multilobular tumour of bone at an unusual location in the axilla of a dog. *Journal of Small Animal Practice* **35** 633–636.

Kuntz, C.A., Dernell, W.S., Powers, B.E. and Withrow, S. (1998) Extraskeletal osteosarcomas in dogs: 14 cases. *Journal of the American Animal Hospital Association* **34** 26–30.

McEvoy, F.J., Peck, G.J., Hilton, G.S. and Webbon, P.M. (1994) Normal venographic appearance of the pelvic limb in the dog. *Veterinary Record* **134** 641–643.

Shah, Z.R., Crass, J.R., Oravec, D.C. and Bellon, E.M. (1992) Ultrasonographic detection of foreign bodies in soft tissues using turkey muscle as a model. *Veterinary Radiology and Ultrasound* **33** 94–100.

Stimson, E.L., Cook, W.T., Smith, M.M., Forrester, S.D., Moon, M.L. and Saunders, G.K. (2000) Extraskeletal osteosarcoma in the duodenum of a cat. *Journal of the American Animal Hospital Association* **36** 332–336.

Warren, H.B. and Carpenter, J.L. (1984) Fibrodysplasia ossificans in three cats. *Veterinary Pathology* **21** 485–499.

Appendix

RADIOGRAPHIC FAULTS

Processing faults are generally more common with manual than with automatic processing, although high-quality manual processing can give extremely good results. However, it should not be assumed that automatic processors are foolproof and always trouble free, as processing faults may arise due to poor maintenance or careless use of the machine. Radiographic faults may also be caused by incorrect use of intensifying screens, film or grids or the use of damaged equipment. The following list gives possible causes and remedies for a variety of radiographic processing faults. Many can occur with both manual and automatic processing; those confined to one or other technique are indicated by (M) or (A) respectively.

Sign	Causes	Remedies
Radiograph too dark Image too dark but area outside primary beam or protected by lead markers normal	Overexposure	Reduce kVp and/or mAs (kVp reduction of 10 is approximately equal to a halving of mAs). Check focus–film distance (FFD), and increase it if it is inadvertently too short
Whole film too dark	Overdevelopment	Reduce developer temperature or developing time; ensure starter solution (restrainer) used where necessary
	Fogging (see below)	See below
Radiograph too light Image of patient too light but background black ("soot and whitewash" film)	Underexposure	Increase kVp to increase penetration of patient. Check FFD and reduce if it is inadvertently too long
Image of both patient and background too light resulting in very low contrast	Underdevelopment	Increase developer temperature or developing time; replenish or replace developer; keep lid on developer tank to delay oxidation (M); check that film is compatible with chemicals used
	Gross underexposure	Increase exposure factors markedly
	Use of incompatible intensifying screens and film (e.g. film not sensitive to light colour emitted by screens)	Check compatibility of intensifying screens and film
Image of patient tolerable (some internal detail) but background is grey not black	Underdevelopment with compensatory overexposure	Correct development and reduce exposure factors
Uneven, marbled appearance to film	Patchy underdevelopment due to uneven developer temperature (M)	Stir developer thoroughly before use to ensure even temperature; use water bath heating method not a direct heater
Fogging (darkening of the film unrelated to the primary beam) – may be generalised or localised	Exposure to white light during storage or processing (exposed area usually black)	Careful storage and use of film; keep lid on developer solution whilst film in (M)

242

APPENDIX: RADIOGRAPHIC FAULTS

Sign	Causes	Remedies
Fogging (contd)	Light leakage into darkroom (film diffusely grey and finger shadows may be seen)	Ensure darkroom is light-proof
	Safelight too bright or faulty	Check by laying film on bench with metal object on it for 30 s, then processing it
	Overdevelopment (chemical fog), including lack of starter (restrainer) solution and incompatibility of developer with film	Check developer is correctly made up and that solution is compatible with the film; use at correct temperature and for correct time
	Exposure to scattered radiation	Keep unexposed film away from the radiography area
	Out-of-date film (storage fog)	Use film chronologically and within its use-by date; store at appropriate temperature
Pale patches on the film	Dried splashes of liquid on the intensifying screens; splashes of water or fixer on the unprocessed film (usually M)	Clean intensifying screens regularly; good darkroom design with wet and dry areas (M); handle films with clean, dry hands
Dark or black patches on the film	Splashes of developer on the unprocessed film (usually M)	As above
White specks and lines on the film	Dirt or animal hairs on the intensifying screens; damage to the screens or film emulsion	Clean intensifying screens regularly; handle screens and film carefully; replace screens when damaged
Parallel white or black lines		
Fine lines, close together	Grid faults: damaged grid; grid not perpendicular to primary beam; focused grid used at wrong FFD or upside down; moving grid not activated	Correct use of the grid
Lines of variable width and further apart	Scratches from automatic processor – e.g. damaged rollers (A)	Regular servicing and cleaning of the automatic processor
Crescentic black lines	Crimp marks from careless handling of the film before processing	Careful handling of unprocessed film
Branching black lines	Static electricity	Handle film carefully; use anti-static screen cleaner; use a darkroom humidifier
Film background grey and not transparent	Incomplete fixing – fixer exhausted or fixing time too short	Periodically change fixer; correct fixing procedure
Film becomes brown or yellow with time	Incomplete fixing (film background as above) or washing (film surface dirty in reflected light)	Correct fixing and washing
Blurring of the image	Movement of the patient	Restrain patient effectively; use short exposure times; expose during respiratory pause
	Movement of the X-ray tube head	Ensure X-ray stand is stable, especially if exposure cable is attached to tube head

SMALL ANIMAL RADIOLOGICAL DIFFERENTIAL DIAGNOSIS

Sign	Causes	Remedies
	Poor screen–film contact (test by scattering paper clips on the cassette and making a radiograph)	Replace the cassette
	Large object–film distance	Have part of interest as close to film as possible and largest FFD practicable
	Fogging (see above)	Depending on the cause
	Very rapid film–screen combination used	Use a slower combination consistent with X-ray machine's capabilities
	Movement of the cassette (large animal radiography)	Use a stable cassette holder on a stand and not held freely

ULTRASOUND TERMINOLOGY AND ARTEFACTS

Terminology

Anechoic: tissues producing no echoes, appearing black on the image.

Hypoechoic: tissues producing few echoes, appearing grey on the image.

Hyperechoic: tissues producing strong echoes, appearing bright white on the image.

Most fluids and tissues of homogeneous cellularity produce few or no echoes, and thus appear anechoic or hypoechoic. Gas and mineral interfaces are highly reflective and thus appear hyperechoic. Tissues with a high fibrous tissue or fat content, and tissues containing multiple internal boundaries, tend to produce more echoes, and therefore appear brighter, than other soft tissues.

Artefacts

Some artefacts impair image interpretation and need to be avoided or minimised, while others are incidental features, or may even aid interpretation. It is helpful to be able to recognise all common artefacts to prevent their misinterpretation.

Poor transducer contact

Multiple concentric (sector) or straight (linear) lines running across the image, parallel to the scanning surface, obscuring detail. This is usually due to poor preparation of the scanning surface or inadequate use of acoustic gel, but may also occur due to poor congruence between the transducer and body surfaces.

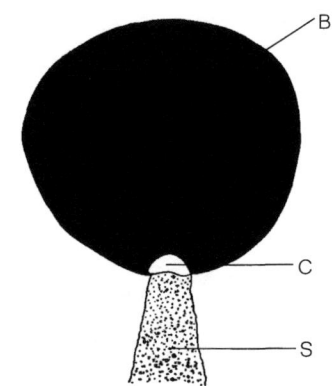

Figure A.1 Acoustic shadowing deep to a urinary bladder calculus. (B = urinary bladder; C = highly echogenic cystic calculus; S = acoustic shadow.)

Acoustic shadowing

Seen at highly reflective or absorptive interfaces, such as those involving bone or gas. A very strong echo is produced at the interface, but little or no sound passes beyond the interface into deeper tissues. Thus a black 'shadow' is seen deep to the hyperechoic surface. May be useful in recognising small mineral or gas accumulations (e.g. renal calculi) but can also impair visualisation of tissues (e.g. rib shadowing may obscure thoracic structures). As far as possible avoid intervening bone or gas containing structures when selecting the scanning site (Figure A.1).

APPENDIX: RADIOGRAPHIC FAULTS

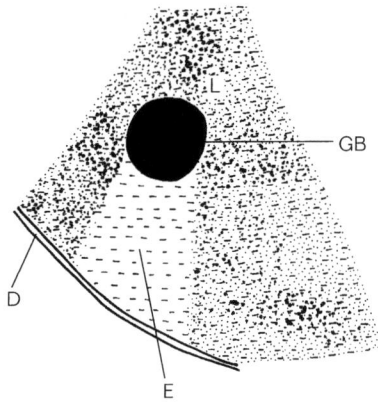

Figure A.2 Acoustic enhancement deep to the gall bladder; liver parenchyma in this area appears artefactually hyperechoic compared with adjacent liver. (D = diaphragm; E = region of acoustic enhancement deep to the gall bladder; GB = gall bladder; L = liver parenchyma.)

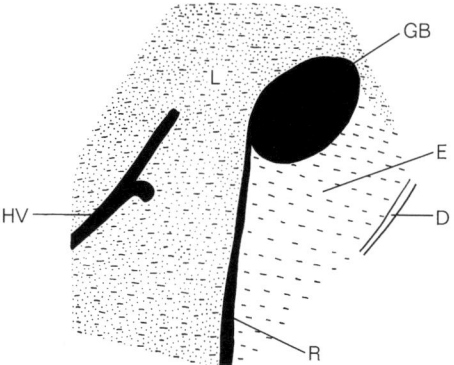

Figure A.3 Refractive shadowing in the liver arising from the edge of the gall bladder. (D = diaphragm; E = acoustic enhancement; GB = gall bladder; HV = hepatic vein; L = liver parenchyma; R = refractive shadowing.)

Acoustic enhancement

Seen deep to fluid-filled structures as an area of increased echogenicity. As sound passes through tissues, it is scattered and absorbed as well as reflected, but little of this occurs as it passes through fluid. Thus the intensity of sound reaching the far side of a fluid focus is greater than that which has travelled to the same depth through soft tissues. Useful in differentiating fluid foci from hypoechoic, but solid, tissues (Figure A.2).

Refractive shadowing

Shadows seen deep to the edges of rounded, fluid-filled structures such as the gall bladder. Occurs due to refraction of those parts of the sound beam impinging on the curved edges of the structure (Figure A.3).

Reverberation artefacts

These are produced at highly reflective interfaces, such as the surface of air-filled lung, due to rapid reverberation of echoes between the interface and the transducer surface. Streams of bright echoes are seen, comprising small, equidistant, parallel lines which eventually trail off (Figure A.4).

Mirror-image artefact

This is produced at rounded, strongly reflective interfaces, and is most commonly seen at the interfaces between liver/lung and heart/lung. Internal reverberations occur between the interface and the superficial tissues, resulting in spurious reconstructions of superficial tissues at deeper sites. Thus, for example, liver tissue may appear to lie on both sides of the diaphragm, and it is important to recognise that this may be an artefact rather than rupture of the diaphragm (Figure A.4).

Side lobe artefact

These are spurious echoes which originate from tissue outside the path of the primary sound beam. Minor sound beams travel in a number of directions, and these are termed side lobes. If a side lobe interacts with a highly reflective interface, the returning echoes may be erroneously displayed on the image. Such echoes are much weaker than those originating from the primary beam.

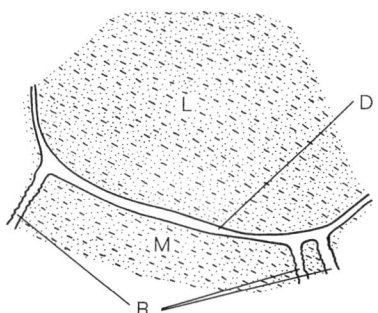

Figure A.4 Mirror image and reverberation artefacts arising at the liver–diaphragm–lung interface. (D = diaphragm; L = liver parenchyma; M = mirror image: illusion of liver beyond the diaphragm; R = reverberations – streams of bright echoes.)

SMALL ANIMAL RADIOLOGICAL DIFFERENTIAL DIAGNOSIS

Slice thickness artefact

The ultrasound beam is very thin but none the less of finite thickness. If part of the thickness of the beam lies within a fluid-filled structure and part lies outside, averaging of the echoes occurs, resulting in the presence of echoes within a fluid-filled structure – "pseudo-sediment". This disappears when the entire thickness of the beam is placed in the fluid-filled structure.

GEOGRAPHIC DISTRIBUTIONS OF DISEASES

Most of the following parasitic and infectious diseases are not found ubiquitously and their approximate geographic distributions are given. For brevity these conditions are indicated throughout the text with *. However, the increased passage of domestic pets between different countries and the possible effects of climate change should be taken into account, as these may result in "exotic" diseases arising in non-endemic areas. Fungal diseases are most often encountered in younger animals, usually those less than 4 years old.

Disease and organism	Type of organism	Species affected	Main geographic distribution
Actinomycosis (*Actinomyces viscosus* and *A. hordeovulneris*)	Bacterium	Dogs – sporadic; cats – infrequent; entry usually via damaged skin	*A. viscosus* – world-wide; *A. hordeovulnaris* – mainly western USA
Aelurostrongylosis (*Aelurostrongylus abstrusus*)–feline lungworm	Helminth	Cats, especially hunting cats as transmitted via gastropods (slugs and snails) +/− small rodents, birds, amphibians and reptiles which have eaten the gastropods and are acting as paratenic hosts	World-wide; mainly Europe (including UK) and USA. Only causes disease occasionally; usually subclinical
Angiostrongylosis (*Angiostrongylus vasorum*)–"French" heartworm	Helminth	Dogs, usually younger dogs kept in confined groups; also foxes. Transmitted via gastropods	Sporadic world-wide, especially western Europe (including UK) in focal areas. Sporadic in USA in imported dogs. Also Africa, Russia, Asia, South America
Aspergillosis (*Aspergillus fumigatus*)	Fungus	Dogs, with systemic form – most often in German Shepherd dog and immunosuppressed patients. Rare in cats	World-wide; saprophyte in soil and decaying vegetation
Babesiosis (especially *Babesia canis* – dog and *B. felis* – cat)	Protozoon	Dogs – *B. canis* transmitted via ticks, mainly *Rhipicephalus sanguineus* (brown dog tick) and *Dermacentor reticulatus*. Cats – *B. felis*; cycle not known	World-wide in tropical, subtropical and warm temperate climes, e.g. southern Europe, North, Central and Southern America, Asia, Africa; increasingly widespread
Blastomycosis (*Blastomyces dermatitidis*) – North American blastomycosis	Fungus	Dogs, especially young, large-breed dogs. Cats – rare	Endemic in North America, mainly close to river valleys and lakes. Sporadic in Central and South America, Europe and Africa. Soil saprophyte

APPENDIX: RADIOGRAPHIC FAULTS

Disease and organism	Type of organism	Species affected	Main geographic distribution
Borrelia burgdorferi – Lyme disease	Spirochaete	Dogs, transmitted via *Ixodes* ticks. Cats may seroconvert but clinical disease is rare	World-wide but focal; North America, Europe (including UK), former USSR, Asia, Australia
Capillariasis (*Capillaria aerophila*; syn. *Eucoleus aerophila*) – fox lungworm	Helminth	Dogs and cats are occasionally affected, but the main host is the fox. Direct life cycle. Recorded as a zoonosis in some countries	Mainly North America, Europe, Middle East, Russia, North Africa
Coccidioidomycosis (*Coccidioides immitis*) – "valley fever" or "San Joaquin Valley fever"	Fungus	Dogs, especially young, medium to large-breed dogs. Cats – rare	Endemic in semi-arid regions of western and south-western USA, Mexico, Central and South America. Soil saprophyte
Crenosomosis (*Crenosoma vulpis*)	Helminth	Dogs affected occasionally, but the main host is the fox. Transmitted via gastropods	World-wide in foxes; occasional in dogs in Europe (including UK), North America and Asia
Cryptococcosis (*Cryptococcus neoformans*) – torulosis or European blastomycosis	Fungus	Cat – the most common systemic mycosis of cats; predisposed to by immunosuppression. Dogs – less common; also predisposed to by immunosuppression	World-wide, especially in warm, humid regions; USA and Australia. Soil saprophyte and found in bird excreta, especially that of pigeons
Dirofilariasis (*Dirofilaria immitis*) – heartworm	Helminth	Dogs – common. Cats – occasionally affected. Transmitted by mosquitoes. Humans occasionally infected; dogs and cats acting as reservoirs	Endemic in tropical, sub-tropical and warm temperate areas (e.g. southern Europe, North and South America, southern Asia, Africa, Australia)
Ehrlichiosis (*Ehrlichia canis*)	Rickettsia	Dogs – transmitted via the brown dog tick *Rhipicephalus sanguineus*.	Most tropical and sub-tropical regions; reported in USA, Africa, the Caribbean and parts of Asia
Filaroidiasis (*Filaroides hirthi* and *F. milksi*)	Helminth	Dogs; *F. hirthi* – sporadic, most often in research colonies or in immunosuppressed or stressed dogs; *F. milksi* – a parasite of wildlife of questionable significance in dogs, although morphologically similar to *F. hirthi*. Both have a direct life cycle	Sporadic world-wide
Francisella (*Pasteurella*) *tularensis* – tularaemia, rabbit fever	Bacterium	Dogs and cats affected occasionally – mainly a disease of rodents and other wildlife. Biting insects can act as reservoirs and hosts	Most virulent Type A strain only in North America; less virulent Type B strain in North America, parts of continental Europe, former USSR, China and Japan
Hepatozoonosis (*Hepatozoon canis*)	Protozoon	Dog and cat, via ingestion of the brown dog tick *Rhipicephalus sanguineus*	World-wide, especially USA, southern Europe, Africa, Middle and Far East
Histoplasmosis (*Histoplasma capsulatum*)	Fungus	Dog – the most common canine systemic mycosis of North America. Cats – reports vary from rare and mild to equal incidence with dogs	Well-defined tropical, sub-tropical and temperate regions: endemic in certain river valleys in USA; also Canada. Sporadic elsewhere. Soil saprophyte.

SMALL ANIMAL RADIOLOGICAL DIFFERENTIAL DIAGNOSIS

Disease and organism	Type of organism	Species affected	Main geographic distribution
Leishmaniasis (*Leishmania donovani*)	Protozoon	Dogs; rare in cats. Potentially communicable to humans. Transmitted via sandflies.	Sporadic in tropical, sub-tropical and temperate climes; mainly between 40° S and 50° N. Endemic in Central and South America, south-eastern USA, southern Europe, Africa and Asia
Nocardiosis (*Nocardia asteroides*)	Bacterium	Sporadic in dogs, especially if immunosuppressed. Less common in cats	World-wide. Soil saprophyte
Oslerus (formerly *Filaroides*) *osleri*	Helminth	Dogs. Direct life cycle	World-wide – present in many countries
Paragonimiasis (mainly *Paragonimus kellicotti*) – lung fluke	Helminth	Dogs and cats. Transmitted via aquatic or amphibian snails with crayfish and crab as intermediate host. Not transmissible directly to man but dogs may act as reservoirs of infection	North America, Latin America, Asia, Africa
Pneumocystosis (*Pneumocystis carinii*)	Fungus, but behaves like a protozoon.	Dogs – sporadic, especially in young Cavalier King Charles Spaniels, Miniature Dachshunds (probably due to immuno-deficiency) and immunosuppressed animals. Cats – asymptomatic.	World-wide but very sporadic.
Pythiosis (*Pythium insidiosum*)	Fungus	Dogs – especially young, large-breed dogs. Cats – rare.	Many subtropical countries (e.g. Australia, south-east Asia, South America, south-eastern USA, Caribbean). Water-borne
Rocky Mountain spotted fever (*Rickettsia rickettsii*)	Rickettsia	Dogs; transmitted via dog ticks *Rhipicephalus sanguineus, Dermacentor variabilis, D. andersoni* and *Amblyomma cajennense*. Humans infected directly or occasionally from dogs.	USA, Canada, Central and South America
Spirocercosis (*Spirocerca lupi*)	Helminth	Dogs – very common in some endemic areas. Cats – seldom reported. Transmitted via dung beetle or by a variety of small vertebrates which have eaten dung beetles and are acting as paratenic hosts.	Most tropical and sub-tropical countries
Sporotrichosis (*Sporothrix schenckii*)	Fungus	Cats – especially male cats. Dogs – less common. The feline disease is zoonotic	Sporadic in southern USA and similar climes; uncommon in Europe. Soil saprophyte
Toxoplasmosis (*Toxoplasma gondii*)	Protozoon	Cats – the definitive host, infected via rodents, birds or raw meat. Dogs – especially if immunosuppressed. Zoonotic.	World-wide

APPENDIX: RADIOGRAPHIC FAULTS

FURTHER READING

Radiography and Ultrasound

Ewers, R.S. (1995) Avoiding errors in radiography. *Veterinary Annual* **35** 47–60.

Kirberger, R.M. and Roos, C.J. (1995) Radiographic artefacts. *Journal of the South African Veterinary Association* **66** 85–94.

Kirberger, R.M. (1995) Imaging artefacts in diagnostic ultrasound – a review. *Veterinary Radiology and Ultrasound* **36** 297–306.

Kirberger, R.M. (1999) Radiographic quality evaluation for exposure variables – a review. *Veterinary Radiology and Ultrasound* **40** 220–226.

Lamb, C.R. (1995) Errors in radiology. *Veterinary Annual* **35** 33–46.

Papageorges, M. (1998) Visual perception and radiographic interpretation. *Compendium of Continuing Education for the Practicing Veterinarian (Small Animal)* **20** 1215–1223.

Papageorges, M. (1990) The Mach phenomenon. *Veterinary Radiology* **31** 274–280.

Penninck, D.G. (1995) Imaging artefacts in ultrasound, in *Veterinary Diagnostic Ultrasound*, pp. 19–29, ed. Nyland, T.G. and Mattoon, J.S. Philadelphia: W.B. Saunders.

Scrivani, P.V., Bednarski, R.M., Myer, C.W. and Dykes, N.L (1996) Restraint methods for radiography in dogs and cats. *Compendium of Continuing Education for the Practicing Veterinarian (Small Animal)* **18** 899–916.

Smallwood, J.E., Shively, M.J., Rendano, V.T. and Hable, R.E. (1985) A standardized nomenclature for radiographic projections used in veterinary medicine. *Veterinary Radiology* **26** 2–9.

Geographic distributions of diseases

Bolt G., Monrad J., Koch J. and Jensen A.L. (1994) Canine angiostrongylosis: a review. *Veterinary Record* **135** 447–452.

Clinkenbeard K.D., Wolf A.M., Cowell R.L. and Tyler R.L. (1989) Canine disseminated histoplasmosis. *Compendium of Continuing Education for the Practicing Veterinarian (Small Animal)* **11** 1347–1360.

Cobb M.A. and Fisher M.A. (1992) *Crensoma vulpis* infection in a dog. *Veterinary Record* **130** 452.

Greene R.T. (1998) Coccidioidomycosis, in *Infectious Diseases of the Dog and Cat*, 2nd ed., pp 391–398, ed. Green, C.E. Philadelphia: W.B. Saunders.

Legendre A. (1998) Blastomycosis, in *Infectious Diseases of the Dog and Cat*, 2nd ed., pp 371–377, ed. Green, C.E. Philadelphia: W.B. Saunders.

Quinn, P.J., Donnelly, W.J.C., Carter, M.E., Markey, B.K.J., Torgerson, P.R. and Breathnach, R.M.S. (1997) *Microbial and Parasitic Diseases of the Dog and Cat*. London: W.B. Saunders.

Torgerson P.R., McCarthy G. and Donnelly W.J.C. (1997) Filaroides hirthi verminous pneumonia in a West Highland white terrier bred in Ireland. *Veterinary Record* **38** 217–219.

Index

Note: Page references in *italics* refer to Figures; those in **bold** refer to Tables

A
abdominal masses 226–32
  caudal abdomen 231–2
  cranial abdomen 227–9
  mid-abdominal 229–31
abdominal wall 210–11
abscess
  malar 75
  prostatic 200, 204, 205
  renal 187, 189, 190, 192
  retrobulbar 79
  retropharyngeal 76
  salivary gland 79
  testicular 205
  ultrasonography 239, *239*
  uterine 203
accessory carpal bone fractures 48, *48*
Achilles tendon, lesions of 59, *60*, *240*
acoustic enhancement 245, *245*
acoustic shadowing 244, *244*
acromegaly, feline, in cranium 67
actinomycosis 87, 113, **246**
acute respiratory distress syndrome (ARDS, shock lung) 111, 112, 118
adamantinoma 68, 69
Addison's disease 120, 121
adenocarcinoma
  anal sac 17
  gastric 172
  hepatic 217
  prostatic 232
  pulmonary 115
  salivary gland 79
  thyroid 122
  tracheal 107
  tympanic bulla 71
adrenal glands 187, 213, 214
  enlargement on ultrasonography 228–9, *229*
  normal appearance on ultrasonography 226
aelurostrongylosis 111, 113, 116, 117, 118, 120, **246**
allergic pulmonary disease 111
alveolar lung pattern 110–12, *110*
ameloblastoma 68, 69
amyloidosis, familial renal *see* Chinese Shar Pei fever syndrome
anaemia
  autoimmune haemolytic 120
  in osteoporosis 14
angiography 135–6, 238–9
  left heart 135
  non-selective 135
  peripheral arteries and veins 238–9

  right heart 136
  selective 135
angiolipoma 97
angiostrongylosis 111, 113, 121, 118, 120, 133, **246**
Angiostrongylus 136
anticoagulant poisoning 97
antibacterium, conditions affecting 45–7
aortic abnormalities 131–2, *132*
aortic body tumour 134
aortic valve 139–40, 136–8
apophysis 1
artefacts 244–6
arteriography 238–9
arthritis *see* osteoarthritis, septic arthritis, rheumatoid arthritis
arthrography 31–2
articular cartilage 2
articular facets, abnormalities of 93
ascites 211, *211*, *213*
aspergillosis 22, 73, *73*, 87, 113, **246**
Aspergillus 73, 92
Aspirated foreign body 107, 111, 113, 122
aspiration pneumonia 111
asteroid hyalosis 78
asthma, feline bronchial 109
astrocytoma 88, 98
ataxia, hereditary 100
atelectasis 110, 111
atlantoaxial instability 89, *89*
atresia ani /coli 180
atrial septal defect (ASD) 120
autoimmune haemolytic anaemia 120
avulsion of the tibial tuberosity 55, *55*
avulsion of tendons, stifle 56, *56*, *57*

B
Baastrup's disease 87
babesiosis 112, 117, **246**
barium burger 153, 154
barium enema 181
barium-impregnated polyethylene spheres (BIPS) 168, 170
barium series 175
benign prostatic hyperplasia 203–205
bicipital tenosynovitis 41
bile peritonitis 211
bilothorax 162
bladder calculi 195, 196
bladder, urinary 194–8
  contrast studies

  abnormal contents 196–7, *197*
  normal appearance 195–6
  wall thickening 197–8
  displacement 194
  masses 231
  non-visualisation 194
  radio-opacity 195
  shape 195
  size 194–5
  tumours 197, *197*
  ultrasonographic examination 198
    contents 198
    cystic structures 198
blastomycosis 22, 79, 113, 117, 152, 205, **246**
bleb, pulmonary 122
block vertebrae 85
bone cysts 12, 20
  aneurysmal 20, 87
  bone fracture and 7
bone lesions, assessment of
  aggressive **7**, *8*
  distribution 5–7
  expansile 20, *20*
  location 7
  non-aggressive **7**, *8*
  number 7
  soft tissue changes 7
  transition zone 7
bone loss (osteolysis) 3
  geographic 4, *4*
  mixed pattern 5, *5*
  moth-eaten 4, *4*
  patterns 4–5
  permeative 4–5, *4*
  presence and type 7
bones 1–28
  altered shape 12
  anatomy, normal 1–2, *2*
  angulation 12
  bowing 12, *12*
  development 2–3
  decreased radiopacity (osteopenia) 16–18
  dwarfism 12–13
  increased radio-opacity 13–14
  metastatic bone tumours 13, 18, *18*, 19, 21
  multifocal diseases 34
  periosteal reactions 14, 15
  primary bone tumours 13, 20, 21, *21*,
  see also fractures; osteogenesis; specific bone or joint
bony masses 16
border effacement 104, 105, *105*
Borrelia burgdorferi 32, 36, **247**
brachycephalic breeds 65, 66

INDEX

brachycephalic obstructive
  syndrome 75, 76
brain, ultrasonography of 67
bronchiectasis 109–10
bronchitis 109
bronchogenic carcinoma 109
bronchopneumonia 109, 110–11
bronchus 109–110
  bronchial lung pattern 109–10, *109*
  lumen opacification 110
  main-stem, changes 108–9, *108*
  wall oedema 109
Brucella canis 92
Budd–Chiari syndrome 216
bulla
  pulmonary 122, *122*
  tympanic 65, 65, 68, *68*, 70, 71, 71, 75, *75*
Borrelia burgdorferi 32, 36
Bursitis, bicipital 41
Butcher's dog disease 17
butterfly vertebra 85, *85*, 88

C

calcification
  abdominal 232
  arterial 132
  external ear canal 71
  intra-thoracic 122–123
  meniscal 37, 57
  metastatic 17, 123, 237
  periarticular 34
  prostatic 205
  renal 192
  soft tissue 18, 77, 118, 147, 158, 237, 239
  thoracic 104
calcifying tendinopathy
  of shoulder joint 41, *41*
  of hip joint 52
calcinosis circumscripta 16, 23, 37, 49, 77, 93, 98, 237, *237*
calcinosis cutis 77, 210, 237
calcium pyrophosphate deposition disease (CPDD) 37, 88, 89, 237
calicivirus, feline 36
calculi
  bladder 195, 196, 197, 198, 232
  prostatic 204, 232
  renal 189, 190, 192
  salivary gland (sialolith) 79
  ureteric 193, 232, 213, 214
  urethral 198, 199, 232
  urinary tract 187, 217
calvarial bones, thickness of 67
cancellous bone 2
canine leucocyte adhesion disorder (CLAD) 22, 26, 69, 74
capillariasis 72, 113, **247**
carcinoma
  bronchiogenic 109, 111, 112, 115
  digital (feline) 35, 50
  larynx 76
  nasal 72
  salivary gland 79
  squamous cell 17, 49, 68, 69, 69, 71, 115, 156, 197
  thyroid 80, 116, 135

cardiogenic pulmonary oedema 110
cardiomegaly
  generalised 128–9
  left-sided 130–1, *131*
  right-sided 132–3, *133*
carotid artery, ultrasonography 80
carpus, conditions affecting 47–9
cauda equina syndrome 94, 194
caudal vena cava abnormalities 134
cavitary lung lesion 122, *122*
central peripheral neuropathy 99
central tarsal bone fractures 59, *59*
cervical (cisterna magna) myelography 93–4
cervical articular facet aplasia 86
cervical vertebral malformation malarticulation syndrome (CVMM, wobbler syndrome) 85–6, *85*
  articular facets in 93
  intervertebral disc space 91
  myelography 96–7, 98
  vertebra in 85, *85*, 88, 89
chalk bones 14
chemodectoma 131, 134, 135
Chinese Shar Pei fever syndrome/familial renal amyloidosis 33, 36, 120
  carpus in 48
  tarsus in 58–9
choke chain injuries 76
cholecystitis, chronic 218
cholecystography 220
choledocholithiasis 218
cholelithiasis (gallstones) 218
cholesteatoma 71
chondrocalcinosis (pseudogout, calcium pyrophosphate deposition disease) 37, 88, 89, 237
chondrodysplasias (dyschondroplasias) 7, 12, 13, 20, 24, 25, 26
  joints and 36
  zinc-responsive 13
chondrodystrophic conformation 16, *17*
chondromatosis, osseous 20
chondrometaplasia 23, 35, 37, 57
chondrosarcoma 39, 50, 90, 107, 135
chordae tendineae 126
chorioretinitis 78
chronic obstructive pulmonary disease (COPD) 109
chylothorax 162
cisterna magna 93–4
coccidioidomycosis 22, 87, 113, 117, 129, 152, **247**
Codman's triangle 6, 22
coeliac/cranial mesenteric arteriography 220
coeliography (peritoneography) 220
colitis 181, 182, *182*
colon *see* large intestine
consolidated lung lobe 114, *114*
constipation 182
Coonhound paralysis 100
copper deficiency 13
cor pulmonale 132, 133
cor triatriatum dexter 134

cortex 2
corticosteroid responsive meningitis 100
Corynebacterium 113
Corynebacterium diphtheria 92
coxofemoral joint 51–2
cranial cavity 66–7
craniomandibular osteopathy (CMO) 15, 16, 26, 68, 68
  radius and ulna in 47
cranium/cranial cavity 66–7
Crenosoma vulpis 109, **247**
cruciate ligament damage 55–6
cryptococcosis 22, 72, 79, 113, 117, 152, 205, **247**
Cushing's disease/syndrome 17, 90, 109, 118, 120, 121, 123, 187, 210
cyst
  bone 7, 12, 20, 87
  bronchogenic 122
  dentigerous 68, 69
  dermoid 99
  epidermoid 99
  ovarian 200
  paraprostatic 204, *204*, 205, *205*
  pericardial 130
  pulmonary 122, *122*
  renal 187
  salivary gland 79
  solitary bone 47, 98
  synovial 33
cystadenocarcinoma 187, 189, 192
cystitis 197–8
  chronic 197, *197*
  emphysematous 195, *195*
cystography 195
  abnormal bladder contents 196–7
  double contrast 196
  following IVU 196
  filling defects *197*
  pneumocystography 196
  positive contrast 196
  reflux following 196
  wall thickening 197–8

D

dacryocystorhinography 77
Dandy–Walker syndrome 88
dens agenesis 89, *89*
dens fracture 89
dens hypoplasia 89
dental formulae **74**
dentigerous cyst 68, 69
dentinogenesis imperfecta 18, 75
dermoid cysts 99
dextrocardia 126–7, *127*
diabetes mellitus 18, 78, 90, 155, 195, 217, 218
diaphragm 160–1
  normal appearance 160, *160*
  ultrasonography 161–2
diaphragmatic hernia 161, 172, 217
diaphragmatic rupture 145, 161, 172, 217
diaphysis 2
  lesions affecting 27–8
digital neoplasia 49, *49*

INDEX

dirofilaria (heartworm) 98, 111, 113, 118, 119, 121, 133, 134, 136, **247**
disc disease 96, *96*, 97
discography 95
discospondylitis 88, 89, 90, 91–2, *92*, 97
disseminated idiopathic skeletal hyperostosis (DISH) 12, 16
  joints and 35, 36
  vertebra in 87
disseminated intravascular coagulation (DIC) 111, 116, 118
distemper, canine 79, 111
distractio cubiti/dysostosis enchondralis 44, 45
distraction index (DI) in hip radiography 51, *51*
doliocephalic breeds *65*, 66
doppler echocardiography 139–40
dorsal acetabular rim view (DAR) 52
double contrast crystography 196
double contrast enema 181–2
double contrast gastrography *168*, 169
double cortical line 5, 6
dwarfism 12–13
dyschondroplasia *see* chondrodysplasias
dyskinesia, primary ciliary 72, 109–10
dysostosis enchondralis 44, 45

E

ear, conditions of 71
Ebstein's anomaly 132
echocardiography 136–40, *137*
ectopic ureters 193, *193*
ehrlichiosis 32, 36, **247**
Eisenmenger's syndrome 133, 136
Elbow, conditions affecting 42–5, *44*, *45*
  International Elbow Working Group (IEWG) grading system 43–5
emphysema
  abdominal wall 211
  bladder 195, *195*
  pulmonary 111, 118, 120, 121, 144, 149, 216
  thoracic wall 157, 159, 160, 211
  soft tissues 7, 10, 76, 236, *238*, 239
emphysematous cystitis 195, *195*
enchondromatosis 12, 20, 23, 25, 28
endocarditis 126
endometritis 203
endophthalmitis 78
endosteum 2
enthesiopathies 12, 16
  carpus 48, *48*
  elbow 43, *43*
ependymoma 88, 98
epicardial tumours 135
epidermoid cysts 99
epididymitis 206
epidurography 94
epiphysiolysis, femoral 52
epiphysis 2
  lesions affecting 23–4
Escherichia coli 92
extra kidney sign 201
extrapleural sign 146, *146*
eye, ultrasonography of 77–9, 77, 78

F

faecolithiasis 181
false pneumothorax 144, *144*
feline infectious peritonitis (FIP) 79, 107, 116, 117, 129, 146, 189, 192
feline leukaemia (FeLV), medullary osteosclerosis in 13, 90
femoral metaphyseal osteopathy, proximal 52
femur, conditions affecting 53
fibrodysplasia ossificans 237
fibroma 16, 135
fibrosarcoma 90, 135
fibula, conditions affecting 57–8
Filaroides 107, 110, 111, 113, 116, 118, 148, **247**
fimbriation 175
fistula, contrast study of 238
'flat pup' syndrome 159
flexor tendon enthesiopathy 43, *43*
foetal death 202
foramen magnum 66
forearm, conditions affecting 45–7
fractures
  assessment
    postoperative radiographic 9–10
    subsequent examinations 10
    at time of injury 9
  atrophic non-union 11, *11*
  causes 7–8
  classification 9
  disease 11
  folding *18*
  healing 10, *10*
  complications 11
  primary bone 10
  secondary bone 10
  hypertrophic non-union 11, *11*
  malunion 11, *11*
  pathological 9, *9*
  radiographic signs 8
  radiography 8
  Salter–Harris classification 9, *9*, 24
  see also under individual bones
fragmented medial coronoid process (FCP) 42, *42*
Francisella (Pasteurella) tularensis 111, 116, **247**
free gas 213
frontal sinuses 73–4
fungal granulomata 116
fungal pneumonia 111

G

gastric dilation/volvulus 166, *166*
gastric ulcer 169, *170*, 172
gastritis 169, *169*, 172
gastric tumours *167*, 168
gastrogram 168, 169
geographic distribution **246–8**
giant axonal neuropathy, canine 99
giant cell granuloma, mandibular 69
giant cell tumour (osteoclastoma) 20, 23, 47
glaucoma 78
globoid cell leukodystrophy 100
glomerulonephritis 187
gonitis, juvenile 54–5
granuloma
  bacterial 19, 113, 115, 116, 152
  diapragm 161
  eosinophilic 107, 115, 152
  foreign body 115, 116
  fungal 115, 116
  hepatic 217, 218, 220, 221, 232
  intraocular 78
  lymphatoid 113, 116
  mandibular giant cell 69
  mediastinal 150, 151, 152
  oesophageal 154, 155, 156, *156*
  parasitic 98, 115, 131, 150, 151, 152, 187, 232
  pleural 146, 147
  prostate 205
  pulmonary 112, 113, 115, 116, 117, 122
  renal 187, 189, 190, 192, 232
  soft tissue 76, 77, 93, 236, 239
  splenic 224
  tracheal 107
  uterine 201, 203
granulomatous meningoencephalomyelitis (GME) 99, 100
gravel sign 166, 167, *167*, 173
greenstick fractures 14, 27
ground glass appearance 211
growth plate closures *see* physis 2–3, **3**
  delayed 13

H

haemangiosarcoma 90, 97, 118, 129, 130, 132, 134, 135, 146, 153, 159, 217, 223
haemarthrosis 35
haematoma 116
  renal 187
  subperiosteal vertebral 97
haemometra 201, 202, 203
haemopericardium 129–30
haemoperitoneum 211
haemophilia 97, 99, 111
haemopneumothorax 145, 162
haemothorax 162
Hansen disc disease
  Type I 91, 96, *96*
  Type II 91, *96*, 97
Heart *see* specific heart chambers and major vessels 125–140
  base tumours 134–5
  dorsal displacement 127
  enlargement, generalised 128–9
  malposition 126–7
  neoplasia 134–5
  normal radiographic appearance 125–6
  normal silhouette with cardiac pathology 126
  size, reduction in 127–8
  ultrasonography 136–40
    contrast echocardiography 139

253

INDEX

Heart (continued)
  Doppler flow abnormalities 138–40
  left heart two-dimensional 136–8
  right heart two-dimensional 138–9
heartworm 98, 111, 113, 118, 119, 121, 133, 134, 136, **247**
hemimelia 12, 45
hemivertebrae 84, *85*, 88
hepatozoonosis 15, 87, **247**
hernia
  diaphragmatic 165
  hiatal 165
  inguinal 210, *210*
  perineal 194
  peritoneopericardial diaphragmatic (PPDH) 130, 165, 172
  scrotal 206
  umbilical 210
high rise syndrome 69
hiatal hernia 165
hilar masses 123, 151, *151*, 152
hip, conditions affecting 51–2
histiocytosis 112, 116, 122
histoplasmosis 22, 113, 116, 117, 123, 152, **247**
hock (tarsus), conditions affecting 58–60
hound ataxia 100
humerus, conditions affecting 41
hydrocephalus, congenital 66, *66*
hydrometra 201, 202
hydromyelia 88, 99, 100
hydronephrosis 187, 189, 190, 191, *191*
hydroperitoneum 211
hydrophthalmos 78
hydropneumothorax 145
hyperadrenocorticism *see* Cushing's disease
hyperparathyroidism (osteitis fibrosa cystica; fibrous osteodystrophy) 12, 17, 72, 90, 187
  nutritional secondary (juvenile osteoporosis) 13, 17, *18*, 87, 88
  primary 12, 17, 90
  pseudo 12, 17, 90
  renal secondary (rubber jaw) 17, 68, *68*, 69
  secondary 12, 17
hyperthyroidism 90
hypertrophic osteodystrophy *see* metaphyseal osteopathy
hypertrophic (pulmonary) osteopathy (HPO, Marie's disease) 7, 15, *15*, 27, 47, 49, 53, 58
hypertrophied annulus fibrosis/disc protrusion (Hansen Type II disc disease) 91, 97
hypertrophied ligamentum flavum 97
hypervascular lung pattern 119, *119*, 120
hypovascular lung pattern 119, *119*, 120
hypervitaminosis A 13, 15, 18, 23, 237

elbow in 44
joints and 35, 36
of stifle 54
vertebra in 87, 90
hypervitaminosis D 13, 18, 188, 237
hypoadrenocorticism (Addison's disease) 120, 121, 128, 155
hypoplasia
  dens 89
  trachea 107
hypothyroidism
  bowing of bones in 12
  congenital 24, 25, 86
  dwarfism and 13
  joints and 36
  radius and ulna in 47
  vertebrae in 90
  vertebral opacity 90
hypovitaminosis D 25

I

immotile cilia syndrome 72, 73, 110, 127
inguinal hernia 210, *210*
interstitial lung pattern 117–119, *117*, *118*
intertarsal subluxation 59, *59*
intervertebral disc space, abnormalities of 91–2
intervertebral foramen, abnormalities of 92–3
intradural extramedullary spinal cord compression on myelography 98
intramedullary spinal cord enlargement on myelography 98–9
intraocular granuloma 78
intraocular tumour 78
intrathoracic mineralised opacities 122–3
intravenous urography (IVU) 188–9
  bolus 188
  infusion 188
  nephrogram/pyelogram phase 188, *188*
intravertebral disc herniation 88, 90
intussusception 176, *176*,178, *179*
involucrum 21

J

joints 31–37
jugular vein, ultrasonography 80
juvenile osteomalacia *see* rickets
juvenile osteoporosis 17, *18*, 87, 88

K

Kartagener's syndrome (immotile cilia syndrome) 72, 73, 110, 127
kidneys 186–93
  contrast studies 188–9, *188*
  enlargement 230, *230*
  non-visualisation 186
  normal appearance 186
  pyelogram, variations in 189–90
  radio-opacity 187–8
  size and shape 186–7, *186*
  tumours 190

  ultrasonographic examination 190
  diffuse parenchymal abnormalities 192–3
  focal parenchymal abnormalities 192
  normal 191, *191*
  perirenal fluid 193
  renal pelvis distension 191
kyphosis 89

L

large intestine 179–83
  colitis 181, 182, *182*
  contents 181
  contrast studies 181–2
  dilation 180
  displacement 179–80
  luminal filling defects 182
  mass 230, 231
  mucosal pattern 182
  normal radiographic appearance 179, *180*
  tumour 182, *182*
  ultrasonographic examination 183
  wall opacity 181
  wall thickness 182
larval migrans 113, 116
larynx 75–6
lateral patellar luxation 54
lead poisoning 14, 18, 26, 91
left atrium
  abnormalities 136–7
  enlargement 130–1
  pressure overload 130–1
  volume overload 130
left ventricle
  abnormalities on echocardiography 137–8
  enlargement 131
Legg–Calvé–Perthe's disease 20, 24, 33, 36, 52, *52*
leiomyoma 172
leiomyosarcoma 172
leishmaniasis 13, 15, 19, 22, 23, 27, **248**
joints and 35, 36
leucoencephalomyelopathy 100
levocardia 126, 127
linear foreign body 174, *174*, 176, *176*
lipoma 238
  of abdominal wall 211
  of chest wall 157
  of thigh 53
liver 215–22
  contrast studies 218–20, *219*
  displacement 216
  enlargement 216–17, *216*, 227–8, *227*, *228*
  mass 229
  radio-opacity 218
  reduced size 217, *217*
  shape 218
  size 216–18
  ultrasonography
    biliary tract abnormalities 221–2
    normal appearance 220, *220*
    parenchymal abnormalities 220–1, *221*
    vascular abnormalities 222

INDEX

lordosis 88
lumbosacral instability 89
lung 109–123
  increased visibility 123
  lobe torsion 112
  opacity, artefactual increase 110
  pattern
    alveolar 110–112, *110*
    bronchial 109–110, *109*
    diffuse, unstructured
      interstitial 117–18, *117*
    linear or reticular interstitial
      118–19, *118*
    mixed 120–1
    normal *109*
    nodular 115–116, *115*
    vascular 119–20, *119*
luxation *see* specific joint
Lyme disease (*Borrelia burgdorferi*)
  32, 36
lymphadenopathy 26, 105, 109,
  111, 112, 113, 116, 118,
  119, 121, 122, 146, 147,
  151, 152, 153, 194, 212,
  222
lymph nodes of head and neck,
  ultrasonography 80
lymphangiography 238
lymphography 238
lymphosarcoma 6, 17, 23, 19, 76,
  97, 98, 99, 107, 109,
  116, 118, 128, 135, 152

M

M-mode echocardiography 137,
  137, 138
mandible 68–69
marble bones 14
Marie's disease *see* hypertrophic
  (pulmonary) osteopathy
  (HPO)
maxilla 67–8
medial epicondylar spur (flexor
  tendon enthesiopathy)
  43, *43*
medial patellar luxation 54, *54*
mediastinum 148–53
  anatomy and radiography 144,
    148–9, *148*
  lymphadenopathy 152
    hilar region 152
    sternal 152
  masses 150–2, *151*
  mediastinal shift 149
  pneumomediastinum 121,
    149–150, *149*
  radio-opacity 149–50
    fat 150
    increased 150
    reduced 149–50
  ultrasonography 152–3
  widening 150
medullary cavity 2
megaoesophagus 121, 154–5, *154*
melanoma, malignant 50
meningioma 67, 92, 97, 98
meningitis 97
meningocoele 86
mesaticephalic breeds 66
mesentery, mass 230
mesothelioma 128, 130, 135, 147
metacarpus, conditions affecting
  49–50

metallosis 11
metaphyseal condensation 14
metaphyseal osteomyelitis 23, 26,
  26
metaphyseal osteopathy
  (hypertrophic
  osteodystrophy; skeletal
  scurvy; Moller–Barlow's
  disease) 6, 12, 14, 15,
  20, 23, 25, 26, *26*, 41,
  47, 53, 57
metaphysis 2
  lesions affecting 25–6
metatarsus, conditions affecting
  49–50
microcardia 120, 127–8, *128*
microphthalmos, congenital 78
mirror-image artefacts 245, *245*
mitral valve 137, 139
mixed lung pattern 120–121
Moller–Barlow's disease *see*
  metaphyseal
  osteopathy
Mono-ostotic lesions 7
Monteggia fracture 45
mucolipidosis 12, 18, 24
mucometra 201, 202, 203
mucopolysaccharidoses 13, 15,
  18, 24, 92
  hip dysplasia in 52
  joints and 35, 36
  vertebra and 86, 87, 88, 90
multiple cartilaginous exostoses
  (multiple
  osteochondromata) 16,
  16, 20, 23
multiple epiphyseal dysplasia
  (stippled epiphyses) 24
multiple myeloma *see* myeloma
muscles, ultrasonography 240
Mycobacteria 35
mycobacterial pneumonia 116
Mycobacterium tuberculosis 15
Mycoplasma
  pneumonia 117
  polyarthritis 35, 36
myelodysplasia 180
myelography
  cervical 93–4
  complications 94
  extradural spinal cord
    compression on 96–8,
    96
  intradural extramedullary spinal
    cord compression on
    98, *98*
  lumbar 94
  normal appearance 94, *94*
  technical errors 95–6, *95*
myeloma
  multiple 4, 6, 12, 18, 19, *19*,
    50
  vertebral solitary plasma cell
    90
myelomalacia 99
myelomeningocoele 86
myelopathy, hereditary 100
myocardial failure 133
myocardial tumours 135
myocarditis 126
myositis ossificans 37, 237, *237*
myxoma 97, 98, 135
myxosarcoma 97, 98, 135

N

nasal cavity 72–3
nasal neoplasia 72–3, *72*
nasolacrimal duct
  contrast studies
    (dacryocystorhinography)
    77
  cysts 68
nasopharyngeal polyp 75, *75*
necrotising vasculitis 97
nephritis 186, 187
nephroblastoma 98, 189
nephrocalcinosis 187, 192
nephrogram 188–9, *188*
nephrolithiasis 187, 192
neuroaxonal dystrophy 99, 100
neurofibroma 92, 97, 98, 99
neurofibrosarcoma 98
nocardiosis 113, 146, **248**
nodular lung pattern 115–16,
  115
Norberg angle 51, *51*
nutrient foramen 2
nutritional secondary
  hyperparathyroidism *see*
  hyperparathyroidism

O

occipitoatlantoaxial malformation
  86
odontoid peg *see* dens
odontoma, complex 68, 69, *69*
oesophagram 153–4
oesophagus, thoracic 153–7
  contrast studies 153–4
  dilation 154–6
  generalised 154–5, *154*
  localised 155–6, *155*
  foreign bodies 157
  masses 156
    extraluminal 156
    intraluminal 156
    intramural 156
  normal radiographic appearance
    153
  redundancy 155
  variations in radio-opacity 156
oligodendroglioma 98
Ollier's disease *see*
  enchondromatosis
omentum, mass 230
optic neuritis 79
orbit, ultrasonography of 77–9
orchitis 205
Oslerus osleri 107, 110, **248**
ossification 2–3
  delayed 13
osteitis fibrosa cystica *see*
  hyperparathyroidism
osteoarthritis 23, 35, *35*, 36, 41,
  45, *45*, 48, *51*, 57, 60,
  70
osteochondrodysplasia 47, 57
  osteochondroma 12, 16, 25
  multiple 20, 23
  of pelvis 50
  trachea in 107
osteochondrosis (OC) 7, 23, 33,
  36, 37
  hip joint 52
  tarsal 58, *58*
  shoulder 40, *40*
  elbow 42, *42*

INDEX

osteochondrosis (OC) (continued)
  sacral 88
  stifle 53–4, 53
osteochondrosis dissecans (OCD) 40
osteoclastoma 20, 20, 23, 47
osteodystrophy
  fibrous see hyperparathyroidism
  hypertrophic see metaphyseal osteopathy
  idiopathic 13
  in Scottish Fold cat (chondro–osseous dysplasia) 47, 49, 58
osteogenesis 3–4
  continuous periosteal reactions 5–6, 5
  interrupted periosteal reactions 6, 6
  presence and type 7
osteogenesis imperfecta 12, 18, 75, 90
osteolysis see bone loss
osteolytic joint disease 33–5
osteolytic lesions 18–20, 18, 19
osteolytic/osteogenic lesions, mixed 20–3
  cf malignant bone neoplasia from osteomyelitis 22–3
osteoma 16, 69
osteomalacia 3, 17
  juvenile see rickets
osteomyelitis 12, 13, 15, 19, 21, 21, 22
  bone fracture and 7
  fracture healing and 11
  haematogenous 7, 23, 28
  of mandible 68–9
  of maxilla and premaxilla 67–8
  metaphyseal 26, 26
  osteolysis in 4, 5
  of osteomyelitis from malignant bone neoplasia 22–3
osteopathy
  craniomandibular 6, 26, 68, 68, 71
  metaphyseal (hypertrophic osteodystrophy) 7, 25, 26, 26, 41, 47, 53, 57
osteopenia 3, 5, 12, 14, 16–18, 27
  bone fracture and 8
  coarse trabecular pattern 18
  joints and 35
osteopetrosis 14, 18, 23, 27, 28, 90
osteoporosis 3, 16
  juvenile 13, 17, 18, 87, 88
  senile 90
osteosarcoma 14, 20, 21, 21, 25
  of cranium 67
  extraskeletal 237
  of femur 53
  of humerus 41
  of metacarpus/metatarsus 49
  of oesophagus 156
  parosteal 16, 53
  of radius and ulna 21, 47
  of ribs 159
  of trachea 107
  of vertebrae 87, 90
osteosclerosis fragilis 14
otitis externa 71
otitis media 71, 71

ovaries 200–1
  cyst 200
  enlargement 200, 230–1
  ultrasonography 200–1

P

pachymeningitis 92
pancreas 225–6
  disease 225, 225
  enlargement 228
  ultrasonography 225–6
panosteitis 7, 14, 14, 15, 18, 23, 27, 28, 41, 47, 53, 57
Paragonimus kellicotti 113, 116, 122, **248**
paraprostatic cyst 204, 204, 205, 205
paraquat poisoning 118, 121
  pseudomediastinum in 149, 149
parasitic pneumonia 111
parathyroid gland, ultrasonography 79–80
paravertebral soft tissues, lesions in 93
paronychia 49, 49
parosteal osteosarcoma 16, 53
patella cubiti 44
patent ductus arteriosus (PDA) 120, 130, 131, 134, 135, 136, 137, 139, 140
pectus carinatum (pigeon breast) 159
pectus excavatum (funnel chest) 127, 159
pelvis, conditions affecting 50
Penicillium 73
PennHIP scheme 51
pericardial cyst 130
pericardial disease 129–30
  ultrasonography 130
pericardial effusion 129, 129
pericarditis 126
perineal hernia 194
periodontal disease 68, 75, 75
periosteal proliferative polyarthritis (Reiter's disease) 36
periosteal reactions 5, 5, 6, 6
periosteum 2, 14–15
perirenal pseudocyst 187, 192, 193
peritoneal cavity 211–13
peritoneal effusion 211, 211, 212, 213
peritoneal fluid 212
peritoneopericardial diaphragmatic hernia (PPDH) 130, 165, 172
peritonitis 212
  pancreatic disease and 225, 225
perocormus 86
persistent hyperplastic primary vitreous (PHPV) 78
persistent right aortic arch (PRAA) 132, 154, 155, 155
Perthe's disease see Legg–Calvé–Perthe's disease
phaeochromocytoma 97, 134, 226
phalanges, conditions affecting 49–50
pharynx 75–6, 75
  breed and conformational variations 65–6

phthisis bulbi 78
physis see growth plate 2
  lesions affecting 24–5
physometra 202
pituitary dwarfism 13, 24, 25, 36, 86
pleural cavity 143–148
  anatomy and radiography 143–4, 144
  increased radiolucency 144–5
  increased radio-opacity 145–6
  pleural and extrapleural nodules and masses 146, 146
  pleural thickening 147–8
  ultrasonography of pleural and extrapleural lesions 146–7
pleural effusion 145, 145, 146
pneumobilia 218
pneumocolon 181
pneumoconiosis 116, 118
Pneumocystis carinii 111, 117, **248**
pneumocystography 196
pneumogastrography 168–9
pneumomediastinum 121, 149–50, 149
pneumonia 111
pneumopericardium 130
pneumothorax 121, 144–5, 144, 162
polioencephalomyelitis, feline 100
polyarteritis nodosa (stiff Beagle disease) 33, 36
polyarthritis
  feline 36
  in Japanese Akita 36
  meningitis syndrome 32, 36
polycystic kidney disease 187, 189, 190, 192
polydactyly, congenital 49
polyostotic lesions 7
polyp
  bladder 196, 198
  nasopharangyeal 71, 73, 75, 75, 121
  tracheal 108
polyradiculoneuritis 100
portal venography (operative portography) 218–19, 219
positive contrast gastrogram 168, 169
post caval syndrome 216
premature closure
  of distal femoral growth plate 54
  of distal ulnar growth plate 46, 46
  of proximal tibial growth plate 54, 54
premaxilla 67–8
progressive haemorrhagic myelomalacia 99
prostate 203–5
  location 203
  mass 231
  radio–opacity 204
  shape and outline 204
  size 203–4, 203
  tumour 200, 200, 204, 205
  ultrasonographic examination 204–5
prostatitis 205

INDEX

pseudogout 37, 88, 89, 237
pseudohyperparathyroidism 12, 17, 90
pulmonary artery trunk
 abnormalities 134, *134*
pulmonary haemorrhage 111
pulmonary hyperlucency
 focal areas 121–2
 generalised 121
pulmonary hypoperfusion 121
pulmonary infiltrate with eosinophilia (PIE) 109, 111, 116
pulmonary lymphomatoid granulomatosis 112, 116, 118
pulmonary nodules or masses, ultrasonography 116–17
pulmonary oedema
 cardiogenic 110
 non–cardiogenic 112
pulmonary opacities, poorly marginated 112–13, *112*
pulmonary osteomata 104, 115, 122
pulmonic valve 140
pyelogram 189–90, *188*
pyelonephritis 187, 190, 191
pyloric stenosis 167, *167*, 170, *170*
pyometra 201, *201*, 202, *202*, 203
pyopneumothorax 145
pythiosis **248**

R

radiation pneumonitis 111
radiographic faults **242–4**
radius curvus syndrome 46, *46*
radius, conditions affecting 45–7
redundant colon 179
redundant oesophagus 155
refractive shadowing 245, *245*
Reiter's disease 36
renal amyloidosis, familial *see* Chinese Shar Pei fever syndrome
renal calculus (nephrolith) 187, 189, 190, 191, 192
renal osteodystrophy 17
renal rickets 17
renal secondary hyperparathyroidism *see* hyperparathyroidism
retained cartilaginous core, ulna 45, 46, *46*
retinal detachment 78
retrobulba abscess 79
retroperitoneal masses 231
retroperitoneal space 213–15
 enlargement 213–14, *213*
retropharyngeal abscess 76
reverberation artefacts 245, *245*
reverse fissure lines 150, *150*
rhabdomyosarcoma 128, 135
rheumatoid arthritis 34, *34*, 36
 of carpus *34*, 47
 of tarsus 58
rhinitis 72, *72*, 73, *73*
rhino horn callus 11, 16
ribs 158, 159, *159*
rickets (juvenile osteomalacia) 7, 12, 13, 18, 25, *25*, 26
 dwarfism and 13
 of radius and ulna 47
 renal 17
 of tibia and fibula 57–8
Rickettsia rickettsii infection 36, 117
right atrium
 abnormalities on echocardiography 138
 enlargement 132
 wall tumours 134
right ventricle
 abnormalities on echocardiography 139
 enlargement 132–3
Rocky Mountain spotted fever 36, 117, **248**
rubber jaw 17, 68, *68*, 69

S

sacralisation 84, *85*
sacrococcygeal (sacrocaudal) dysgenesis 86
salivary ducts 79
salivary glands 79
Salter–Harris growth plate fractures 9, 23, 40–1, 45, 46, 52, 55, 59
sarcoma, synovial 34, *34*, 44, 55
scapula, conditions affecting 39
Schmorl's nodes 88, 90
schwannoma 98
scleritis 78
sclerosis 3–4, 13
scoliosis 88
scrotal hernia 206
sensory neuropathy 100
sentinel loop 173
septic arthritis 23, 33, 36
sequestrum 21, *22*
sesamoids 2, 49, *49*
shock lung (acute respiratory distress syndrome) 112, 118
short urethra syndrome 194
shoulder, conditions affecting 39–41
sialography 79
side lobe artefact 245
silhouette sign 104, 105, *105*
sinus tracts, contrast study of 238
situs inversus 126, *127*
situs solitus 126
skeletal scurvy *see* metaphyseal osteopathy
skull
 anatomy 65
 breed and conformational variations 65–6
 conditions affecting 66–75
 radiographic technique 65
slice thickness artefact 246
slipped epiphysis 52
small intestine 172–9
 contents 174–5
 contrast studies 175
  technical errors with 175–6
 displacement 172–3
 intestinal loops
  number 172
  bunching 173
  width 173–4
 lumen dilation *174*, *175*, 178
 luminal diameter 176, *176*, *177*
 luminal filling defects 176
 mass 230
 normal radiographic appearance 172
 transit time 177
 ultrasonographic appearance *171*, 177–9
 wall thickness 176, *177*
soft tissues 236–41
 of head and neck 76–80
 thickening 76
 variations in radio–opacity 76–7
 joint tumour 34, *34*, 36
 radio-opacity 236–8
 thickness 236
 tumours 7, 19, *19*, 21, 34, *34*, ultrasonography 239
solitary bone cyst 47
solitary plasma cell myeloma, vertebral 90
solitary pulmonary nodules or masses 114–15
Spalding's sign 202
spina bifida 86, 99, 180
spinal arachnoid cyst 98
spinal contrast studies 93–5
spinal cord
 atrophy 99
 lesions affecting, on myelography 96–99
 neurological deficits 99–100
spinal dysraphism 88, 99, 100
spinal muscular atrophy 100
spine
 conditions affecting 84–100
 radiographic technique 83–4, *83*
Spirocerca lupi 87, 97, 98, 123, 131, 132, 150, 151–2, 156, *156*, 157, **248**
spleen 222–5
 absence of shadow 222
 enlargement 229–30, *230*
 radio-opacity 224
 size and shape 2234
 tail 222–3
 ultrasonographic examination 224–5, *224*
splenoportography 219–20
spondylarthrosis 93
spondylitis 87, *87*, 90
spondylosis 86, *86*, 90
sporotrichosis 113, **248**
squamous cell carcinoma
 of ear 71
 of mandible 69
 of nail bed 49
 of premaxilla 68, 69
Staphylococcus aureus 92
Staphylococcus intermedius 92
steatitis 128
sternal dysraphism 159
sternal spondylosis 159
sternum 159
stiff Beagle disease 33, 36
stifle, conditions affecting 53–7
stifle joint effusion *32*
stifle osteoarthritis *35*, 36, 57
stippled epiphyses 24

INDEX

stomach 165–172
    abnormal gastric mucosal pattern 169–70
    contents 167
    contrast studies 168–9, *168*
    displacement 165–6
    emptying time 170
    enlargement 228
    gastric luminal filling defects 169
    gastrogram technical errors 169
    normal appearance 165, *165*
    size variations 166
    ultrasonographic examination 170–2, *171*
    wall 167–8, 171–2
Streptococcus 92
stress protection 8
subchondral bone 2
sublumbar mass 231, *231*, 232
subperiosteal vertebral haematoma 97
subretinal haemorrhage 78
'swimmers' sternum 159
syndesmitis ossificans 86
synovial cysts 33
synovial osteochondromatosis (chondrometaplasia) 23, 35, 37, 57
synovial sarcoma 34, *34*, 44, 55
syringomyelia 88, 99, 100
systemic lupus erythematosus 32, 35, 36

T

tarsus (hock), conditions affecting 58–60
teeth 74–5, *74*
telangiectasia
    hepatic 221
    renal 188
temporomandibular joint 70, *70*
tendinopathy, calcifying 41, *41*, 52
tendon avulsions, stifle 56–7, *56*
tendons 239–40, *240*
tenosynovitis 41
tentorium osseum 66
testes 205–6
    retained 231
tetralogy of Fallot 120, 132, 136, 139

thoracic trauma 162–3
thoracic wall 157–62
    ribs 158–9
    soft tissue components 157–8
    sternum 159
    vertebrae 159
    ultrasonography 159–60
thorax, radiographic technique 103–4
thrombocytopenia 97, 99
thyroid carcinoma, ectopic 135
thyroid gland, ultrasonography 79–80
tibia, conditions affecting 57–8
tibial plateau deformans 54, *54*
Toxocara canis 187
toxoplasmosis 79, 109, 113, 116, 117, **248**
trachea 105–108
    diameter, variations in 106–7, *107*
    displacement 105–6, *106*
    ultrasonography 108
    wall visibility 108
tracheal collapse syndrome 107, 109
tracheal lumen opacification 107–8
tracheal polyp 108
tracheobronchitis 111
tracheo-oesophageal stripe sign 108, 154
transitional vertebrae 84, *85*
tricuspid valve 132, 133, 134, 136, 138–9, 140
tuberculosis 111, 113
    feline 15, 22, 35, 36, 37
tularaemia 111, 116
tympanic bulla 71, *71*
typhlitis 181

U

ulna, conditions affecting *12*, 45–7
ultrasound, terminology and artefacts 244–6, *244*, *245*
umbilical hernia 210
ununited anconeal process (UAP) 42–3, *43*
ununited medial epicondyle 43
ureteral diverticula 194

ureterocoele 194
ureters 193–4
    dilated 193–4, *193*
    normal appearance 193, *193*
    ultrasonographic appearance 194
urethra 198–200
    contrast studies 199–200, *199*, *200*
    ultrasonography 200
urethritis 200
urethrography, retrograde 199, *199*
uroabdomen 211
uterus 201–3
    contents 202
    dystocia 202
    enlargement 201, *201*, 231
    foetal death 202
    masses 231
    radio-opacity 201–2
    ultrasonography 202–3
    wall thickening 203

V

vaginourethrography, retrograde 199, *199*
vascularising anomaly 155, *155*
vascular lung pattern 119–20, *119*
venography 238–9
ventricular septal defect (VSD) 120, 130, 131, 133, 134, 136, 139, 140
vertebrae
    alignment 88–9
    number 84
    opacity
        diffuse changes in 89–90
        localised changes 90–1
    size and shape 84–8
vertebral heart score 125, *126*
villonodular synovitis (VNS) 33, 35, 36
von Willebrand's disease 15, 111, 118

W

Wobbler syndrome *see* cervical vertebral malformation malarticulation syndrome

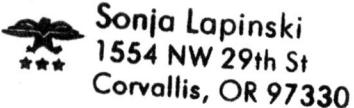
Sonja Lapinski
1554 NW 29th St
Corvallis, OR 97330